NEUROSCIENCE RESEARCH PROGRESS

DEEP BRAIN STIMULATION

NEUROSCIENCE RESEARCH PROGRESS

Additional books in this series can be found on Nova's website under the Series tab.

Additional e-books in this series can be found on Nova's website under the e-book tab.

NEUROSCIENCE RESEARCH PROGRESS

DEEP BRAIN STIMULATION

RAJA MEHANNA, MD
EDITOR

NOVA BIOMEDICAL
New York

Library of Congress Cataloging-in-Publication Data

ISBN: 978-1-63483-282-3

Published by Nova Science Publishers, Inc. † New York

To my parents
For love and education

To my wife
For patience and support

To my children
My pride and joy

To my mentors
For teaching and guidance

And to the Almighty
For all the above.

CONTENTS

PREFACE

Deep brain stimulation (DBS) is now a well-established treatment of Parkinson's disease, essential tremor, dystonia and obsessive compulsive disorders. Because of its success, it is constantly investigated in other conditions, and the list of FDA approved indications is likely to grow soon.

Its success stems essentially from its reversible nature compared to the destructive lesions created during thalamotomy and pallidotomy, and from its flexibility through programming that allows modification of the energy delivered to the specific brain targets in order to obtain maximal benefit with minimal side effects.

This book was conceived as a comprehensive, yet practical guide for any physician interested in this life changing therapy. It covers all the aspects of DBS including: a historical review; the underlying neurophysiologic mechanism of treatment; intra-operative details from the neurosurgical and the neurophysiologic standpoint; a review of the evidence supporting the use of deep brain stimulation for each disorder; algorithms for patient selection, programming strategies; and troubleshooting and prospective indications.

Written by experts in the field from different world renowned institutions, it gives a unique and comprehensive insight into the universe of DBS.

We hope it will be a valuable resource for all healthcare professionals involved in the management of patients with DBS.

CONTRIBUTORS

Pornpimol Anprasertporn MD, Department of Neurology, University of Alabama at Birmingham, Birmingham, Alabama.

Alberto Bona MD, Department of Neurology, Center for Movement Disorders and Neurorestoration, University of Florida, Gainesville, Florida.

Allison Boyle MD, Assistant Professor of Neurology, UT MOVE, University of Texas Health Science Center at Houston, Houston, Texas.

Scott E. Cooper MD, PhD. Professor of Neurology,, Center for Neurological Restoration, Cleveland Clinic, Cleveland, Ohio. Present address: Professor of Neurology, University of Minnesota, Minneapolis, Minessota.

Albert Fenoy MD, Assistant Professor of Neurosurgery, University of Texas Health Science Center at Houston, Houston, Texas.

Hubert H. Fernandez, MD. Professor of Neurology, Center for Neurological Restoration, Cleveland Clinic, Cleveland, Ohio.

Erin Furr-Stimming MD, Assistant Professor of Neurology, UT MOVE, University of Texas Health Science Center at Houston, Houston, Texas.

Neda Hidarilak MD, Department of Neurology, University of Alabama at Birmingham, Birmingham, Alabama.

Raja Mehanna MD. Assistant Professor of Neurology, UT MOVE, University of Texas Health Science Center at Houston, Houston, Texas.

William Ondo MD, Professor of Neurology, UT MOVE, University of Texas Health Science Center at Houston, Houston, Texas.

Neepa Patel MD, Assistant Professor of Neurology and Neurotherapeutics, Clinical Center for Movement Disorders, University of Texas-Southwestern, Dallas, Texas

Mya Schiess MD, Professor of Neurology, UT MOVE, University of Texas Health Science Center at Houston, Houston, Texas.

Aasef G. Shaikh, MD, PhD. Department of Neurology, Center for Neurological Restoration, Cleveland Clinic, Cleveland, Ohio.

Jessika Suescun MD, Department of Neurology, UT MOVE, University of Texas Health Science Center at Houston, Houston, Texas.

Sebastian J. Villarreal MD, Department of Neurosurgery, University of Texas Health Science Center at Houston, Houston, Texas.

Aparna Wagle Shukla MD, Assistant Professor of Neurology, Center for Movement Disorders and Neurorestoration, University of Florida, Gainesville, Florida.

Harrison Walker MD, Associate Professor of Neurology, University of Alabama at Birmingham, Birmingham, Alabama.

Roger Walz MD, Department of Neurology, Center for Movement Disorders and Neurorestoration, University of Florida, Gainesville, Florida; and Center for Applied Neurosciences (CeNAp) and Department of Internal Medicine, University of Santa Catarina, Brazil.

In: Deep Brain Stimulation
Editor: Raja Mehanna

ISBN: 978-1-63483-282-3

Chapter 1

DEEP BRAIN STIMULATION: A HISTORICAL REVIEW

Raja Mehanna, MD
University of Texas Health Science Center at Houston, Houston, TX, US

ABSTRACT

While the general opinion is that deep brain stimulation was born in the late 1980's, its conception actually started as early the late 1940's. In this chapter, we report the main earlier works that led to the development of DBS as we know it today, and the 4 fields in which this development happened: psychiatry, pain, epilepsy and movement disorders. We then briefly review the evolution of neurostimulators, the decrease in size of which was instrumental in making DBS a viable therapeutic option for many disorders.

INTRODUCTION

It is widely recognized that the modern era of deep brain stimulation (DBS) was inaugurated by the work of Benabid, Pollak and their colleagues in Grenoble, France, through their landmark paper published in 1987, reporting improvement of tremor after thalamic DBS contralateral to thalamotomy [1]. Since then, case series, open label studies and randomized controlled trial have multiplied, reporting the impact of DBS in different subcortical structures on various movement disorders [2]. More recently, application of this therapy is being sought in psychiatric disorders, pain and epilepsy [3]. Current Food and Drug Administration approved applications for DBS are presented in Table 1.

However, the fascinating genesis of DBS started well before 1987, and involved psychiatry, pain and epilepsy as much, if not more than movement disorders [3]. While the evidence for this therapy in each of its current application will be detailed in the following chapters, we will here review the evolution of deep brain stimulation, from adjuvant to stereotactic ablation to a therapy in its own right.

Table 1. FDA approved indication for DBS as of April 2015

Indication	Year approved
Thalamic DBS for essential tremor and PD-related tremor	1997
STN and GPi DBS for PD	2003
STN DBS and GPi DBS for primary generalized dystonia, hemidystonia and segmental dystonia (humanitarian device exemption).	2003
DBS of the anterior limb of the internal capsule for obsessive- compulsive disorder (humanitarian device exemption)	2009

Legend: FDA: Food and Drug Administration; DBS: deep brain stimulation; PD: Parkinson's disease, STN: subthalamic nucleus, GPi: globus pallidus interna.

The (Very) Early Days

In 1947 in Philadelphia, in an attempt to avoid the side effect of crude frontal lobotomy in psychiatric patients, Speigel et al. described a stereotactic frame to perform ablative procedures [4]. Their first target was the medial nucleus of the thalamus, and intraoperative electrical stimulation was used to explore the brain target prior to lesioning [4-6]. The same year, Talairach et al. developed a grid system to implant chronic electrodes in medial temporal structures for recording and stimulation in patients with epilepsy [7]. A few years later, Speigel et al. applied their stereotactic technique to the treatment of movement disorders, by performing pallidoansotomies in patient with Huntington chorea and choreoathetosis, then with Parkinson's disease (PD) [8].

In the 1950's, Heath, Delgado and Bechtereva individually reported on chronic stimulation of various brain targets including the septal area, the caudate, the cingulum and the sensory thalamus for the treatment of chronic pain [3].

The first application of DBS was thus in psychiatry, as a systematic adjuvant to stereotactic ablation through intraoperative electrical stimulation. Within a decade, its use spread to movement disorders, pain and epilepsy. Afterwards, it evolved at different speed in these different areas.

DBS in Psychiatry

In 1950, Heath and his colleagues of the University of Tulane, in New Orleans, started studying the impact of chronic stimulation of the septal area in psychotic patients [9]. Very quickly, Heath also expanded the application of this technique to pain and epilepsy. Soon after, Bickford et al. [10] expanded on the work of Delgado et al. [11] and reported improvement of several psychotic patients after stimulation lasting several days. This was presented as a more focal, thus more safe and effective, form of electroshock.

In 1979, Laintinen reported that intra-operative prelesioning stimulation of rostral and middle cingulum, anterior internal capsule, or subcaudate region of the substantia innominate modulated emotional response in 135 psychiatric patients [12]. He further noted that a stimulation frequency of 60 Hz was the most effective in producing emotional responses while a frequency of 3 to 6 Hz rarely elicited such responses.

From the 1950's to the 1970's, Sem-Jackobsen intensively utilized chronic outpatient deep brain stimulation lasting weeks to months in an attempt to improve the leucotomy operation [13]. He would perform intermittent chronic stimulation of various brain targets prior to subsequent lesioning, but still did not see in deep brain stimulation more than an adjunct to leucotomy.

In the late 1960's and early 1970's, Delgado developed a technique of subcortical stimulation using chronically implanted electrodes and a subcutaneous "Stimoceiver," implanted in the scalp, that could be controlled by radio waves. This could be seen as the first model of modern deep brain stimulation [14-16]. In the late 1970's, reviewing the work already done, Latinen suggested that "it may even be possible to treat the patient with repeated electrical stimulation without macroscopic destruction of brain tissue" [17].

Table 2. Milestones in the development of DBS in psychiatry

1947	Spiegel et al.	Description of a stereotactic frame to perform ablative procedures, in an attempt to replace frontal lobotomy [4].
1947	Spiegel et al.	Medial thalamotomy for psychiatric disorders, with intraoperative electrical stimulation to explore the brain target prior to lesioning [4-6].
1950	Heath	Evaluation of chronic stimulation of the septal area in psychotic patients [9].
1952	Delgado et al.	Suggestion of electrode implantation for chronic recording and stimulation to evaluate therapeutic value in psychotic patients [11].
1953	Bickford et al.	Improvement of several psychotic patients after stimulation lasting several days [10].
1963	Heath	Evaluation of the effect of stimulation in caudate, septal area, amygdala, central medial thalamus, and various areas of the hypothalamus on "rewarding" and "aversive" reactions [93].
1963	Sem-Jacobsen	Transient improvement or resolution of psychotic symptoms with chronic electrical stimulation of the ventro-medial part of the frontal lobe [94].
1968-1977	Delgado	Development of subcortical stimulation using chronically implanted electrodes and a "Stimoceiver" that could be controlled by radio waves, for use in psychiatric patients [14-16].
1972	Escobedo et al.	2 patients with epilepsy, mental retardation, and destructive aggressive behavior implanted in the head of the caudate [95].
1979	Dieckman	Unilateral stimulation of non-dominant thalamus improved phobia in one woman [18].
1979	Laitinen	Intra-operative prelesioning stimulation of rostral and middle cingulum, anterior internal capsule, or subcaudate region of the "substantia innominata" modulated emotional response in 135 psychiatric patients [12].
1999	Nuttin et al.	First report on DBS for obsessive compulsive disorder [19].

Legend: DBS: deep brain stimulation.

Only a handful of psychiatric patients treated with DBS were afterwards reported (Table 2). Among these, Dieckman reported disappearance of phobia after unilateral stimulation of the non-dominant thalamus at a frequency of 5 Hz in one patient. He further noted that stimulation with 50 Hz caused a disagreeable sensation [18]. The use of DBS in psychiatric patients then fell in limbo until Nuttin first reported on its impact in OCD [19], paving the way for the approval of DBS of the anterior limb of the internal capsule for obsessive-compulsive disorder by the FDA in 2009 (Table 1). The current evidence of DBS in various psychiatric disorders will be reviewed in Chapter 9.

DBS in Pain

Since the 1950's, Heath, Delgado, Bechtereva and others reported on chronic stimulation of various brain targets including the septal area, the caudate, the cingulum and the sensory thalamus for the treatment of chronic pain [3]. However, its benefit was less impressive than for psychiatric or movement disorders, and the interest for DBS in chronic pain did not resurface until 1969, when Reynolds reported that rats exposed to electrical stimulation of the periaqueductal gray region could undergo laparotomy without anesthesia [20]. He was among the first to suggest that brain stimulation could induce selective pain inhibition in the absence of concomitant emotional or affective side effects [21].

In the early 1970's, Mazars et al. in France [22-24] and Hosobuchi et al. [25] in the US successfully treated chronic deafferentation pain with stimulation of the sensory thalamus. Later on, Adams et al. reported 50 to 100% reduction in pain in 5 patients treated with internal capsule DBS, but this target never gained popularity [26].

In addition to the thalamus and the internal capsule, the periventricular and periaqueductal gray matter was suggested as a DBS target for pain in rat models by Reynolds in 1969 and in humans by Richardson et al. in 1977 [27-28]. This was further supported by Hosobuchi et al. who demonstrated a loss of the periventricular and periaqueductal gray matter DBS benefit on pain after administration of the opioid antagonist Naloxone, supporting the concept that these cerebral structures play a role in the processing of painful sensations [29]. In the early 1980's, Mazars reported that stimulation of the ventroposterolateral (VPL) nucleus of the thalamus could control both the pain and the abnormal movement in patients with post-amputation pain and a spontaneous myoclonus within the painful area, that he called "jumping stump"[30, 31]. However, VPL stimulation for parkinsonism, intention tremor, and other dyskinesia not associated with sensory deafferentation did not improve the abnormal movements [30-32].

The popularity of thalamic or central grey matter DBS for pain became such that Medtronic trademarked the term "DBS" with respect to chronic subcortical stimulation for pain in the mid-1970s [3, 33]. However, because of lack of randomized control trials proving its efficacy, DBS was never approved for pain by the FDA [3, 21, 34, 35]. Nevertheless, it continued to be used in Europe [36] and, between 2001 and 2005, Leone et al. in Italy, reported on a total of 24 patients with medication resistant cluster headache who markedly improved after DBS of the posterior hypothalamic gray matter [37-40]. In the US, DBS became again the object of attention as an adjunct to pain treatment more recently, with its success in movement disorders [41].

Table 3. Milestones in the development of DBS in pain disorders

1950's	Heath, Delgado, Bechtereva	Chronic stimulation of various brain targets including the septal area, the caudate, the cingulum and the sensory thalamus for the treatment of chronic pain [3].
1973-1975	Mazars et al., Hosobuchi et al.	Mazars et al. in France [22-24] and Hosobuchi et al. [25] in the US successfully treat chronic deafferentation pain with stimulation of sensory thalamus.
1974	Adams et al.	Reports on internal capsule DBS for pain [26].
1977	Richardson et al.	Reports on stimulation of periventricular and periaqueductal gray matter for chronic pain [27, 28].
2001-2005	Leone et al.	Reports marked improvement of medication resistant cluster headache in 24 patients after DBS of the posterior hypothalamic gray matter [37-40].

Legend: DBS: deep brain stimulation.

DBS in Epilepsy

As mentioned above, Talairach developed a grid system to implant chronic electrodes in medial temporal structures for recording and stimulation in patients with epilepsy as early as 1947 [7, 42, 43]. Cooper stimulated the cerebellum with good results in 1972. His combined experience over the following years reported that 18 of 32 patients had their seizures reduced by half or more after cerebellar stimulation [44-45]. Chronic DBS was then introduced as a treatment of epilepsy, targeting thalamic, cerebellar as well as other brain structures [3]. As early as 1979, Cooper targeted the anterior nucleus of the thalamus in patient with refractory complex partial seizures with good results, while Velasco et al. targeted the center median thalamic nucleus later on (Table 3). The interest of DBS in epilepsy then cooled down until 2002, when Hodaie et al. reported a mean reduction of 54% in seizure frequency in five patients with medically refractory epilepsy after bilateral DBS of the anterior thalamus [46]. In 2007, Boon et al. reported an open label study on 10 patients with DBS in the medial temporal lobe (MTL) structures in patients with MTL epilepsy. Seven had more than 50% seizure frequency reduction and only one did not respond [47]. The first blinded randomized control trial was published by Fisher et al. in 2010 and reported favorable results of anterior thalamic nucleus DBS on epilepsy [48] possibly opening the way for FDA approval in the future.

The current evidence of DBS in epilepsy will be reviewed in Chapter 9.

DBS in Movement Disorders

In the late 1930's, neurosurgeon E. Jefferson Browder luckily observed that caudate nucleus extirpation improved parkinsonian symptoms, which led Russell Meyer to advocate targeting of the basal ganglia for the treatment of tremor [49, 50]. In the 1950's, Spiegel et al. reported improvement of movement disorders after stereotactic pallidoansotomies in

Table 4. Milestones in the development of DBS in epilepsy

1947	Talairach	Developed grid system to implant chronic electrodes in medial temporal structures for recording and stimulation in patients with epilepsy [7].
1972	Escobedo et al.	Reports on 2 patients with epilepsy, mental retardation, and destructive aggressive behavior implanted in the head of the caudate [95].
1973	Cooper et al.	Promising results of cerebellar stimulation in 7 patients [44].
1978	Cooper and Upton	Cerebellar stimulation produced marked improvement in 18 of 29 patients, but there was rebound after stopping stimulation [45].
1979	Cooper et al.	5 out of 6 patients with refractory complex partial seizures improved with DBS of the anterior nucleus of the thalamus [73, 96].
1987	Velasco et al.	5 patients with refractory generalized or multifocal epilepsy improved with DBS of the center median thalamic nucleus, and psychological performance improved beyond that expected by reduction in seizure activity [97].
2002	Hodaie et al.	5 patients with medically refractory epilepsy improved with bilateral DBS of the anteriorthalamus [46].
2007	Boon et al.	9 out of 10 patients withrefractory medial temporallobe MTL epilepsy improve after DBS in the MTL [47].
2010	Fisher et al.	Benefit of anterior thalmic nucleus DBS on epilepsy demonstrated in a multicenter blinded randomized controlled trial [48].

Huntington's and Parkinon's disease (PD) [8], then reported improvement of motor symptoms after interruption of pallidofugal fibers [51]. In parallel, Meyers experimented on surgery on the pallidofugal fibers in PD patients [52].

In 1953, Cooper accidentally injured the choroidal artery of a PD patient and noted a resolution of the patient‘s tremor and rigidity without other deficits [53, 54]. Because the choroidal artery vascularizes the pallidum, Cooper postulated that a lesion of that structure would be beneficial in the treatment of tremor, which gave birth to the surgical method of pallidotomy. Later on, when anatomical controls showed that the efficient lesion was actually situated in the thalamus, thalamotomy was conceived [55, 56], and stereotactic ventrolateral thalamotomy for PD was successfully developed by Hassler and Riechertas well as Talairach [57, 58].

It isn't until the 1960's that stereotactic stimulation for movement disorders was introduced, albeit only as an intraoperative mean to confirm the location of the lead before creating the therapeutic lesion. One should remember that the advanced imaging techniques we enjoy today were not available at that time. During these pre-lesioning stimulation sessions, Alberts el al described a modification of PD tremor with stimulation of the globus pallidus interna (GPi) or the ventro-intermediate nucleus of the thalamus (Vim) at 60 HZ [59], while Albe Fessard reported suppression of PD tremor with stimulation of the Vim at 100 to 200 Hz [60]. Several authors similarly reported that low frequency stimulation of the thalamus, subthalamic nucleus, or zona incerta could worsen tremor while high frequency stimulation would improve it [3, 61-65].

In 1965, the Norwegian neurophysiologist Sem-Jacobsen implanted multiple electrodes in the thalamus of PD and tremor patients and delivered chronic stimulation for weeks. This allowed him to determine the most suitable site for thalamotomy: the electrode yielding the best stimulation result was then used to create the lesion [66, 67]. The development of chronic deep brain stimulation stopped one step short of becoming a therapy of its own for tremor and PD. At that time, the introduction of Levodopa and its remarkable success in the treatment of parkinsonian symptoms lead to the decline of stereotactic surgery in this domain [68].

Table 5. Milestones in the development of DBS in movement disorders

1890	Horsley	Extirpation of the motor cortex for treatment of athetosis [98].
1930's	Browder	Fortuitous observation that caudate nucleus extirpation improved parkinsonian symptoms [49, 50].
1950	Spiegel et al.	Reports of stereotactical pallidoansotomies for Huntington chorea and choreoathetosis, then PD [8].
1950	Spiegel et al.	Intentional interruption of pallidofugal fibers improved bradykinesia, rigidity, and tremor in PD patients [51].
1953	Cooper	Accidental lesion of the anterior choroidal artery while attempting to section the cerebral peduncle in PD patient. That artery was ligated and this lead to disappearance of rigidity and tremor with preserved motor and sensory function [53-54].
1954	Hassler and Riechert	Lesions of the VL nucleus of the thalamus to treat PD [57]
1957	Talairach et al.	Lesions of the VL nucleus of the thalamus to treat PD [58].
1961	Alberts et al.	Intraoperative pre-lesioning stimulation of the GPi or Vim in 62 patients with PD can elicit or disrupt tremor [59].
1963	AlbeFessard et al.	Improvement of PD tremor with high frequency (100-200 HZ) stimulation of the Vim prior to ablation [60].
1965	Sem-Jacobsen	Extraoperative chronic thalamic stimulation through multiple electrodes, to identify the most suitable site of thalamotomy for PD and tremor [66, 67].
1969	Nashold et al.	Intra-operative prelesioning tremor suppression during stimulation of various subcortical structures at frequencies of 120-300 Hz [63].
1969	Cotzias et al.	Decline of stereotactic surgery because of the success of Levodopa in the treatment of parkinsonian symptoms [68].
1972-1977	Bechtereva	First to suggest chronic subcortical stimulation as a permanent therapy for movement disorders. No implantable stimulator available in USSR, so stimulation was in fact used to select best target for lesioning [3, 69-71].
1977	Mundinger	Reports positive results of DBS in ZI, ventral oral anterior and ventral oral internal nuclei of the thalamus for cervical dystonia [72].
1980-1982	Cooper et al.	DBS of the thalamus and the internal capsule for various movement disorders [73, 74].
1980	Brice and McLellan	Report on DBS of the subthalamic area in 3 patients with multiple sclerosis induced intention tremor [75].
1983	Andy	Reports fair to excellent results of DBS targeting Vim and other areas of the thalamus and subthalamus, in 9 patients with movement disorders [76].
1987	Benabid et al.	Improvement of tremor with thalamic DBS contralateral to thalamotomy. Beginning of modern DBS era [1].

Table 5. (Continued)

1991	Benabid et al.	Complete or almost complete tremor suppression in PD and ET after bilateral Vim DBS. Good safety profile [77].
1992	Laitinen et al.	Reintroduction of the Leksell pallidotomy technique for patients with advanced PD and severe adverse effects from levodopa. Contrary to Vim DBS, this improved all motor symptoms of PD, not just tremor [99].
1993	Pollak et al.	First case of STN DBS in a PD patient [86].
1994	Siegfried et al.	First use of GPi DBS in PD [87].
1998	Limousin et al.	Open label documentation of safety and efficacy of bilateral STN DBS in advanced PD [101].
1998	Kumar et al.	First blinded evaluation of STN DBS in PD, showing similar results than open label studies [88].
1999	Burchiel KJ et al.	Similar improvement in PD symptoms after Gpi or STN DBS in a randomized comparison [101].
1999	Coubes et al.	First case report of GPi DBS for dystonia [89].
1999	Vandewalle et al.	First reports on DBS for Tourette syndrome [102].
2000	Coubes et al.	GPi DBS effective in treating DYT1 primary generalized dystonia [103].
2003	Sydow et al.	50% persistent suppression at 6 years in essential tremor patients with Vim DBS [104].
2003	Krack et al.	50% improvement in motor and activities of daily living scores at 5 y in PD patients with STN DBS [105].
2003	Krauss et al.	GPi DBS effective in generalized non-DYT1 dystonia [106].
2005	Vidailhet et al.	50% improvement of dystonia in double-blinded evaluation after GPi DBS [107].
2006	Deuschl et al.	STN DBS superior to optimal medical management in patients with advanced PD and levodopa-related motor complications [108].
2006	Kupsch et al.	First randomized, double-blind, sham-controlled trial of GPi DBS in primary segmental or generalized dystonia [109].
2007	Kiss et al.	40% improvement in cervical dystonia after GPi DBS in single blinded study [110].
2009	Vidailhet et al.	Variable effect of Gpi DBS on dystonia-choreoathetosis in cerebral palsy [111].

Legend: PD: Parkinson's disease; VL: ventrolateral; GPi: globus pallidus interna; Vim: ventro-intermedius nucleus of the thalamus; USSR: Union of Soviet Socialist Republics; ZI: zona incerta.

The development of deep brain stimulation for movement disorders was slow over the following 2 decades. In the 1970's, the soviet neurophysiologist Bechtereva was the first to suggest chronic subcortical stimulation as a permanent therapy for movement disorders [3, 69]. She implanted electrodes in the ventrolateral and the centromedian thalamus and performed intermittent sessions of high frequency stimulation for up to 1.5 years [70], naming this technique "therapeutic electrostimulation" [71]. However, the Union of Soviet Socialist Republics did not have access to implantable neurostimulators at that time, and these stimulation sessions were ultimately used to select the best target for lesioning, like Sem Jacobsen had done 10 years earlier. In the Western world, the first battery powered neuropacemaker was developed in the early 70s, allowing implantation of the system and the use of DBS as a chronic therapy rather than an adjunct to ablative surgery.

In the late 1970'sGerman neurosurgeon Mundinger implanted electrodes unilaterally in the ventral oral anterior and ventral oral internal nuclei of the thalamus as well as in the zona incerta in patients with cervical dystonia, delivering intermittent stimulation with frequencies of up to 390 Hz [72]. In the US, Cooper and his team performed chronic stimulation in the thalamus and the internal capsule for various movement disorders. He might have been the first to use the term "DBS" in the context of neurosurgery for movement disorders [73], and, like Mundinger, underlined the reversibility of this therapy and it's advantage over stereotactic ablation [73, 74].

In 1980, Brice and McLellan reported improvement of multiple sclerosis induced intention tremor in 2 out of 3 patients treated with high frequency (75-150Hz) DBS of the subthalamic area [75]. Three years later, Andy reported on high frequency (50-200 HZ) DBS targeting the Vim and other areas of the thalamus and subthalamus, in 9 patients with movement disorders [76].

At that time, refractory tremor was treated with unilateral thalamotomy, bilateral stereotactic lesions being too dangerous. As a result, some PD patients were left with a severe untreated unilateral tremor. Benabib and Pollack, in Grenoble, France, offered DBS contralateral to the thalamotomy for these patients, with marked success [1]. Their article, published in 1987, is considered the beginning of the modern area of DBS. Shortly after, they reported on the marked benefit of bilateral Vim DBS for tremor in PD or essential tremor [77]. Subsequently, Vim DBS virtually replaced thalamotomy as a first-hand procedure for essential tremor [78-80]. In addition, the movement disorders community started facing the late effects of levodopa therapy. Indeed, motor fluctuations and dyskinesia are closely associated with the use of levodopa, particularly at higher dosages and after prolonged use [81]. These side effects led to a renewed interest in surgical therapies. However, contrary to pallidotomy, Vim DBS did not improve bradykinesia or rigidity in PD patients. For that reason, Leskell's old posteroventral pallidotomy was revived by Laitinen et al. and overshadowed DBS for PD during the 1990s [82, 83].

Using the model of basal ganglia developed by Albin et al. [84] and De Long [85], which was based on the hypothesis that there were segregated circuits within the basal ganglia thalamocortical network, each serving a different function; the Grenoble's team implanted DBS in the subthalamic nucleus (STN) of a PD patient for the first time in 1993, with marked improvement of all cardinal motor symptoms [86]. The following year, Siegfried et al. reported improvement of PD symptoms with DBS to the GPi (Siegfried et al., 1994) [87]. The first blinded evaluation of STN DBS for PD was published by Kumar et al. in 1998, showing similar results than open label studies [88]. In 1999, Coubes et al. reported the first case of GPi DBS for dystonia with dramatic improvement of the symptoms, adding another movement disorders on the list of applications of DBS (Table 5) [89].

Case series and open label studies multiplied, showing the benefit, safety and reversibility of DBS for various movement disorders including dystonia, Tourette's syndrome, essential tremor, and cerebral palsy (Table 5). In addition to its benefits in psychiatry, pain, epilepsy and movement disorders, there are case reports of using DBS for the treatment of vegetative state, addiction, obesity, dementia, and stroke recovery [2, 90].

The evidence of DBS for each disorder will be reviewed in Chapters 6 through 9.

Neurostimulators: From the Operating Room to under the Skin

Because the development of fully implantable neurostimulators and handheld programmers contributed to the increasing popularity of DBS versus previously used destructive procedures [32], it is important to summarize this evolution.

Implantable radiofrequency stimulators were already invented in the early 1930'sand were used for stimulation of the phrenic nerve for artificial respiration as early as 1963 [91]. In 1960, the first battery-powered cardiac pacemaker was implanted. This technology was then adapted and further developed, leading to the implantation of the first battery powered neuropacemaker in the early 1970s [32, 91]. However, these first neurostimulators were not yet fully implantable. Only the receiver was implanted, and patients had to carry the cigarette pack-sized 9 volts battery-driven stimulator on their belt and an antenna placed on the skin over the receiver area, in order to achieve stimulation. The antenna was held in place by a double sided adhesive disk. The stimulator had patient-adjustable amplitude and frequency dials as well as a physician-adjustable screw to adjust the pulse width [21]. However, the selection of electrode contacts and polarity at the time of surgery was final. Indeed, the brain leads were hardwired to an external stimulus generator for several days, during which test stimulation was performed. Out of the 4 available, the 2 most favorable electrode contacts were then selected and attached by the surgeon to the positive and negative poles of the stimulator extension cable at the time of system internalization. The two unused pins on the connector were then clipped off and discarded, and the connector assembly was sealed permanently [21].

Fully implantable neurostimulators (FINS) became available in the mid 1980's, initially as spinal cord stimulators that were then adapted for DBS [92]. Earlier FINS required the same briefcase-sized physician programmer as used by cardiologists for pacemakers, but with a special software cartridge for DBS. In the 1990's, programmers finally became small enough to fit into the pocket of a doctor's white coat [21].

Conclusion

The development of DBS spans over more than a half century. Although currently essentially known as a major part of the armamentarium against movement disorders, DBS had its first steps in the fields of psychiatry, pain and epilepsy but did not evolve much in these fields until recently. Indeed, because of its success in movement disorders therapy, DBS is now re-evaluated rigorously for the management of many other disorders, with some promising results.

References

[1] Benabid A. L., Pollak P., Louveau A., Henry S., de Rougemont J. Combined (thalamotomy and stimulation) stereotactic surgery of the VIM thalamic nucleus for bilateral Parkinson's disease. *Appl Neurophysiol*. 1987; 50:344-346.

[2] Miocinovic S. L, Somayajula S., Chitnis S., Vitek J. L. History, applications, and mechanisms of deep brain stimulation. *JAMA Neurol.* 2013; 70(2):163-71.
[3] Hariz M. I. L., Blomstedt P., Zrinzo L. Deep brain stimulation between 1947 and 1987: The untold story. *Neurosurg Focus.* 2010; 29:E1.
[4] Spiegel EA, Wycis HT, Marks M, Lee AJ. Stereotaxic apparatus for operations on the human brain. *Science.* 1947; 106:349-350.
[5] Gildenberg P., History repeats itself. *Stereotact Funct Neurosurg* 2003; 80:61-75.
[6] Gildenberg P. L., Evolution of neuromodulation. *Stereotact Funct Neurosurg.* 2005; 83:71-79.
[7] Talairach J., Hecaen H., David M., Monnier M., De Ajuriaguerra J. Recherches sur la coagulation thérapeutique des structures sous-corticales chez l'homme. *Rev Neurol* 1949; 81:4-24.
[8] Spiegel E. A., Wycis H. T., Pallidothalamotomy in chorea. *Arch Neurol Psychiatry* 1950; 64:295-296.
[9] Heath R. G., *Depth recording and stimulation studies in patients*, in Winter A. (ed): The Surgical Control of Behavior. Springfield, IL: Charles C. Thomas, 1971, pp. 21-37.
[10] Bickford R. G., Petersen M. C., Dodge H. W. Jr., Sem-Jacobsen C. W. Observations on depth stimulation of the human brain through implanted electrographic leads. *Proc Staff Meet Mayo Clin.* 1953; 28:181-187.
[11] Delgado J. M., Hamlin H., Chapman W. P., Technique of intracranial electrode implacement for recording and stimulation and its possible therapeutic value in psychotic patients. *Confin Neurol.* 1952; 12:315-319.
[12] Laitinen L. V., Emotional responses to subcortical electrical stimulation in psychiatric patients. *Clin Neurol Neurosurg.* 1979; 81:148-157.
[13] Sem-Jacobsen C. W., Styri O. B., *Depth-electrographic stereotaxic psychosurgery*, in Hitchcock E., Laitinen L., Vaernet K. (eds): Psychosurgery. Springfield, IL: Charles C. Thomas, 1972, pp. 76-82.
[14] Delgado J. M., Mark V., Sweet W., Ervin F., Weiss G., Bach-Y-Rita G. et al., Intracerebral radio stimulation and recording in completely free patients. *J Nerv Ment Dis.* 1968; 147:329-340.
[15] Delgado J. M. R., Obrador S., Martín-Rodríguez J. G., *Two-way radio communication with the brain in psychosurgical patients*, in Laitinen L. V., Livingstone K. E. (eds): Surgical Approaches in Psychiatry. Lancaster, UK: Medical and Technical Publishing Co, 1973, pp. 215-223.
[16] Delgado J. M. R., *Therapeutic programmed stimulation in man*, in Sweet W. H., Obrador S., Martín-Rodríguez J. G. (eds). Neurosurgical Treatment in Psychiatry, Pain, and Epilepsy. Baltimore: University Park Press, 1977, pp. 615-637.
[17] Laitinen L. V., *Ethical aspects of psychiatric surgery*, in Sweet W. H., Obrador S., Martín-Rodríguez J. G. (eds): Neurosurgical Treatment in Psychiatry, Pain, and Epilepsy. Baltimore: University Park Press, 1977, pp. 483-488.
[18] Dieckmann G., *Chronic mediothalamic stimulation for control of phobias*, in Hitchcock E. R., Ballantine H. T. Jr., Meyerson B. A. (eds): Modern Concepts in Psychiatric Surgery. Amsterdam: Elsevier, 1979, pp. 85-93.
[19] Nuttin B., Cosyns P., Demeulemeester H., Gybels J., Meyerson B., Electrical stimulation in anterior limbs of internal capsules in patients with obsessive-compulsive disorder. *Lancet* 1999; 354:1526.

[20] Reynolds D. V., Surgery in the rat during electrical analgesia induced by focal brain stimulation. *Science* 1969; 164:444-445.

[21] Coffey R. J., Deep brain stimulation devices: a brief technical history and review. *Artif Organs*. 2009; 33:208-220.

[22] Mazars G., Mérienne L., Ciolocca C., Intermittent analgesic thalamic stimulation. Preliminary note. *Rev Neurol* 1973; 28:273-279.

[23] Mazars G., Mérienne L., Cioloca C., Treatment of certain types of pain with implantable thalamic stimulators. *Neurochirurgie* 1974; 20:117-124.

[24] Mazars G. J., Intermittent stimulation of nucleus ventralisposterolateralis for intractable pain. *Surg Neurol* 1975; 4:93-95.

[25] Hosobuchi Y., Adams J. E., Rutkin B., Chronic thalamic stimulation for the control of facial anesthesia dolorosa. *Arch Neurol*. 1973; 29:158-161.

[26] Adams J. E., Hosobuchi Y., Fields H. L., Stimulation of internal capsule for relief of chronic pain. *J Neurosurg*. 1974; 41:740-744.

[27] Richardson D. E., Akil H., Pain reduction by electrical brain stimulation in man. Part 1: Acute administration in periaqueductal and periventricular sites. *J Neurosurg*. 1977; 47:178-183.

[28] Richardson D. E., Akil H., Pain reduction by electrical brain stimulation in man. Part 2: Chronic self-administration in the periventricular gray matter. *J Neurosurg*1977; 47:184-194.

[29] Hosobuchi Y., Adams J. E., Linchitz R., Pain relief by electrical stimulation of the central gray matter in humans and its reversal by naloxone. *Science* 1977; 197:183-186.

[30] Mazars G., Merienne L., Cioloca C., Control of dyskinesias due to sensory deafferentation by means of thalamic stimulation. *Acta Neurochir Suppl* (Wien) 1980; 30:239e43.

[31] Merienne L., Mazars G., Treatment of various dyskinesias by intermittent thalamic stimulation. *Neurochirurgie* 1982; 28:201e6.

[32] Blomstedt P., Hariz M. I., Deep brain stimulation for movement disorders before DBS for movement disorders. *Parkinsonism Relat Disord*. 2010; 16:429-433.

[33] Coffey R. J., Deep brain stimulation devices: a brief technical history and review. *Artif Organs* 2009; 33:208-220.

[34] Coffey R. J., Deep brain stimulation for chronic pain: the results of two multi-center trials and a structured review. *Pain Med* 2001; 2:183-192.

[35] Hamani C., Schwalb J. M., Rezai A. R., Dostrovsky J. O., Davis K. D., Lozano A. M., Deep brain stimulation for chronic neuropathic pain: long-term outcome and the incidence of insertional effect. *Pain* 2006; 25:188-196.

[36] Hariz M. I., Bergenheim A. T. Thalamic stereotaxis for chronic pain: ablative lesion or stimulation? *Stereotact Funct Neurosurg*. 1995; 64:47-55.

[37] Leone M., Franzini A., Bussone G., Stereotactic stimulation of posterior hypothalamic gray matter for intractable cluster headache. *N Engl J Med*. 2001; 345; 1428-1429.

[38] Leone M., Franzini A., Broggi G., May A., Bussone G., Long-term follow up of bilateral hypothalamic stimulation for intractable cluster headache. *Brain* 2004; 127; 2259-2264.

[39] Leone M., Franzini A., Broggi G., Bussone G., Hypothalamic stimulation for intractable cluster headache: long-term experience. *Neurology* 2006; 67:150-152.

[40] Leone M., Deep brain stimulation in headache. *Lancet Neurol*. 2006; 5:873-877.

[41] Bittar R. G., Kar-Purkayastha I., Owen S. L., Bear R. E., Green A., Wang S. et al., Deep brain stimulation for pain relief: a meta-analysis. *J Clin Neurosci*. 2005; 12:515-519.

[42] Mazoyer B., In memoriam: Jean Talairach (1911-2007): a life in stereotaxy. *Hum Brain Mapp* 2008; 29:250-252.

[43] Talairach J., Bancaud J., Bonis A., Szikla G., Tournoux P., Functional stereotaxic exploration of epilepsy. *Confin Neurol*. 1962; 22:328-331.

[44] Cooper I. S., Amin I., Gilman S., The effect of chronic cerebellar stimulation upon epilepsy in man. *Trans Am Neurol Assoc*. 1973; 98:192-196.

[45] Cooper I. S., Upton A. R., Effects of cerebellar stimulation on epilepsy, the EEG and cerebral palsy in man. *Electroencephalogr Clin Neurophysiol Suppl*. 1978; 34:349-354.

[46] Hodaie M., Wennberg R. A., Dostrovsky J. O., Lozano A. M., Chronic anterior thalamus stimulation for intractable epilepsy. *Epilepsia* 2002; 43:603-608.

[47] Boon P., Vonck K., De Herdt V. et al., Deep brain stimulation in patients with refractory temporal lobe epilepsy. *Epilepsia* 2007; 48:1551-1560.

[48] Fisher R., Salanova V., Witt T., Worth R., Henry T., Gross R. et al., SANTE Study Group. Electrical stimulation of the anterior nucleus of thalamus for treatment of refractory epilepsy. *Epilepsia*. 2010; 51:899-908.

[49] Gabriel E. M., Nashold B. S., Jr. Evolution of neuroablative surgery for involuntary movement disorders: an historical review. *Neurosurgery* 1998; 42:575-590.

[50] Wagle Shukla A., Okun M. S., Surgical treatment of Parkinson's disease: patients, targets, devices, and approaches. *Neurotherapeutics*. 2014; 11:47-59.

[51] Spiegel E. A., Wycis H. T., Szekely E. G. et al., Stimulation of Forel's field during stereotaxic operations in the human brain. *Electroencephalogr Clin Neurophysiol*. 1964; 16:537-548.

[52] Meyers R., Surgical experiments in the therapy of certain "extrapyramidal" diseases: a current evaluation. *Acta Psychiatr Neurol Suppl* 1951; 67:1-42.

[53] Cooper I. S., Ligation of the anterior choroidal artery for involuntary movements: Parkinsonism. *Psychiatr Q*. 1953; 27:317-319.

[54] Cooper I. S., Surgical alleviation of Parkinsonism; effects of occlusion of the anterior choroidal artery. *J Am Geriatr Soc* 1954; 2:691-718.

[55] Cooper, I. S., An investigation of neurosurgical alleviation of parkinsonism, chorea, athetosisand dystonia. *Annales Medicinae Internae Fenniae* 1956;45:381-392.

[56] Benabid A. L., Chabardes S., Torres N., Piallat B., Krack P., Fraix V. et al., Functional neurosurgery for movement disorders: a historical perspective. *Prog Brain Res* 2009; 175:379-391.

[57] Hassler R., Riechert T., Indikationen und lokalisationsmethode der gezieltenhirnoperationen. *Nervenarzt*. 1954; 25:441-447.

[58] Talairach J., David M., Tournoux P., Corredor H., Kvasina T. *Atlas d'anatomie stereotaxique*. Paris, France: Masson; 1957.

[59] Alberts W. W., Wright E. W. Jr., Levin G., Feinstein B., Mueller M., Threshold stimulation of the lateral thalamus and globuspallidus in the waking human. *Electroencephalogr Clin Neurophysiol*. 1961; 13:68-74.

[60] Albe Fessard D., Arfel G., Guiot G. et al., Characteristic electric activities of some cerebral structures in man. *Ann Chir*. 1963; 17:1185-1214.

[61] Hassler R., Riechert T., Mundinger F., Umbach W., Ganglberger J. A., Physiological observations in stereotaxic operations in extrapyramidal motor disturbances. *Brain* 1960; 83:337-350.

[62] Hullay J., Velok J., Gombi R., Boczàn G., Subthalamotomy in Parkinson's disease. *Confin Neurol*. 1970; 32:345-348.

[63] Nashold B. S., Slaughter D. G., *Some observations on tremor,* in Gillingham F. J., Donaldson I. M. L. (eds): Third Symposium on Parkinson's Disease. Edinburgh: Livingstone, 1969, pp. 241-246.

[64] Rümler B., Schaltenbrand G., Spuler H., Wahren W., Somatotopic array of the ventro-oral nucleus of the thalamus based on electrical stimulation during stereotactic procedures. *Confin Neurol.* 1972; 34:197-199.

[65] Siegfried J., *Deep brain stimulation for movement disorders*, in Gildenberg P. L., Tasker R. R. (eds): Textbook of Stereotactic and Functional Neurosurgery. New York: McGraw-Hill, 1996, pp. 1081-1085.

[66] Sem-Jacobsen C. W., Depth electrographic stimulation and treatment of patients with Parkinson's disease including neurosurgical technique. *Acta Neurol Scand Suppl.* 1965; 13 Pt 1:365-377.

[67] Sem-Jacobsen C. W., Depth-electrographic observations related to Parkinson's disease. Recording and electrical stimulation in the area around the third ventricle. *J Neurosurg.* 1966; 24:388-402.

[68] Cotzias G. C., Papavasiliou P. S., Gellene R., Modification of Parkinsonism: chronic treatment with L-dopa. *N Engl J Med.* 1969; 280:337-345.

[69] Bekhtereva N. P., Bondarchuk A. N., Smirnov V. M., Meliucheva L. A., [Therapeutic electric stimulation of deep brain structures.] *Vopr Neirokhir* 1972; 36:7-12 (Russian).

[70] Bechtereva N. P., Bondartchuk A. N., Smirnov V. M., Meliutcheva L. A., Shandurina A. N. Method of electrostimulation of the deep brain structures in treatment of some chronic diseases. *Confin Neurol.* 1975; 37:136-140.

[71] Bechtereva N. P., Kambarova D. K., Smirnov V. M., Shandurina A. N., *Using the brain's latent abilities for therapy: Chronic intracerebral electrical stimulation*, in Sweet B. W., Obrador S., Martín-Rodríguez J. G. (eds): Neurosurgical Treatment in Psychiatry, Pain, and Epilepsy. Baltimore: University Park Press, 1977, pp. 581-613.

[72] Mundinger F., [New stereotactic treatment of spasmodic torticollis with a brain stimulation system.] *Med Klin* 1977; 72:1982-1986.

[73] Cooper I. S., Upton A. R. M., Amin I. Reversibility of chronic neurologic deficits. Some effects of electrical stimulation of the thalamus and internal capsule in man. *Appl Neurophysiol.* 1980; 43:244-258.

[74] Cooper I. S., Upton A. R. M., Amin I. Chronic cerebellar stimulation (CCS) and deep brain stimulation (DBS) in involuntary movement disorders. *Appl Neurophysiol.* 1982; 45:209-217.

[75] Brice J., McLellan L., Suppression of intention tremor by contingent deep-brain stimulation. *Lancet* 1980; 1:1221-1222.

[76] Andy O. J., Thalamic stimulation for control of movement disorders. *Appl Neurophysiol.* 1983; 46:107-111.

[77] Benabid A. L., Pollak P., Gervason C., Hoffmann D., Gao D. M., Hommel M. et al., Long-term suppression of tremor by chronic stimulation of the ventral intermediate thalamic nucleus. *Lancet.* 1991; 337:403-406.

[78] Koller W., Pahwa R., Busenbark K., Hubble J., Wilkinson S., Lang A. et al., High-frequency unilateral thalamic stimulation in the treatment of essential and parkinsonian tremor. *Ann Neurol.* 1997; 42:292-299.

[79] Limousin P., Speelman J. D., Gielen F., Janssens M., Multicentre European study of thalamic stimulation in parkinsonian and essential tremor. *J Neurol Neurosurg Psychiatry* 1999; 66: 289-296.

[80] Schuurman P. R., Bosch D. A., Bossuyt P. M., Bonsel G. J., van Someren E. J., de Bie R. M. et al., A comparison of continuous thalamic stimulation and thalamotomy for suppression of severe tremor. *N Engl J Med.* 2000; 342:461-468.

[81] Mehanna R., Lai E. C., Deep brain stimulation in Parkinson's disease. *Transl Neurodegener.* 2013; 18; 2(1):22.

[82] Laitinen L. V., Bergenheim A. T., Hariz M. I., Leksell's posteroventral pallidotomy in the treatment of Parkinson's disease. *J Neurosurg* 1992; 76:53-61.

[83] Hariz M. I., From functional neurosurgery to "interventional" neurology: Survey of publications on thalamotomy, pallidotomy, and deep brain stimulation for Parkinson's disease from 1966 to 2001. *Mov Disord* 2003; 18:845-53.

[84] Albin R. L., Young A. B., Penney J. B., The functional anatomy of basal ganglia disorders. *Trends Neurosci.* 1989; 12:366-375.

[85] De Long M. R. Primate models of movement disorders of basal ganglia origin. *Trends Neurosci.* 1990; 13:281-285.

[86] Pollak P., Benabid A. L., Gross C., Gao D. M., Laurent A., Benazzouz A. et al., Effects of the stimulation of the subthalamic nucleus in Parkinson disease. *Rev Neurol* (Paris) 1993; 149:175-176.

[87] Siegfried J., Lippitz B., Bilateral chronic electrostimulation of ventroposterolateral pallidum: A new therapeutic approach for alleviating all parkinsonian symptoms. *Neurosurgery.* 1994; 35:1126-1129, discussion 1129-1130.

[88] Kumar R., Lozano A. M., Kim Y. J. et al., Double-blind evaluation of subthalamic nucleus deep brain stimulation in advanced Parkinson's disease. *Neurology.* 1998; 51:850-855.

[89] Coubes P., Echenne B., Roubertie A., Vayssiere N., Tuffery S., Humbertclaude V. et al., Treatment of early-onset generalized dystonia by chronic bilateral stimulation of the internal globus pallidus. Apropos of a case. *Neurochirurgie* 1999; 45:139-144.

[90] Shah S. A., Schiff N. D., Central thalamic deep brain stimulation for cognitive neuromodulation: a review of proposed mechanisms and investigational studies. *Eur J Neurosci.* 2010; 32:1135-1144.

[91] Davis R., *Chronic stimulation of the central nervous system.* In: Gildenberg P. L., Tasker R., (eds). Textbook of stereotactic and functional neurosurgery. McGraw-Hill; 1996. pp. 963-969.

[92] Shatin D., Mullett K., Hults G. Totally implantable spinal cord stimulation for chronic pain: design and efficacy. *Pacing Clin Electrophysiol* 1986; 9:577-83.

[93] Heath R. G., Electrical self-stimulation of the brain in man. *Am J Psychiatry* 1963; 120:571-577.

[94] Sem-Jacobsen C. W. Depth-electrographic observations in psychotic patients. *Proc Gaustad Ment Hospital* (Oslo) 1963; 412-416.

[95] Escobedo F., Fernández-Guardiola A., Solís G., *Chronic stimulation of the cingulum in humans with behaviour disorders.* In Laitinen, L. V., Livingstone K. E. (eds): Surgical

Approaches in Psychiatry. Lancaster, UK: Medical and Technical Publishing Co, 1973, pp. 65-68.

[96] Rosenow J., Das K., Rovit R. L., Couldwell W. T. Irving S. Cooper and his role in intracranial stimulation for movement disorders and epilepsy. *Stereotact Funct Neurosurg,* 2002; 78:95-112.

[97] Velasco F., Velasco M., Ogarrio C., Fanghanel G., Electrical stimulation of the centromedian thalamic nucleus in the treatment of convulsive seizures: A preliminary report. *Epilepsia* 1987; 28:421-430.

[98] Horsley V., Remarks on the surgery of the central nervous system. *BMJ.* 1890; 2:1286-1292.

[99] Laitinen L. V., Bergenheim A. T., Hariz M. I. Ventroposterolateral pallidotomy can abolish all parkinsonian symptoms. *Stereotact Funct Neurosurg* 1992; 58:14-21.

[100] Limousin P., Krack P., Pollak P., Benazzouz A., Ardouin C., Hoffmann D. et al., Electrical stimulation of the subthalamic nucleus in advanced Parkinson's disease. *N Engl J Med.* 1998; 339:1105-1111.

[101] Burchiel K. J., Anderson V. C., Favre J., Hammerstad J. P., Comparison of pallidal and subthalamic nucleus deep brain stimulation for advanced Parkinson's disease: results of a randomized, blinded pilot study. *Neurosurgery.* 1999; 45:1375- 1382, discussion 1382-1384.

[102] Vandewalle V., van der Linden C., Groenewegen H. J., Caemaert J. Stereotactic treatment of Gilles de la Tourette syndrome by high frequency stimulation of thalamus. *Lancet* 1999; 353:724.

[103] [Coubes P., Roubertie A., Vayssiere N., Hemm S., Echenne B. Treatment of DYT1-generalised dystonia by stimulation of the internal globus pallidus. *Lancet.* 2000; 355:2220-2221.

[104] Sydow O., Thobois S., Alesch F., Speelman J. D. Multicentre European study of thalamic stimulation in essential tremor: a six year follow up. *J Neurol Neurosurg Psychiatry.* 2003; 74:1387-1391.

[105] Krack P., Batir A., Van Blercom N. et al., Five-year follow-up of bilateral stimulation of the subthalamic nucleus in advanced Parkinson's disease. *N Engl J Med.* 2003; 349:1925-1934.

[106] Krauss J. K., Loher T. J., Weigel R., Capelle H. H., Weber S., Burgunder J. M. Chronic stimulation of the globuspallidusinternus for treatment of non-dYT1 generalized dystonia and choreoathetosis: 2-year follow up. *J Neurosurg.* 2003;98:785-792.

[107] Vidailhet M., Vercueil L., Houeto J. L. et al., French Stimulation du Pallidum Interne dans la Dystonie (SPIDY) Study Group. Bilateral deep-brain stimulation of the globuspallidus in primary generalized dystonia. *N Engl J Med.* 2005; 352:459-467.

[108] Deuschl G., Schade-Brittinger C., Krack P. et al., German Parkinson Study Group, Neurostimulation Section. A randomized trial of deep-brain stimulation for Parkinson's disease. *N Engl J Med.* 2006; 355:896-908.

[109] Kupsch A., Benecke R., Muller J. et al., Deep-Brain Stimulation for Dystonia Study Group.Pallidal deep-brain stimulation in primary generalized or segmental dystonia. *N Engl J Med.* 2006; 355:1978-1990.

[110] Kiss Z. H., Doig-Beyaert K., Eliasziw M., Tsui J., Haffenden A., Suchowersky O. Functional and Stereotactic Section of the Canadian Neurosurgical Society; Canadian

Movement Disorders Group. The Canadian multicentre study of deep brain stimulation for cervical dystonia. *Brain.* 2007; 130:2879-2886.

[111] Vidailhet M., Yelnik J., Lagrange C. et al., French SPIDY-2 Study Group. Bilateral pallidal deep brain stimulation for the treatment of patients with dystoniachoreoathetosis cerebral palsy: a prospective pilot study. *Lancet Neurol.* 2009;8:709-717.

In: Deep Brain Stimulation
Editor: Raja Mehanna

ISBN: 978-1-63483-282-3

Chapter 2

Basal Ganglia Physiology and DBS for Parkinson's Disease: Introduction and Postulated Mechanisms

Pornpimol Anprasertporn MD, Neda Hidarilak MD and Harrison Walker MD
University of Alabama at Birmingham, Birmingham, AL, US

Abstract

After reviewing the historical development of deep brain stimulation (DBS) as a therapy in the first chapter, and before we dive into its clinical applications in different disorders, we will here review the motor circuitry of the basal ganglia, how it is dysfunctional in Parkinson's disease, then the postulated mechanism of action of DBS.

Introduction

The basal ganglia are a somatotopically organized group of nuclei located beneath the cerebral cortex, above the midbrain, and surrounding the thalamus.

Although the basal ganglia are classically regarded as playing roles in modulating movements, there are anatomic and functional connections between many regions of the cerebral cortex, basal ganglia, and thalamus, which have given rise to the idea of segregated closed loops with parallel circuits implicated in motor, oculomotor, limbic and prefrontal circuits [1-3].

Depicted schematically in Figure 1, these largely segregated networks are known as "cortico-striato-pallido-thalamocortical loops."

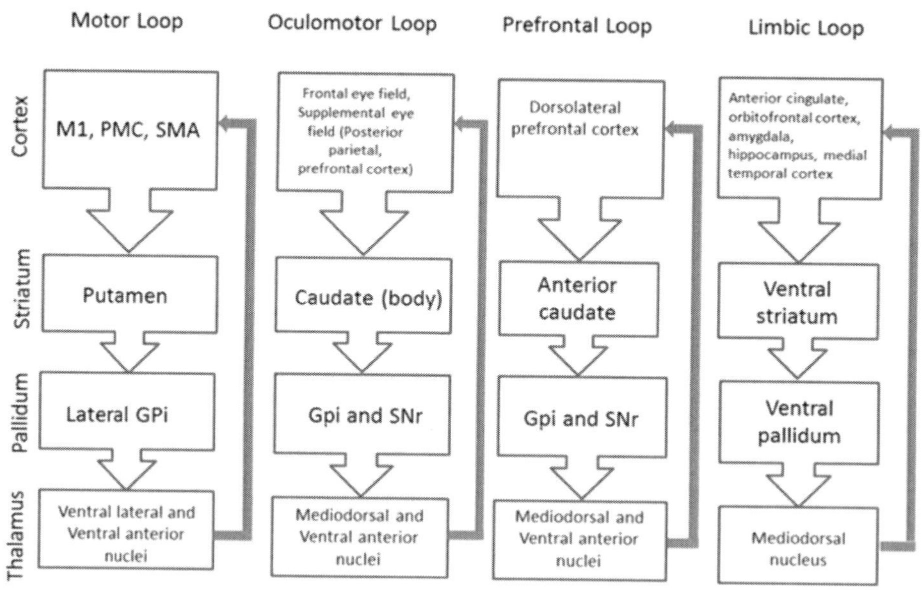

M1 = Primary motor cortex, PMC = Premotor cortex, SMA = Supplemental motor area.

Figure 1. 4 parallel basal circuit schemes.

ANATOMY AND PHYSIOLOGY OF THE MOTOR CIRCUITRY OF THE BASAL GANGLIA

The basal ganglia consist of four groups of interconnected nuclei as follows: (1) the striatum (caudate and putamen) receives cortical input, (2) the globus pallidus (internal and external segments), (3) the substantia nigra (pars compacta and pars reticulata), and (4) the subthalamic nucleus (STN). The globus pallidus interna and substantia nigra pars reticulata are the primary output nuclei of the basal ganglia. The structural/anatomical relationships among these nuclei are illustrated schematically in Figure 2. We will use the motor pathway as a prototype to describe the basal ganglia network as shown in Figure 3. In the classical view, circuitry of the basal ganglia is thought to consist of two opposing circuits, the direct and indirect pathways. The direct pathway refers to the direct projection from striatum and the globus pallidus interna, one of the main output nuclei of the basal ganglia. The indirect pathway refers to the projection from striatum to the globus pallidus externa, STN, and ultimately the globus pallidus interna. In the classical view, these pathways originate from separate populations of striatal medium spiny neurons (MSN), the activity of which is differentially modulated by dopamine. In the motor circuit, primary motor cortex, precentral cortex (especially Brodmann areas 4 and 6), and postcentral somatosensory cortical regions provide glutamatergic projections to putaminal activating MSNs. These neurons in turn project to basal ganglia output structures via the direct and indirect pathways. The output structures of the basal ganglia then project largely to motor subdivisions of the thalamus (the ventral anterior nucleus and the anterior portion of ventral lateral anterior nucleus), then back to corresponding cortical areas.

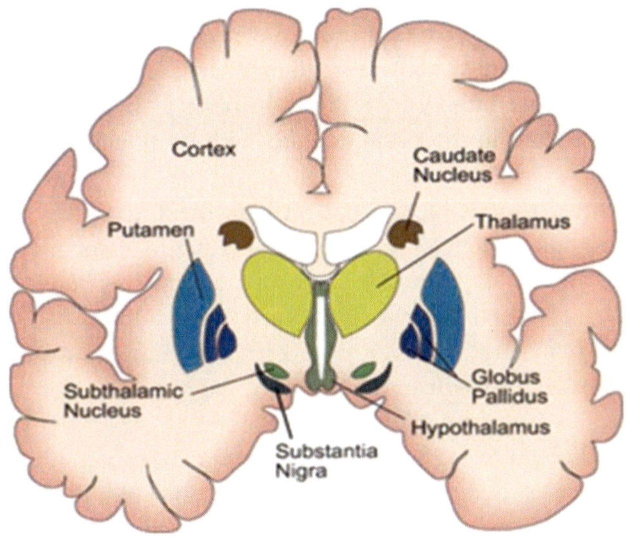

Figure 2. Basal Ganglia Anatomy.

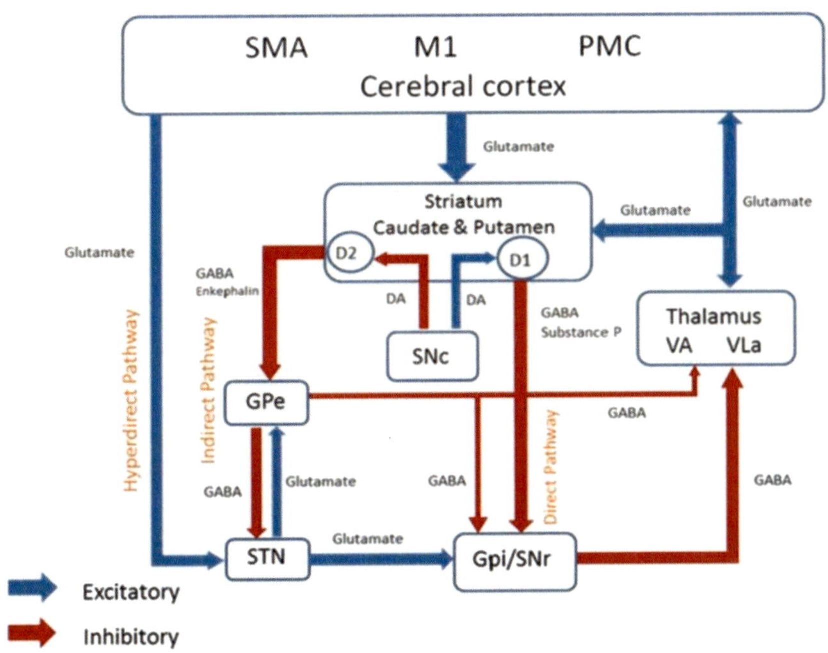

M1 = Primary motor cortex, PMC = Premotor cortex, SMA = Supplemental motor area, DA = Dopamine, GPe = Globus pallidus externa, Gpi = Globus pallidus internal, STN = Subthalamic nucleus, SNc = Substantia nigra pars compacta, SNr = Substantia nigra pars reticularis, VA = Vental anterior nucleus of thalamus, VLa = Anerior portion of vental lateral nucleus of thalamus, GABA = Gamma-aminobutyric Acid.

Figure 3. Motor circuit of basal ganglia.

The anatomic segregation of these output structures likely confers functional specialization for various aspects of motor control. Corticostriatal, thalamocortical, and STN neurons are excitatory, utilizing glutamate as their neurotransmitter. In contrast, the other nuclei in the basal ganglia are largely inhibitory, utilizing GABA. The substantia nigra pars compacta plays a critical role in the basal ganglia with its dopaminergic projections to the striatum.

The core of the model resides in the concept that direct and indirect striatal projections modulate the main output structures of the basal ganglia (globus pallidus interna and substantia nigra pars reticulata) to exert opposing effects on movement. These output structures are GABAergic, discharging in either a rhythmic (globus pallidus interna) or tonic (substantia nigra pars reticulata) manner on their projections. Activation of the direct pathway is therefore thought to result in inhibition of the output nuclei, which disinhibits the thalamic relay nuclei, allowing activation of motor cortical areas. Conversely, activation of the indirect pathway is thought to inhibit the globus pallidus externa, which in turn disinhibits the STN. The STN has an excitatory projection to the globus pallidus interna which inhibits the motor thalamus, which in turn inhibits motor cortical areas. This final negative feedback to cerebral cortex is thought to reduce or eliminate undesired motor activity. The coordinated activity of the direct and indirect pathways is critical for the appropriate timing and synchrony of the basal ganglia circuits during movement.

The two pathways are structurally and functionally intertwined at least at two distinct levels: in the striatum, where the direct and indirect pathways communicate via complex networks of interneurons, and outside of the striatum, where GPe collaterals may bridge the two pathways, potentially allowing the direct pathway to modulate the indirect pathway. In these respects, the direct and indirect pathways might not be viewed as independent systems.

Beyond these anatomic distinctions, the MSNs of the direct and indirect pathway are thought to differentially express dopamine receptors. Striatonigral MSNs of the direct pathway express D1 receptors, whereas striatopallidal MSNs of the indirect pathway express D2 receptors. These two dopamine receptor subtypes are associated with distinct sets of G proteins that are linked to different intracellular signaling pathways, leading to different intracellular responses following dopamine receptor activation [4].

The D1 receptors receive dopaminergic input from SNc and results in an excitatory effect via the projections of MSNs to output nuclei using substance P and dynorphin, whereas D2 receptors receive dopaminergic input from substantia nigra pars compacta and results in an inhibitory effect via the projections of striatal neurons to GPe using encephalin [2, 4].

As suggested previously, the anatomy and physiology of these interconnected pathways is likely oversimplified in the classical model. Among some of the many additional anatomic connections that have been described, the STN also sends excitatory projections to GPe and the pedunculopontine nucleus (PPN), and GPe sends an inhibitory input directly to the output nuclei and to the thalamus. Additionally, there are dense excitatory thalamic projections back to the striatum. In primates, the intralaminar nuclei in the thalamus project to the dorsolateral striatum, whereas the midline and medial parafascicularis nuclei project to ventral or limbic striatum [5, 6]. Different groups of thalamic nuclei project to corresponding striatal and cortical areas, presumably to maintain the functional properties of the different striatal and cortical regions.

How specific regions of cerebral cortex interact with the basal ganglia in humans is poorly understood. One anatomic projection that has gained recent interest is the hyperdirect (or corticosubthalamic) pathway which connects cerebral cortex to the STN. This pathway bypasses the traditional direct and indirect pathways within the basal ganglia [7-9]. It was first described in primates using anatomic tracer methods, and a later electrophysiological study by Nambu et al. confirmed the existence of this hyperdirect pathway [9]. The hyperdirect pathway conveys excitatory signals from cortex to the STN, likely over faster conduction times than are possible via either the direct or indirect pathways. In this way, the hyperdirect pathway was initially proposed to participate in action selection by defining the temporal boundaries for an intended movement. More recently, single cell recordings and anatomic methods have added complexity ideas about its function, particularly with the demonstration of projections from functionally distinct cortical areas into the various subdivisions of the STN [5, 7].

ABNORMALITIES OF THE BASAL GANGLIA PHYSIOLOGY IN DIFFERENT STATES

Despite decades of research, the role of the basal ganglia in movement disorders pathophysiology is complex and defies simple explanations. Several models have been hypothesized to explain changes following dopaminergic depletion in Parkinson's disease (PD), primarily focusing on abnormal discharge rates and/or patterns in the basal ganglia, as well as beta frequency hypersynchrony in the motor network [2, 10]. The rate model proposes that modulation of the direct and indirect pathways produces functionally opposite effects in the thalamic neurons receiving basal ganglia output. As mentioned earlier, increased activity of the direct pathway leads to reduced inhibition of neurons in the thalamus. In contrast, increased activity of the indirect pathway leads to an increase in the inhibition of thalamic nuclei. Microelectrode recordings in 1-methyl-4-phenyl-1,2,3,6-tetrahydropyridine (MPTP)-treated monkeys and PD patients undergoing stereotactic movement disorder surgery have reported decreased mean discharge rates in GPe and VLa and increased mean discharges rates in the STN and GPi [2]. The rate model alone does not explain the full spectrum of PD motor symptoms and their response to different forms of therapy. Although PD is regarded as the prototypical hypokinetic movement disorder, a variety of PD symptoms such as rest tremor, "off" dystonia, and levodopa-induced dyskinesias are hyperkinetic.

Although akinesia and bradykinesia might conceivably relate to dopamine loss in the striatum and subsequent alteration of either discharge rate or pattern in the internal pallidum, how this relates to these other motor symptoms from PD is more speculative. Indeed, in the original descriptions of the classical model, the authors conceded that it did not explain rest, action, or postural tremor, nor did it explain some of the paradoxical observations from stereotactic surgeries. To date, the anatomic origin and mechanisms underlying tremor in and other movement disorders remains poorly understood. If one considers rest tremor a hyperkinetic disorder, dopamine replacement might be expected to worsen this symptom, yet it typically improves or even abolishes it.

Similarly, muscle rigidity is defined as an increase in muscle tone upon passive joint manipulation. In this sense, it might be regarded as a kind of hyperkinetic movement, because an abnormal number of motor units are recruited during the passive joint movement to generate the opposing force. Similar to its effects on tremor, dopamine replacement typically improves muscle rigidity as well. With respect to stereotactic surgeries, the classical model predicts that pallidotomy or pallidal DBS should worsen levodopa-induced dyskinesias, various forms of tremor, and primary dystonia, yet DBS and lesions abolish these symptoms [2]. Furthermore, according to the rate model, a decrease in the discharge rate in VLa should result in bradykinesia, such that stereotactic lesions would be predicted to worsen this symptoms in PD patients. In contrast to this prediction, stereotactic lesions in the motor thalamus improve tremor associated with PD, without worsening bradykinesia. On balance, the role of the basal ganglia with respect to the planning and execution of movements seems to primarily reflect a modulatory role that can become particularly deranged in certain disease states. Patients with DBS or with large basal ganglia lesions of various types are typically able to select actions (motor or otherwise), and they usually retain remarkable abilities to perform intricate and complex motor acts despite altered or absent basal ganglia modulation of the motor system. In many ways, these observations suggest that no basal ganglia is preferable to an unhealthy one.

Beyond its effects on the motor system, selective activation of the direct and indirect pathways in the striatum has been postulated in mechanisms of reinforcement learning in the context of reward and punishment. According to this hypothesis, activation of D1-expressing neurons causes persistent reinforcement, whereas activation of D2-expressing neurons induces transient punishment [11]. In the context of specific behaviors, alterations of these processes could drive or at least modulate symptoms related to psychiatric disorders and drug addiction [12]. In addiction, the direct pathway seems to be involved in reward learning and cocaine sensitization. Additionally, the indirect pathway is implicated in aversive behavior such that the disruption of indirect pathway MSNs facilitates behavioral sensitization, while the decrease of excitability of direct pathway MSNs impairs the persistence of behavioral sensitization following drug exposure. The role of the basal ganglia in reward/punishment and behavioral sensitization might be relevant both for psychiatric diseases such as depression and obsessive-compulsive disorder, and also in impulse control disorders in PD patients. The dopamine dysregulation syndrome is seen with some regularity in PD patients, in which dopamine replacement to improve motor symptoms drives nascent, pathological interest in gambling, hypersexuality, compulsive shopping, compulsive eating, and excessive engagement in hobbies [13-15].

Mechanism of Action of DBS in PD

Deep brain stimulation (DBS) is a remarkable therapy for movement disorders that has driven resurgent interest in systems neuroscience in patients with movement disorders. As detailed in chapter 1, the basal ganglia began to emerge as a target for neuromodulation in patients with movement disorders as by Russel Meyers as early as the late 1930s. He removed the anterior two-thirds of the caudate head under the hypothesis that abnormal movements were mediated by the neopallidum. This idea arose from a chance observation by Browder that a patient with parkinsonism who had received a frontal lobectomy noted cessation of his tremor following the procedure [2]. In 1952, Irving Cooper reported a patient with parkinsonism who experienced the disappearance of tremor and rigidity without weakness following anterior choroidal artery ligation [2]. Spiegel and Wycis used stereotactic surgery for movement disorders in 1947, and Hassler investigated ventrolateral (VL) thalamus as a target, as well. Pallidotomies were performed for decades for a variety of different movement disorders, most commonly PD, until the advent of levodopa in 1967. Upon its initial usage, levodopa was viewed as almost as a cure for PD, such that pallidotomy lost favor. Its utility was later appreciated again for improving dyskinesia and wearing off, as motor fluctuations emerged as a result of chronic levodopa therapy. The ventrolateral GPi was used as a target by Laitinen in early 1990's [16]. Then the STN began to come into vogue as a target in the 1990's [17]. DBS has advantages over pallidotomy or thalamotomy in that it is less destructive, reversible, and adjustable. The preferred targets for DBS in PD patients are GPi and the STN. Evidence from randomized trials indicates that both stimulation sites are effective for motor symptoms of advanced PD with similar safety profiles, and this will be discussed in detail in chapter 6. Interestingly, GPi and STN DBS both help tremor, bradykinesia, rigidity, wearing off, and levodopa-induced dyskinesias, whereas DBS of the ventral intermediate nucleus of the thalamus helps tremor alone, and as such this target is typically not the first recommendation for PD patients.

The therapeutic mechanism of DBS is poorly understood. A consistent, unexplained observation across indications is that high frequency stimulation (>100 Hz) is typically most effective for motor symptoms, although there can be considerable variability in individual responses. Early hypotheses suggested that DBS inhibits local neuronal elements, based on the phenomenological similarity of DBS to stereotactic lesions [2, 10, 18]. These ideas center on various forms of functional inactivation including depletion of neurotransmitters, depolarization block, or the activation of inhibitory afferents to decrease the output of the target structure. In 1991, Benabid et al. hypothesized that DBS interacts with the diseased network to eliminate or subdue the underlying pathological neural activity; this later became known as "jamming" [10]. Paradoxically, however, subsequent studies suggest that DBS drives neuronal activity, both at the stimulation site and at downstream nodes in the motor network. Additionally, computer models suggest more complex phenomena, such that stimulation decouples the soma from the axon. In this way, the cell body is depolarized or inactivated, yet activity in the axon on the same neuron is driven by stimulation [10, 19-21]. Evidence from functional imaging studies generally agree that DBS increases blood flow at the stimulation site, using both positron emission tomography (PET) and single-photo emission computed tomography (SPECT) [19]. Hershey et al. in 2003 measured the cerebral blood flow responses to STN stimulation using PET scans with DBS off and on. They found that STN stimulation increased blood flow in midbrain including the STN, globus pallidus, and thalamus, primarily on the left side, and concomitantly reduced blood flow in the bilateral frontal, parietal, and temporal cortices. Their interpretation was that high frequency STN stimulation increases firing of STN output neurons, which increases inhibition of thalamocortical projections, and ultimately decreasing blood flow in cortical targets [22]. However, a qualification of the imaging studies is that they have limited temporal resolution (on the order of seconds) and they measure changes in blood flow as a surrogate for brain activity.

Interest has grown in understanding the role of motor cortical areas, including the hyperdirect pathway projection, in the therapeutic mechanism of DBS. Recent work in animal models has fueled interest in whether DBS interacts with hyperdirect pathway axons [18, 23, 24], demonstrating retrograde (antidromic) activation of cortical neurons with single unit recordings during electrical stimulation in the STN. In particular, Gradinaru et al. showed improvement in movement in a mouse model of Parkinson's disease (PD) during selective optical stimulation of frontal cortex neurons and electrical stimulation of the STN region but not during selective photic stimulation or inhibition of STN neurons alone [25]. Similarly, multiple groups have demonstrated antidromic activation of cortical layer V neurons by STN DBS, including the suppression of beta frequency oscillations during stimulation [18, 23, 26]. Recordings of both single-unit activity and local field potentials in the motor cortex of freely moving rats with hemiparkinsonism during STN DBS found that the antidromic spikes generation decreased with increasing stimulation frequencies, and that the maximum number of antidromic spikes was elicited at around 125 Hz stimulation, the frequency that produced the optimal improvement in parkinsonian motor symptoms. Thus, these studies with single unit recordings demonstrate that STN DBS can potentially generate widespread and heterogeneous effects, both at local and distal sites including cerebral cortex [23, 27].

A number of recent studies in PD patients have focused on interactions between cerebral cortex and basal ganglia, in the context of DBS therapy. Many of these studies focus on measuring the suppression of beta oscillations as a proxy for outcome in PD patients. Suppression of beta oscillations during DBS in PD patients was described by Eusebio et al. in 2014. They performed EEG recordings in 16 patients with PD who had undergone STN DBS and found that DBS progressively suppressed pathological peaks in local field potential activity at frequencies between 11 and 30 Hz [28]. Kuriakose et al. used transcranial magnetic stimulation to measure cortical excitability at various latencies relative to the STN stimulus pulse [27]. They found that motor cortex excitability was increased at specific intervals following STN stimulation at clinically effective contacts. They interpreted short latency cortical activation as a manifestation of antidromic activation of the hyperdirect (corticosubthalamic) pathway, whereas medium latency activation was associated with the output of the classical basal ganglia-thalamocortical loop. Walker et al. used EEG methods to directly visualize antidromic activation of the hyperdirect pathway during STN DBS in PD patients. They found short latency activation of the cortex across a range of stimulation voltages and frequencies, including clinically effective frequencies, demonstrating activation of the hyperdirect pathway in humans during clinically effective high frequency stimulation [29].

Cortical signals over the estimated origin of the hyperdirect pathway also demonstrated attenuation of beta hypersynchrony during DBS in the STN region, whereas signals from non-specific regions of motor cortex were not attenuated [30]. Whitner et al. also measured the local field potentials dorsal to and within the STN of PD patients and in the motor cortex in a subset of these patients. They used diffusion tensor imaging (DTI) to guide the placement of subdural cortical surface electrodes over the DTI identified origin of the hyperdirect pathway. They found the local beta power was attenuated during high-frequency DBS both dorsal to and within the DBS. In 2013, de Hemptinne et al. note phase-amplitude coupling in motor cortical areas. They analyzed the local field potentials recorded from the primary motor cortex (M1) arm area in patients undergoing DBS surgery. In PD, coupling between the phase of beta waves (13-30 Hz) and the amplitude of gamma waves (50-200Hz) in M1 was exaggerated compared with patients with craniocervical dystonia and patients without movement disorders who underwent neurosurgery for severe epilepsy. In addition, therapeutic STN stimulation reduced this excessive coupling. Peaks in gamma frequency in primary motor cortex were also found to be coupled to the beta frequency trough, suggesting that cortical local field potentials could be used as a control signal for automated programming of DBS [31]. Future studies are needed to further elucidate systems-level connections between cortex and basal ganglia in DBS patients with PD and other diseases [9, 32-41].

Together, these studies have led to the conclusion that an important potential mechanism of STN DBS involves an interaction with cerebral cortex, possibly via the hyperdirect pathway. The results of these and other investigations promise to produce methods to optimize outcomes in patients who undergo DBS for PD and to guide innovation as DBS is investigated for new indications in neurology and psychiatry.

Conclusion

It is still unclear how DBS exactly affects the firing rate and pattern of neurons and how these changes actually modify the symptoms of Parkinson's disease. However, the effects of DBS should be considered at the level of circuits rather than the specific brain structure where the lead is implanted.

Many questions are still unanswered, but exciting continuous discoveries carry the promise of ever improving technology, allowing better symptom control.

References

[1] Everitt, B. J., Robbins, T. W. Neural systems of reinforcement for drug addiction: from actions to habits to compulsion. *Nat. Neurosci.* 2005;8:1481-1489.

[2] Kopell, B. H., Rezai, A. R., Chang, J. W., Vitek, J. L. Anatomy and physiology of the basal ganglia: implications for deep brain stimulation for Parkinson's disease. *Mov. Disord.*, 2006;21 Suppl. 14:S238-S246.

[3] Albin, R. L., Young, A. B., Penney, J. B. The functional anatomy of basal ganglia disorders. *Trends Neurosci.*, 1989;12:366-375.

[4] Gerfen, C. R., Surmeier, D. J. Modulation of striatal projection systems by dopamine. *Annu. Rev. Neurosci.*, 2011;34:441-466.

[5] McFarland, N. R., Haber, S. N. Convergent inputs from thalamic motor nuclei and frontal cortical areas to the dorsal striatum in the primate. *J. Neurosci.* 2000;20:3798-3813.

[6] Smith, Y., Raju, D. V., Pare, J. F., Sidibe, M. The thalamostriatal system: a highly specific network of the basal ganglia circuitry. *Trends Neurosci.* 2004;27:520-527.

[7] Braak, H., Del Tredici, K. Cortico-basal ganglia-cortical circuitry in Parkinson's disease reconsidered. *Exp. Neurol.* 2008;212:226-229.

[8] Monakow, K. H., Akert, K., Künzle, H. Projections of the precentral motor cortex and other cortical areas of the frontal lobe to the subthalamic nucleus in the monkey. *Exp. Brain Res.* 1978;33:395-403.

[9] Nambu, A., Takada, M., Inase, M., Tokuno, H. Dual somatotopical representations in the primate subthalamic nucleus: evidence for ordered but reversed body-map transformations from the primary motor cortex and the supplementary motor area. *J. Neurosci.* 1996;16:2671-2683.

[10] McIntyre, C. C., Hahn, P. J. Network perspectives on the mechanisms of deep brain stimulation. *Neurobiol. Dis*. 2010;38:329-337.

[11] Kravitz, A. V., Tye, L. D., Kreitzer, A. C. Distinct roles for direct and indirect pathway striatal neurons in reinforcement. *Nat. Neurosci*. 2012;15:816-818.

[12] Koob, G. F., Volkow, N. D. Neurocircuitry of addiction. *Neuropsychopharmacology*. 2010;35:217-238.

[13] Hikida, T., Kimura, K., Wada, N., Funabiki, K., Nakanishi, S. Distinct roles of synaptic transmission in direct and indirect striatal pathways to reward and aversive behavior. *Neuron* 2010;66:896-907.

[14] Ferguson, S. M., Eskenazi, D., Ishikawa, M., Wanat, M. J., Phillips, P. E., Dong, Y., Roth, B. L., Neumaier, J. F. Transient neuronal inhibition reveals opposing roles of indirect and direct pathways in sensitization. *Nat. Neurosci*. 2011;14:22-24.

[15] Voon, V., Fernagut, P. O., Wickens, J., Baunez, C., Rodriguez, M., Pavon, N., Juncos, J. L., Obeso, J. A., Bezard, E. Chronic dopaminergic stimulation in Parkinson's disease: from dyskinesias to impulse control disorders. *Lancet Neurol*. 2009;8:1140-1149.

[16] Laitinen, L. V., Bergenheim, A. T., Hariz, M. I. Leksell's posteroventral pallidotomy in the treatment of Parkinson's disease. *J. Neurosurg*. 1992;76:53-61.

[17] Alvarez, L., Macias, R., Lopez, G., Alvarez, E., Pavon, N., Rodriguez-Oroz, M. C., Juncos, J. L., Maragoto, C., Guridi, J., Litvan, I., Tolosa, E. S., Koller, W., Vitek, J., DeLong, M R., Obeso, J. A. Bilateral subthalamotomy in Parkinson's disease: initial and long-term response. *Brain* 2005;128:570-583.

[18] Li, Q., Ke, Y., Chan, D. C., Qian, Z. M., Yung, K. K., Ko, H., Arbuthnott, G. W., Yung, W. H. Therapeutic deep brain stimulation in parkinsonian rats directly influences motor cortex. *Neuron* 2012;76:1030-1041.

[19] Mehanna, R. and E. C. Lai, Deep brain stimulation in Parkinson's disease. *Transl. Neurodegener*., 2013;2:22.

[20] Vitek, J. L. Mechanisms of deep brain stimulation: excitation or inhibition. *Mov. Disord*. 2002;17 Suppl. 3:S69-72.

[21] Okun, M. S., Oyama, G. Mechanism of action for deep brain stimulation and electrical neuro-network modulation (ENM). *Rinsho Shinkeigaku*, 2013;53:691-694.

[22] Hershey, T., Revilla, F. J., Wernle, A. R., McGee-Minnich, L., Antenor, J. V., Videen, T. O., Dowling, J. L., Mink, J. W., Perlmutter, J. S. Cortical and subcortical blood flow effects of subthalamic nucleus stimulation in PD. *Neurology* 2003;61:816-821.

[23] Li, Q., Qian, Z. M., Arbuthnott, G. W., Ke, Y., Yung, W. H. Cortical effects of deep brain stimulation: implications for pathogenesis and treatment of Parkinson disease. *JAMA Neurol*. 2014;71:100-103.

[24] Li, S., Arbuthnott, G. W., Jutras, M. J., Goldberg, J. A., Jaeger, D. Resonant antidromic cortical circuit activation as a consequence of high-frequency subthalamic deep-brain stimulation. *J. Neurophysiol*. 2007;98:3525-3537.

[25] Gradinaru, D., Minn, A. L., Artur, Y., Minn, A., Heydel, J. M. Drug metabolizing enzyme expression in rat choroid plexus: effects of in vivo xenobiotics treatment. *Arch. Toxicol*. 2009;83:581-586.

[26] Wichmann, T., Dostrovsky, J. O. Pathological basal ganglia activity in movement disorders. *Neuroscience* 2011;198:232-244.

[27] Kuriakose, R., Saha, U., Castillo, G., Udupa, K., Ni, Z., Gunraj, C., Mazzella, F., Hamani, C., Lang, A. E., Moro, E., Lozano, A. M., Hodaie, M., Chen, R. The nature

and time course of cortical activation following subthalamic stimulation in Parkinson's disease. *Cereb. Cortex* 2010;20:1926-1936.

[28] Eusebio, A., Thevathasan, W., Doyle Gaynor, L., Pogosyan, A., Bye, E., Foltynie, T., Zrinzo, L., Ashkan, K., Aziz, T., Brown, P. Deep brain stimulation can suppress pathological synchronisation in parkinsonian patients. *J. Neurol. Neurosurg. Psychiatry* 2011;82:569-573.

[29] Walker, H. C., Huang, H., Gonzalez, C. L., Bryant, J. E., Killen, J., Cutter, G. R., Knowlton, R. C., Montgomery, E. B., Guthrie, B. L., Watts, R. L. Short latency activation of cortex during clinically effective subthalamic deep brain stimulation for Parkinson's disease. *Mov. Disord.* 2012;27:864-873.

[30] Whitmer, D., de Solages, C., Hill, B., Yu, H., Henderson, J. M., Bronte-Stewart, H. High frequency deep brain stimulation attenuates subthalamic and cortical rhythms in Parkinson's disease. *Front. Hum. Neurosci.* 2012;6:155.

[31] de Hemptinne, C., Ryapolova-Webb, E. S., Air, E. L., Garcia, P. A., Miller, K. J., Ojemann, J. G., Ostrem, J. L., Galifianakis, N. B., Starr, P. A. Exaggerated phase-amplitude coupling in the primary motor cortex in Parkinson disease. *Proc. Natl. Acad. Sci. US* 2013;110:4780-4785.

[32] Leblois, A., Boraud, T., Meissner, W., Bergman, H., Hansel, D. Competition between feedback loops underlies normal and pathological dynamics in the basal ganglia. *J. Neurosci.* 2006;26:3567-3583.

[33] Nakano, K. Neural circuits and topographic organization of the basal ganglia and related regions. *Brain Dev.* 2000;22 Suppl. 1:S5-16.

[34] Bateup, H. S., Santini, E., Shen, W., Birnbaum, S., Valjent, E., Surmeier, D. J., Fisone, G., Nestler, E. J., Greengard, P. Distinct subclasses of medium spiny neurons differentially regulate striatal motor behaviors. *Proc. Natl. Acad. Sci. US*, 2010; 107: 14845-14850.

[35] Kravitz, A. V., Freeze, B. S., Parker, P. R., Kay, K., Thwin, M. T., Deisseroth, K., Kreitzer, A. C. Regulation of parkinsonian motor behaviours by optogenetic control of basal ganglia circuitry. *Nature* 2010;466(7306):622-626.

[36] Baron, M. S., Vitek, J. L., Bakay, R. A., Green, J., Kaneoke, Y., Hashimoto, T., Turner, R. S., Woodard, J. L., Cole, S. A., McDonald, W. M., DeLong, M. R. Treatment of advanced Parkinson's disease by posterior GPi pallidotomy: 1-year results of a pilot study. *Ann. Neurol.* 1996;40:355-366.

[37] Dybdal, D., Forcelli, P. A., Dubach, M., Oppedisano, M., Holmes, A., Malkova, L., Gale, K. Topography of dyskinesias and torticollis evoked by inhibition of substantia nigra pars reticulata. *Mov. Disord.* 2013;28: 460-468.

[38] Sabatini, U., Boulanouar, K., Fabre, N., Martin, F., Carel, C., Colonnese, C., Bozzao, L., Berry, I., Montastruc, J. L., Chollet, F., Rascol, O. Cortical motor reorganization in akinetic patients with Parkinson's disease: a functional MRI study. *Brain* 2000;123:394-403.

[39] Alonso-Frech, F., Zamarbide, I., Alegre, M., Rodríguez-Oroz, M. C., Guridi, J., Manrique, M., Valencia, M., Artieda, J., Obeso, J. A. Slow oscillatory activity and levodopa-induced dyskinesias in Parkinson's disease. *Brain* 2006;129:1748-1757.

[40] Forstmann, B. U., Keuken, M. C., Jahfari, S., Bazin, P. L., Neumann, J., Schäfer, A., Anwander, A., Turner, R. Cortico-subthalamic white matter tract strength predicts interindividual efficacy in stopping a motor response. *Neuroimage* 2012;60:370-375.

[41] Alexander, G. E., DeLong, M. R. and Strick, P. L. Parallel organization of functionally segregated circuits linking basal ganglia and cortex. *Annu. Rev. Neurosci.* 1986;9:357-381.

In: Deep Brain Stimulation
Editor: Raja Mehanna

ISBN: 978-1-63483-282-3

Chapter 3

BASICS OF NEUROSTIMULATION

Aasef G. Shaikh, MD, PhD
and Hubert H. Fernandez, MD
Center for Neurological Restoration,
Cleveland Clinic, Cleveland, Ohio, US

ABSTRACT

Deep brain stimulation is one of the most important inventions of the 20th century. It has not only revolutionized how we treat numerous movement disorders including Parkinson's disease, essential tremor, and dystonia. Deep brain stimulation, without any debate, dramatically treats these movement disorders and substantially improved quality of life. Cutting edge neuroscientific research focusing on the animal models, neurophysiology, neuroanatomy, and computational neuroscience has explained rationale for the function of deep brain stimulators.

This chapter will discuss contemporary scientific hypothesis delineating the neurophysiology of deep brain stimulation and cutting edge neuromodulation technology. Finally we will speculate the future of neuromodulation and will discuss investigational technology for selective neurostimulation.

INTRODUCTION

Neuromodulation and its application for the treatment of movement disorders is an ideal example of the successful application of technical advances in basic neuroscience, clinical neurology, and stereotactic neurosurgery. The resultant technology of deep brain stimulation is a modern way to treat patients with medically refractory movement disorders. Deep brain stimulation is an FDA-approved treatment of essential tremor and Parkinson's disease, and has a humanitarian device exemption for dystonia and obsessive-compulsive disorders. This chapter will briefly review the anatomy and physiology of basal ganglia pertinent to the principles of deep brain stimulation and the basics of neuromodulation for the treatment of movement disorders, that were detailed in chapter 2, before discussing the clinically pertinent information about the hardware that comprises the deep brain stimulation system.

The history of surgical treatment of movement disorders interestingly dates back to the 19th century. Horsley (1890) was the first to perform extirpation of motor cortex for the treatment of athetosis [1]. About half a century later, as detailed in the first chapter of this book, Spiegel described the stereotactic frame and made pallidal fiber lesions in patients with Parkinson's disease to treat bradykinesia and tremor [2]. Around the same time, Hassler, Riechert, and Talaraich made lesions in the human thalamus to treat tremor [3, 4]. The inadvertent ligation of the anterior choroidal artery led to the significant improvement of rigidity and tremor in a patient with Parkinson's disease [5]. Approximately a decade later, Albe-Fessard stimulated thalamus at high frequencies, in the range of 100-200 Hz, and found improvement in tremor in a Parkinson patient [6]. In 1989 Benabid and colleagues heralded the contemporary era of deep brain stimulation in patients with essential tremor [7]. Discovery of a model of basal ganglia function, primarily based on direct and indirect circuits, gave a new insight into the current strategies for deep brain stimulation for Parkinson's disease [8].

Finally in 1998, the first report of successful treatment of Parkinson's disease with subthalamic nucleus deep brain stimulation was published [9]. Subsequently, numerous studies, including larger trials have consistently reported efficacy of the deep brain stimulation for the treatment of essential tremor, dystonia, and Parkinson's disease.

How does deep brain stimulation work? What improves tremor, bradykinesia, rigidity, and dystonia? What is target specificity in treatment of various movement disorders?

The subsequent sections will outline basic principles of deep brain stimulation with pertinent anatomy and physiology of motor circuits in the basal ganglia.

Basic Principles

There is little debate that deep brain stimulation offers a dramatic response in the motor symptoms of medically refractory Parkinson's disease, essential tremor, and dystonia. However, the physiological mechanism for deep brain stimulation remains unclear. The current hypotheses are only speculations for its mechanism of action.

The initial hypothesis came from the pallidotomy experience. High-frequency stimulation of the prospective area for pallidotomy led to a transient improvement in parkinsonian symptoms during the surgery.

The development of deep brain stimulator devices allowed this principle to be converted into clinical practice. The rationale for its success was consistent with the physiological model of Parkinson's disease, emphasizing that the symptoms are likely due to increased activity of the subthalamic nucleus and globus pallidus interna. It was, therefore, hypothesized that deep brain stimulation improves clinical symptoms by suppressing the outflow of the basal ganglia. In other words, deep brain stimulation "physiologically ablates" the output of the basal ganglia [10, 11].

There is a lack of consensus about the physiological effects of deep brain stimulation for the treatment of movement disorders. While some investigators believe that deep brain stimulation works through the inhibition, others are in favor of excitation [12-17].

The caveat for the hypotheses proposing the inhibition of basal ganglia outflow is that the same stimulation parameters also treat dystonia, a disorder known to have reduced firing response in globus pallidus and subthalamic nucleus.

Contemporary studies suggest *hypersynchronization* of spontaneous neural activity as a cause of tremor and rigidity. Naturally, desynchronization of such activity might immediately resolve these symptoms. Desynchronization is possible by lesioning the parts of hypersynchronized circuit (e.g. pallidotomy or thalamotomy), or electrically stimulating (thereby suppressing) parts of that circuit (e.g., deep brain stimulation) [18, 19].

Anatomy and Physiology of the Basal Ganglia Relevant to Deep Brain Stimulation

The contemporary concepts of surgical planning, intra-operative mapping, and post-operative programming of deep brain stimulation heavily relies on the concepts of basic anatomical organization of the basal ganglia and their relationship to the thalamo-cortical circuits. The conceptual framework of such organization was laid out by studies in the 1980s [20, 21]. These investigations viewed the cortico-striato-pallido-thalaamocortical loop as an isolated network involving projections from the cerebral cortex to the areas in the basal ganglia and back to the cerebral cortex via the thalamic relay nuclei [22]. In this grand scheme of organization, the caudate and putamen are the designated input nuclei, while the globus pallidus interna and substantia nigra pars reticulata serve at the output stage [23].

This overview pioneered by DeLong is depicted in Figure 1. In this diagram, the motor circuit from the pre-central motor area and post-central somatosensory areas project to the putamen. The putamen then projects to the output structures of venterolateral globus pallidus interna and the caudolateral subtantia nigra pars reticulata via direct and indirect pathways.

The projections from these output tracks reach the thalamic relay nuclei [24]. Such anatomical segregation of this output carries functional significance. Pallidal projections to the thalamus are essential for sequencing and execution of movements, while substantia nigra pars reticulata projections dictate planning of the action [25]. Therefore, the output from the globus pallidus interna serves as an important target for the treatment of Parkinson's disease and dystonia. The separate ventral intermediate nucleus in the thalamus receives cerebellar projection. This area of the thalamus is critical for neuromodulation for essential tremor.

Additional projections within this network were also proposed. The subthalamic nucleus directly connects to the substantia nigra pars compacta, and reciprocally projects to the globus pallidus externa [26, 27].

Additionally, the globus pallidus externa directly projects to the globus pallidus interna, substantia nigra pars reticulata, and the reticularis nucleus of the thalamus [26]. Finally, direct cortical projections to the subthalamic nucleus was also described as the *hyper-direct pathway* [27-29]. Such direct cortical projection to the subthalamic nucleus may carry sensory input to the basal ganglia, which make it critical to synchronize the oscillatory activity in the cortex, the subthalamic nuclei, and the pallidum [30].

Structures other than the basal ganglia, such as the pedunculopontine nucleus and the midbrain extrapyramidal area, can serve to integrate cortical, thalamic, basal ganglia and spinal activity. These structures are potential future targets for neuromodulation.

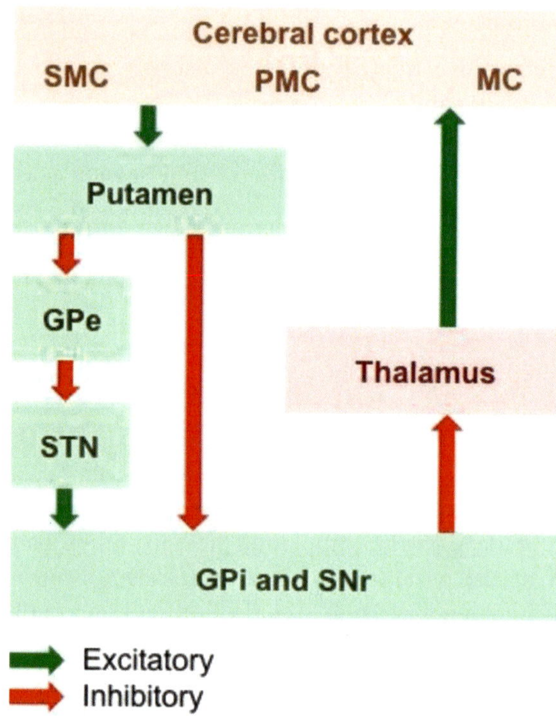

SMC: supplementary motor cortex, PMC: premotor cortex, MC: motor cortex, GPe: globus pallidum extrna, GPi: globus pallidum interna, STN: subthalamic nucleus, SNr: substantia nigra reculata.

Figure 1. Schematic outline of connections of basal ganglia, thalamus, and cerebral cortex.

Lack of dopamine due to degenerative process causes most of the physiological changes in Parkinson's disease. Understanding of these changes is essential to establish the basis for deep brain stimulation, determine changes expected during microelectrode recording while mapping and optimizing therapeutic stimulation.

Two models have tried to explain the neurophysiology of Parkinson's disease. The most accepted model is the *rate model.* According to this hypothesis, due to the paucity in dopaminergic inhibition, there is an increase in the activity of the globus pallidus interna and subthalamic nucleus excitatory output.

This model is consistent with the electrophysiological signature of increased discharge rate in the subthalamic nucleus and globus pallidus interna in patients undergoing stereotactic surgery for the Parkinson's disease, also seen in animal models with 1-methyl-4-phenyl-1,2,3,6-tetrahydropyridine-treated monkeys [31-34]. The rate model hypothesis is also consistent with decreased mean discharge in globus pallidus externa and the thalamus; and it also supports the concept of pallidotomy where the lesion in globus pallidum interna and subsequent reduction in its output disinhibits the thalamus to improve parkinsonian symptoms.

However, pallidal and subthalamic lesions or deep brain stimulation can also disinhibit the thalamus and should therefore promote hyperkinetic side effects such as dyskinesia [35].

The contrary is true for pallidotomy in treatment of dystonia or hemiballismus and deep brain stimulation for the treatment of dystonia [33]. Such contradictory findings led to the development of the *pattern model.*

The *pattern model* emphasizes an alteration in the activity *patterns* in the subthalamic nuclei, globus pallidus interna, and thalamus of Parkinson's disease patients. These neurons have propensity to burst with higher synchronized oscillatory discharge [23]. The bursting pattern of thalamic neurons can be described as the pathological transformation of their tonic (physiological) firing due to lack of dopamine and increased outflow of basal ganglia affecting their resting membrane potential [36].

The alternate view described the thalamic bursts as the transmitted activity of the globus pallidus interna and subthalamic nucleus neurons. It is also believed that the changes in the motor functions in patients with Parkinson's disease could be related to abnormally wide receptive fields of the neurons in the basal ganglia and thalamus. Microelectrode recordings of the subthalamic nucleus, globus pallidus interna, and thalamus supported the predictions of the pattern model [32, 37].

The rate or the pattern of basal ganglia activity may therefore lead to symptoms of Parkinson's disease, the alteration in the pattern of the basal ganglia discharge can cause dystonia, and hypersynchronization might result in essential tremor.

Although these are all hypotheses, it is clear that deep brain stimulation provides a robust motor effect in the treatment of these disorders. In subsequent sections, we will discuss the technology used for chronic high-frequency stimulation for the treatment of movement disorders.

Deep Brain Stimulation Devices and Technology

The deep brain stimulation system is comprised of in vivo and external components. The internal pulse generator, electrode lead, and connector are in vivo while programming devices are external components. Programming devices interface with the internal pulse generator to modulate the parameters of electrical stimulation at the site of the implanted electrode lead.

Internal Pulse Generator (Neurostimulator)

The internal pulse generator is a unit containing vital electronic hardware and battery, enclosed within a titanium casing. The internal pulse generator empowers the deep brain stimulator system. The internal pulse generator is implanted subcutaneously in an easily accessible site; typically in the sub-clavicular region of the chest or occasionally in the abdominal wall. Two major manufacturers of the internal pulse generators are Medtronic™ and St. Jude Medical System™. The Medtronic™ systems are available worldwide, while St. Jude™ products for deep brain stimulation are not yet approved in the United States. Internal pulse generators from both manufacturers are classified into three main categories – *single channel*, *dual channel*, and *rechargeable devices*.

Single Channel Internal Pulse Generator

These devices provide stimulation to one single deep brain stimulation lead. Hence, a single channel internal pulse generator has less volume of hardware and requires a smaller sized battery. Given its compact size, it is most suitable for patients with a lean body mass.

The other advantage of a single channel pulse generator is that, because one internal pulse generator is responsible for modulating one lead, in cases of malfunction of one internal pulse generator during bilateral deep brain stimulation, the second side would remain functional. Additionally, in case the internal pulse generator becomes infected and the infection spreads to involve the lead, which then requires the ablation of the whole system, having 2 single channels IPG will allow to keep the contralateral non-infected system in place. On the contrary, if one dual channel IPFG was connected to both leads and became infected, that would put both leads at risk of infection - and removal. The major drawback of single channel internal pulse generator is the need for double the number of surgeries during IPG implantation as well as during battery replacement.

Dual-Channel Internal Pulse Generator

These are relatively advanced systems empowering two deep brain stimulator leads, typically one on each side of the brain. The patients requiring bilateral deep brain stimulator implantation benefits the most from this type of device. There are two significant drawbacks of dual-channel internal pulse generator. First, it has a significantly larger in size to accommodate the additional hardware and the bigger battery powering the two leads. The larger internal pulse generator units may not be suitable for patients with a lean body mass, particularly when implanted in the chest. The second drawback is the lack of a "backup" contralateral generator in case of hardware or battery failure: complete (bilateral) dysfunction occurs if the dual channel internal pulse generator fails due to battery drainage or infection.

Rechargeable Dual-Channel Internal Pulse Generator

These are the newest generation of internal pulse generators. Their principal advantage is less frequent battery replacements since it can be recharged in vivo. Manufacturers recommend at recharging them at least weekly, but most providers recommend recharging the battery every day. The latter reduces the overall time to recharge the battery and offers longer sustainability of each charge. Both leading manufacturers make all three types of internal pulse generators. Although the general concept is the same, each model and brand has peculiarities as outlined in Table 1 (Medtronic™) and Table 2 (St. Jude Medical System™). Figure 2 shows internal pulse generators from both leading manufacturers.

Deep Brain Stimulator Leads

Two types of deep brain stimulator leads are currently considered standard of care. Both kinds of leads are available through Medtronic™ and St.Jude Medical System™. The standard Medtronic™ lead thickness is 1.27 mm and has four platinum-iridium electrodes.

Each electrode is 1.5 mm long. The inter-electrode spacing is the discriminating feature between the two lead types. The spacing between the electrodes in the longer lead type (labelled 3387) is 1.5 mm while spacing is 0.5 mm in the shorter lead type (labelled 3389). Each lead type has distinct suitabilities. The short lead is most ideal for targets with shorter spans, such as the subthalamic nucleus.

The long lead, however, may be suitable for larger targets such as the globus pallidus internus or thalamus.

Table 1. Medtronic™ internal pulse generators

	Activa PC®	Activa SC®	Activa RC®
Size (height, length, thickness)	65mm, 49 mm, 15 mm	55mm, 60 mm, 11 mm	54mm, 54 mm, 9 mm
Volume/Weight	39 cm^3/67 gm	28 cm^3/45 gm	22 cm^3/40 gm
Power source	6.3 Amp hours, 3.2 V cell	4.5 Amp hours, 3.2 V cell	Lithium ion rechargeable battery (life 9 years)
Amplitude range (current mode)	0 – 25.5 mA (0.1mA resolution)	0 – 25.5 mA (0.1mA resolution)	0 – 25.5 mA (0.1mA resolution)
Amplitude range (voltage mode)	0 – 10.5 V (0.1V resolution)	0 – 10.5 V (0.1V resolution)	0 – 10.5 V (0.1V resolution)
Pulse width	60 – 450 μs	30 – 450 μs	30 – 450 μs
Rate (current mode)	30 – 250 Hz (5 Hz resolution)	30 – 250 Hz (5 Hz resolution)	30 – 250 Hz (5 Hz resolution)
Rate (voltage mode)	2-250 Hz (5Hz resolution)	2-250 Hz (5Hz resolution)	2-250 Hz (5Hz resolution)
Cycling	0.1 s to 24 hr	0.1 s to 24 hr	0.1 s to 24 hr

Table 2. Medtronic electrode lead configuration

	Model 3387	Model 3389
Connector	Quadripolar, in-line	Quadripolar, in-line
Shape	Straight	Straight
Conductor resistance	<100 Ω	<100 Ω
Length	10 – 50 cm	10 – 50 cm
Diameter	1.27 mm	1.27 mm
Number of electrodes	4	4
Electrode shape	Cylindrical	Cylindrical
Electrode length	1.5 mm	1.5 mm
Electrode spacing	1.5 mm	0.5 mm
Electrode distance	10.5 mm	7.5 mm
Distal tip distance	1.5 mm	1.5 mm
Lead contact length	2.3 mm	2.3 mm
Lead contact spacing	4.3 mm	4.3 mm
Lead contact distance	16.6 mm	16.6 mm
Stylet handle length	40.1 mm	40.1 mm

Nevertheless, any model can be used for any target. Specific features and peculiarities of both Medtronic™ models are outlined in Table 3. Figure 3 depicts the schematic diagram of Medtronic™ deep brain stimulator lead.

Extensions and Connectors

The extracranial portion of the lead is connected to an extension wire encased within a silicone coating through a connector typically located over the parietal bone or the mastoid bone. The extension wire is connected to the internal pulse generator.

The extension is tunneled into the skin from the scalp to the neck then the chest. Extensions are available at different lengths to accommodate either abdominal or sub-clavicular positions of the stimulator.

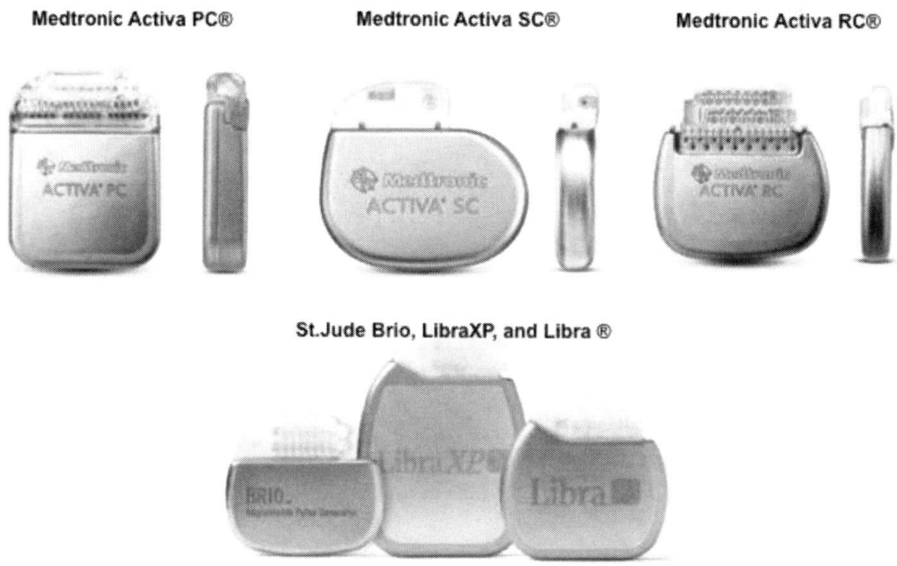

Bottom panel shows three models of St. Jude™ internal pulse generators (with permission from Metronic™ and St.Jude™).

Figure 2. Top panel depicts three models of Medtronic™ internal pulse generators are illustrated in their front and side view.

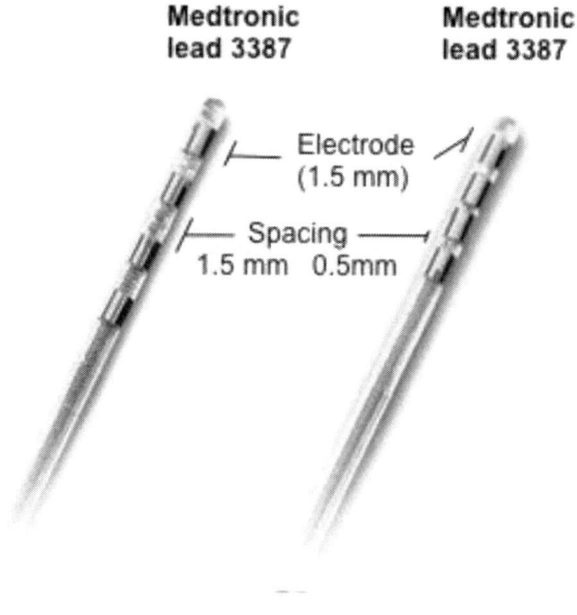

With permission from Medtronic™.

Figure 3. Two models of Medtronic™ deep brain stimulation electrode leads are illustrated.

Table 3. St. Jude™ internal pulse generators

	Brio®	LibraXP®	Libra®
Height	48 mm	76 mm	50 mm
Width	53 mm	58 mm	54 mm
Thickness	0.95 mm	14 mm	14 mm
Weight	29 gm	83 gm	53 gm
Volume	17.7 cm^3	49 cm^3	29 cm^3
Power source	Rechargeable lithium-ion cell	Lithium thionyl chloride	Lithium thionyl chloride
Pulse width (step)	50-500 μs (13 μs)	52-507 μs (13 μs)	52-507 μs (13 μs)
Frequency (step)	2-240 Hz (2 Hz)	2-200 Hz (2 Hz)	2-240 Hz (2 Hz)
Amplitude	0-12.75 mA	0-12.75 mA	0-12.75 mA

Basics of Neurostimulation

Effective DBS programming corresponds to creating a sufficient neuronal response in the intended target without spread of electrical stimulation to unintended nearby structures. This is achieved by a judicious choice of active electrode configuration and by determining an effective combination of electrical parameters in order to obtain tremor control without causing side effects. Each DBS lead has a variety of variables that can be modified in an effort to achieve the most effective treatment. The variables that can be adjusted are the electrode configuration (monopolar or bipolar), voltage, pulse width and rate. The electrical charge generated during the DBS pulse dissipates with distance from the electrode and the electrical charge is highest near the active electrode contact.

The active electrodes can be configured as monopolar, bipolar and multi-polar. The monopolar configuration has a single negative electrode (cathode) and the metal case of the implanted neurostimulator acts as the positive electrode (anode). In the bipolar configuration a single electrode is negative and another electrode is positive. In the multi-polar configuration there are one or more negative electrodes and one or more positive electrodes. The distance between the positive and negative electrodes affects the intensity of the electric field, the closer they are together the more intense the signal. The monopolar configuration is broad resulting in a less intense, but larger electrical field; whereas the bipolar or multipolar configurations lead to a smaller, more intense electrical field (Figures 4 and 5).

The electrical field can be further modified by adjusting the stimulation parameters: voltage, pulse width and rate. The stimulation delivered is usually not continuous but intermittent. The voltage corresponds to the amplitude of the stimulation delivered (in volts), the pulse width corresponds to the duration of each stimulation (in microseconds) and the rate, or frequency, corresponds to the number of stimulations delivered each second (in herz) (Figure 6). The number and location of axons that are stimulated can be adjusted by changes in the voltage. Higher voltages can stimulate more axons by increasing the spatial extent of the electrical field intensities. Within the electrical field, increasing the voltage can increase the number of axons stimulated. The type of axon that is stimulated can be manipulated by changes in the pulse width.

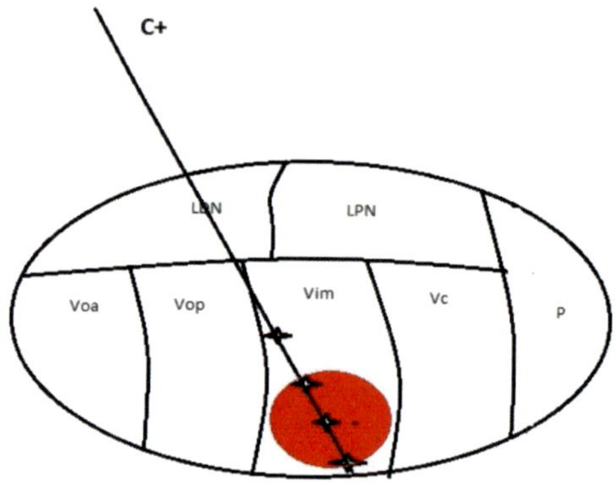

The electrode is here placed in the Vim for illustration. C+: the neurostimulator is used as the anode. LDN: Lateral Dorsal Nucleus, LPN: Lateral Posterior Nucleus, Voa: Ventral oris anterior, Vop: Ventral oris posterior, Vim: Ventral intermedius, Vc: Ventral caudalis, P: pulvinar.

Figure 4. Schematic representation of the field of stimulation in a monopolar configuration.

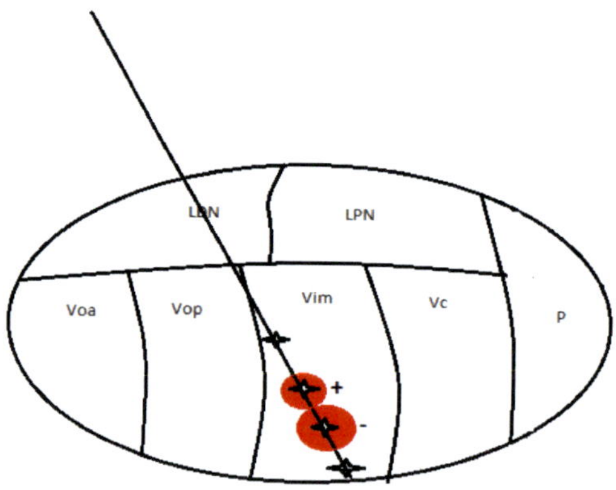

The electrode is here placed in the Vim for illustration. LDN: Lateral Dorsal Nucleus, LPN: Lateral Posterior Nucleus, Voa: Ventral oris anterior, Vop: Ventral oris posterior, Vim: Ventral intermedius, Vc: Ventral caudalis, P: pulvinar.

Figure 5. Schematic representation of the field of stimulation in a bipolar configuration.

Axons with larger diameters are stimulated by shorter pulse widths, whereas small diameter axons are stimulated by longer pulse widths (see below). The effects of different rates (frequency) of DBS on neuronal activities are less straightforward.

In the past, it was thought that high frequency inhibits the stimulated target and low frequency excites the target; however, there are many cases in which low frequency is therapeutic.

Overall, tremor usually responds better to higher frequencies, but this requirement does not seem to exist for dystonia or other signs of Parkinson's disease. In all disorders, the most effective parameter is the electrical charge, which is the multiplication of voltage and pulse width. Increase in either parameter increases the stimulation charge. There are two disadvantages of increasing the charge.

First, it drains the battery faster hence requiring more frequent replacements. Rechargeable neurostimulators conveniently addresses this drawback.

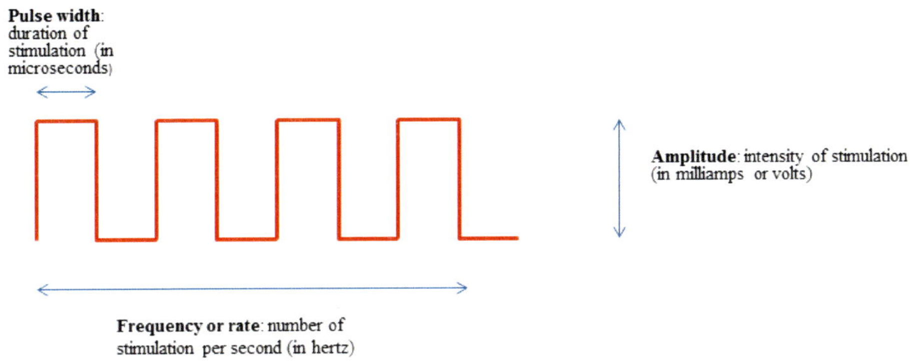

Figure 6. Stimulation parameters for deep brain stimulation.

Second, currently inevitable, drawback is that high charge stimulates large neuronal volume, and the effect is not as selective as anticipated. Higher charge causes stimulation of unwanted targets such as fiber tracts around the basal ganglia leading to unwanted side effects. There is a non-linear relationship between the pulse width and the electrical current that are necessary to stimulate a neural element. The rheobase current is the minimum current that is required to stimulate the neural element with a long pulse width while the chronaxie is the pulse duration that is needed to evoke twice the rheobase current. Typical chronaxie values of myelinated axons range between 30 to 200 microseconds while they are in the range of 1 to 10 milliseconds for unmyelinated fibers and cell bodies. A relatively smaller electrical charge is more likely to stimulate low chronaxie fibers, i.e. the myelinated fibers. As the charge increases, it starts including fibers with broader range of chronaxie values. Such phenomenon results in the stimulation dependent fiber tract stimulation. Inadvertent stimulation of the internal capsule fibers results in unintended muscle stimulation leading to spasm while the stimulation of the medial longitudinal fasciculus can cause paresthesia.

The other unwanted side effect, putatively related to the stimulation of surrounding nuclei such as substantia nigra pars reticulate, results in behavioral side effects ranging from depression to psychosis.

The fiber tract stimulation can often be beneficial. For example, anecdotal evidence suggests that stimulation of dorsal contacts in globus pallidus interna or those at the border of globus pallidus interna and externa results in better control of Parkinson's disease and dystonia. Such benefit also stands true in the case of stimulation of dorsal contacts in the subthalamic nucleus. One speculation for such benefit is that these contacts not only stimulate the neural substrates of the target, but also indirectly affect the projection sites by stimulating the fiber tracts. Thus, the efficacy of the same amount of electrical stimulation is increased.

In consideration of these basic principles, there are certain suggested guidelines. Typical initial programming sessions implement parameters with such guidelines. In Parkinson's disease, initial stimulation frequency is usually between 130 and 185 Hz, and pulse width is 60 or 90 microseconds. In typical programming of dystonia, the initial frequency is around 130 Hz with a pulse width around 60 microseconds. Initial programming in essential tremor is done at the frequency of 185 Hz and pulse width of 60 to 90 microseconds. These suggested guidelines are certainly helpful during initial programming.

However, subsequent programming needs further adjustments that may deviate significantly from the suggested range. This will be detailed further in the following chapters.

Future of Deep Brain Stimulation Technology

Real-Time Adaptively Controlled (Closed-Loop) Deep Brain Stimulation

Conventional deep brain stimulation technology relies on continuous stimulation of the target location. Clinicians will periodically change the stimulation parameters as determined by clinical outcomes. Such technique has helped patients suffering from Parkinson's disease, dystonia, and essential tremor. Programming strategies will be discussed in chapters 6, 7 and 8. There are exciting novel developments that are currently still in the preclinical arena. One novel technology, pioneered by Bergman and colleagues, is called *real-time adaptive control* of deep brain stimulation, or *close-loop* deep brain stimulation [38]. Traditional deep brain stimulation is a constant stimulation or "open-loop," while the "closed-loop" system modifies stimulation parameters in real-time, according to the discharge pattern sampled from the cerebral cortex [38].

This technology has two fundamental aspects. One is the stimulation of output basal ganglia nucleus, such as the globus pallidus, and the second is the sampling of neuronal activity from a reference brain area such as the motor cortex [38]. The novel idea is to modulate the stimulation parameters at the basal ganglia as "dictated" by the activity of the motor cortex. Hence the stimulation of basal ganglia is not constant, but rather "on demand." Figure 7 schematizes the principle of closed-loop technology. This exciting technology has been successfully tested in macaque model of Parkinson's disease [38]. In the macaque model of Parkinson's disease, the closed-loop paradigms were compared with standard deep brain stimulation protocols and the study revealed that closed-loop paradigms with real-time adaptive stimulation had many more clinical benefits compared to conventional deep brain stimulation techniques [38].

Compared to conventional stimulation, closed loop deep brain stimulation led to more pronounced improvement in akinesia in all four limbs, and most notably in the arm contralateral to the stimulation site [38]. Adaptive closed-loop deep brain stimulation also caused reduction in spike rate and oscillatory activity in the globus pallidus [38].

The closed-loop system also led to a decrease in stimulation frequency and increase in the variability of inter-stimulus interval as compared to high-frequency stimulation.

Optogenetic Deep Brain Stimulation

Optogenetics, a contemporary technique used in basic neuroscience research where light with specific wavelength is used to control firing activity of genetically-sensitized neurons, has shown some promise in selectively stimulating specific subsets of neurons participating in a specific function of the nervous system. Current spread and non-selective stimulation are significant pitfalls of the actual deep brain stimulation system using electricity. Optogenetics conveniently addresses this limitation.

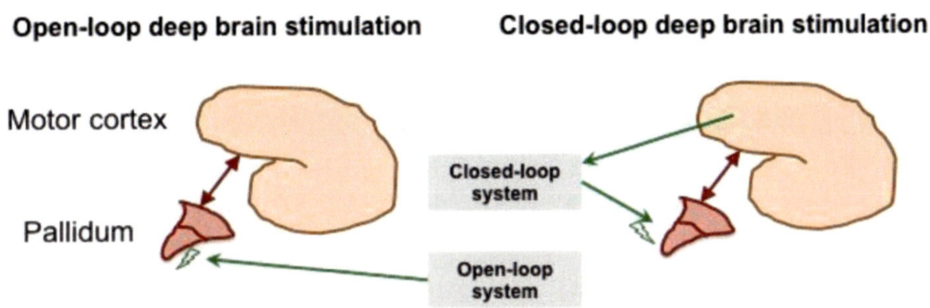

Figure 7. Schematic illustration of open-loop (conventional) and closed-loop deep brain stimulation technologies.

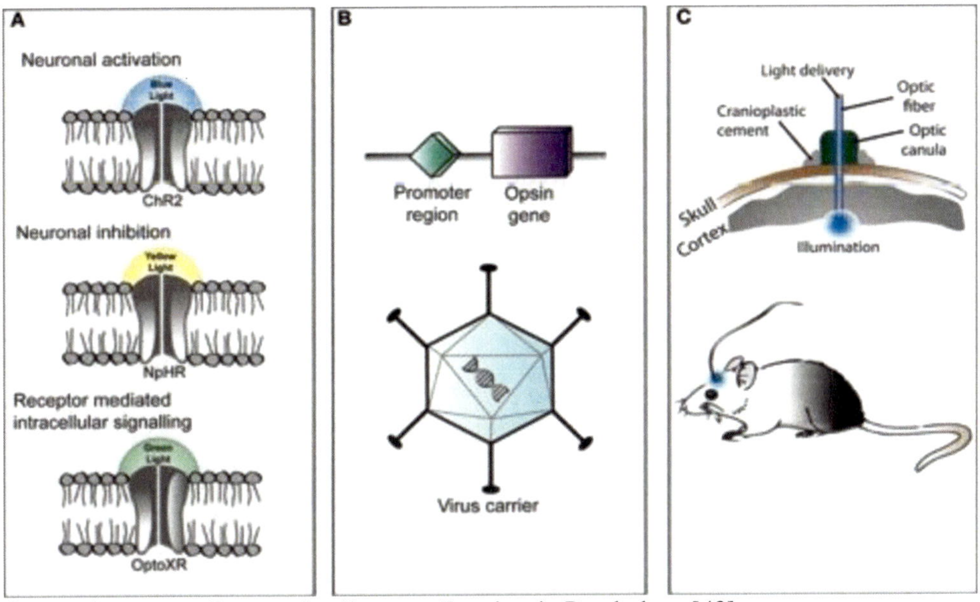

The diagram is courtesy Pama and colleagues, Frontiers in Psychology [42].

Figure 8. Principles of optogenetic neuromodulation.

As the name implies, optogenetics uses light and genetics to control activities of individual neurons in vivo. Optogenetics use light-sensitive proteins, optogenetic actuators, such as channelrhodopsin, halorhodopsin, and archaerhodopsin. The first step of optogenetic stimulation is to determine the specifications of the light-responsive proteins (opsins). The opsins are of several types, each type having a different reaction to light stimulation. The reaction is dependent upon the wavelength.

For example, blue light leads to neuronal depolarization via channelrhodopsin, whereas halorhodopsin causes neuronal hyperpolarization when it reacts with the yellow light. Incorporation of optoXRs in the G-protein pathway leads to the modulation of receptor mediated intracellular signaling (Figure 8A) [39]. The next step is the injection of harmless virus carrying these proteins into the brain (Figure 8B) [40].

Finally, light is delivered straight into the brain using optical fibers through a cannula implanted in the skull (Figure 8C) [39, 40].

The light delivery is then used to selectively modulate neuronal activity [39, 40]. This technique has shown promise in rodent models of Parkinson's disease [41]. Gradinaru and colleagues systematically modulated an array of distinct neural circuit elements in Parkinsonian rodents with optogenetic techniques [41]. More importantly, they found therapeutic effects within the subthalamic nucleus by direct selective stimulation of its afferent neurons [41]. Although such optical approach is far from clinical utilization, its arrival in standard health care may be one of the biggest therapeutic advancements in this area.

Conclusion

Deep brain stimulation is a well-established treatment modality for Parkinson's disease, essential tremor, as well as obsessive compulsive disorders and dystonia. Despite the uncertainty of its mechanism of action its benefits are clear and likely to increase further in light of the technological promises.

References

[1] Horsley, V. Remarks on the Surgery of the Central Nervous System. *British medical journal*. 1890;2:1286-92.

[2] Spiegel, E. A., Wycis, H. T., Marks, M., Lee, A. J. Stereotaxic Apparatus for Operations on the Human Brain. *Science*. 1947;106:349-50.

[3] Hassler, R., Riechert, T. [Indications and localization of stereotactic brain operations] *Der Nervenarzt*. 1954;25:441-7.

[4] Talairach, J., David, M., Tournoux, P., Corredor, H., Kvasina, T. *Atlas d'anatomie stereotaxique*. Paris, France: Masson; 1957.

[5] Cooper, I. S. Ligation of the anterior choroidal artery for involuntary movements; parkinsonism. *The Psychiatric quarterly*. 1953;27:317-9.

[6] Albe Fessard, D., Arfel, G., Guiot, G., Derome, P., Dela, H., Korn, H., et al. [Characteristic Electric Activities of Some Cerebral Structures in Man] *Annales de chirurgie*. 1963;17:1185-214.

[7] Benabid, A. L., Pollak, P., Louveau, A., Henry, S., de Rougemont, J. Combined (thalamotomy and stimulation) stereotactic surgery of the VIM thalamic nucleus for bilateral Parkinson disease. *Applied neurophysiology*. 1987;50:344-6.

[8] DeLong, M. R. Primate models of movement disorders of basal ganglia origin. *Trends in neurosciences*. 1990;13:281-5.

[9] Limousin, P., Krack, P., Pollak, P., Benazzouz, A., Ardouin, C., Hoffmann, D., et al. Electrical stimulation of the subthalamic nucleus in advanced Parkinson's disease. *The New England journal of medicine*. 1998;339:1105-11.

[10] Benazzouz, A., Hallett, M. Mechanism of action of deep brain stimulation. *Neurology*. 2000;55:S13-6.

[11] Dostrovsky, J. O., Levy, R., Wu, J. P., Hutchison, W. D., Tasker, R. R., Lozano, A. M. Microstimulation-induced inhibition of neuronal firing in human globus pallidus. *Journal of neurophysiology*. 2000;84:570-4.

[12] McIntyre, C. C., Grill, W. M. Extracellular stimulation of central neurons: influence of stimulus waveform and frequency on neuronal output. *Journal of neurophysiology*. 2002;88:1592-604.

[13] McIntyre, C. C., Grill, W. M., Sherman, D. L., Thakor, N. V. Cellular effects of deep brain stimulation: model-based analysis of activation and inhibition. *Journal of neurophysiology*. 2004;91:1457-69.

[14] Windels, F., Bruet, N., Poupard, A., Feuerstein, C., Bertrand, A., Savasta, M. Influence of the frequency parameter on extracellular glutamate and gamma-aminobutyric acid in substantia nigra and globus pallidus during electrical stimulation of subthalamic nucleus in rats. *Journal of neuroscience research*. 2003;72:259-67.

[15] Jech, R., Urgosik, D., Tintera, J., Nebuzelsky, A., Krasensky, J., Liscak, R., et al. Functional magnetic resonance imaging during deep brain stimulation: a pilot study in four patients with Parkinson's disease. *Movement disorders: official journal of the Movement Disorder Society*. 2001;16:1126-32.

[16] Hershey, T., Revilla, F. J., Wernle, A. R., McGee-Minnich, L., Antenor, J. V., Videen, T. O., et al. Cortical and subcortical blood flow effects of subthalamic nucleus stimulation in PD. *Neurology*. 2003;61:816-21.

[17] Perlmutter, J. S., Mink, J. W., Bastian, A. J., Zackowski, K., Hershey, T., Miyawaki, E., et al. Blood flow responses to deep brain stimulation of thalamus. *Neurology*. 2002;58: 1388-94.

[18] Groppa, S., Herzog, J., Falk, D., Riedel, C., Deuschl, G., Volkmann, J. Physiological and anatomical decomposition of subthalamic neurostimulation effects in essential tremor. *Brain: a journal of neurology*. 2014;137:109-21.

[19] Herzog, J., Hamel, W., Wenzelburger, R., Potter, M., Pinsker, M. O., Bartussek, J., et al. Kinematic analysis of thalamic versus subthalamic neurostimulation in postural and intention tremor. *Brain: a journal of neurology*. 2007;130:1608-25.

[20] Albin, R. L., Young, A. B., Penney, J. B. The functional anatomy of basal ganglia disorders. *Trends in neurosciences*. 1989;12:366-75.

[21] Alexander, G. E., DeLong, M. R., Strick, P. L. Parallel organization of functionally segregated circuits linking basal ganglia and cortex. *Annual review of neuroscience*. 1986;9:357-81.

[22] Wichman, T., Vitek, J. L. *Physiology of the basal ganglia and pathophysiology of movement disorders*. Totowa, NJ: Humana Press; 2002.

[23] Wichman, T., DeLong, M. R., Vitek, J. L. Pathophysiological considerations in basal ganglia surgery: role of the basal ganglia in hypokinetic and hyperkinetic movement disorders. *Progress in Neurological Surgery*. 2000;15:31-57.

[24] Hirai, T., Jones, E. G. A new parcellation of the human thalamus on the basis of histochemical staining. *Brain research Brain research reviews*. 1989;14:1-34.

[25] Ilinsky, I. A., Jouandet, M. L., Goldman-Rakic, P. S. Organization of the nigrothalamocortical system in the rhesus monkey. *The Journal of comparative neurology*. 1985;236:315-30.

[26] Hazrati, L. N., Parent, A. Projection from the external pallidum to the reticular thalamic nucleus in the squirrel monkey. *Brain research*. 1991; 550:142-6.

[27] Hamani, C., Saint-Cyr, J. A., Fraser, J., Kaplitt, M., Lozano, A. M. The subthalamic nucleus in the context of movement disorders. *Brain: a journal of neurology*. 2004;127: 4-20.

[28] Hamada, I., DeLong, M. R. Excitotoxic acid lesions of the primate subthalamic nucleus result in reduced pallidal neuronal activity during active holding. *Journal of neurophysiology*. 1992;68:1859-66.

[29] Nambu, A., Tokuno, H., Hamada, I., Kita, H., Imanishi, M., Akazawa, T., et al. Excitatory cortical inputs to pallidal neurons via the subthalamic nucleus in the monkey. *Journal of neurophysiology*. 2000; 84:289-300.

[30] Magill, P. J., Bolam, J. P., Bevan, M. D. Relationship of activity in the subthalamic nucleus-globus pallidus network to cortical electroencephalogram. *The Journal of neuroscience: the official journal of the Society for Neuroscience*. 2000;20:820-33.

[31] Miller, W. C., DeLong, M. R. *Altered tonic activity of neurons in the globus pallidus and subthalamic nucleus in the primate MPTP model of parkinsonism*. New York: Plenum Press; 1987.

[32] Filion, M., Tremblay, L. Abnormal spontaneous activity of globus pallidus neurons in monkeys with MPTP-induced parkinsonism. *Brain research*. 1991;547:142-51.

[33] Vitek, J. L., Chockkan, V., Zhang, J. Y., Kaneoke, Y., Evatt, M., DeLong, M. R., et al. Neuronal activity in the basal ganglia in patients with generalized dystonia and hemiballismus. *Annals of neurology*. 1999;46:22-35.

[34] Vitek, J. L., Bakay, R. A., Hashimoto, T., Kaneoke, Y., Mewes, K., Zhang, J. Y., et al. Microelectrode-guided pallidotomy: technical approach and its application in medically intractable Parkinson's disease. *Journal of neurosurgery*. 1998;88:1027-43.

[35] Lozano, A. M., Lang, A. E., Galvez-Jimenez, N., Miyasaki, J., Duff, J., Hutchinson, W. D., et al. Effect of GPi pallidotomy on motor function in Parkinson's disease. *Lancet*. 1995;346:1383-7.

[36] Llinas, R. R. Intrinsic electrical properties of mammalian neurons and CNS function: a historical perspective. *Frontiers in cellular neuroscience*. 2014;8:320.

[37] Bergman, H., Wichmann, T., Karmon, B., DeLong, M. R. The primate subthalamic nucleus. II. Neuronal activity in the MPTP model of parkinsonism. *Journal of neurophysiology*. 1994;72:507-20.

[38] Rosin, B., Slovik, M., Mitelman, R., Rivlin-Etzion, M., Haber, S. N., Israel, Z., et al. Closed-loop deep brain stimulation is superior in ameliorating parkinsonism. *Neuron*. 2011;72:370-84.

[39] Airan, R. D., Thompson, K. R., Fenno, L. E., Bernstein, H., Deisseroth, K. Temporally precise in vivo control of intracellular signalling. *Nature*. 2009;458:1025-9.

[40] Fenno, L., Yizhar, O., Deisseroth, K. The development and application of optogenetics. *Annual review of neuroscience*. 2011;34:389-412.

[41] Gradinaru, V., Mogri, M., Thompson, K. R., Henderson, J. M., Deisseroth, K. Optical deconstruction of parkinsonian neural circuitry. *Science*. 2009;324:354-9.

[42] Pama, E. A., Colzato, L. S., Hommel, B. Optogenetics as a neuromodulation tool in cognitive neuroscience. *Frontiers in psychology*. 2013;4:610.

In: Deep Brain Stimulation
Editor: Raja Mehanna

ISBN: 978-1-63483-282-3

Chapter 4

DEEP BRAIN STIMULATION FROM THE NEUROSURGICAL STANDPOINT

Sebastian J. Villarreal MD and Albert Fenoy MD
University of Texas Medical School at Houston, Houston, TX, US

ABSTRACT

Over the past 30 years, deep brain stimulation (DBS) has become a widely recognized technique for reversible modulation of brain function that is adjunctive to the medical management of movement disorders and obsessive-compulsive disorders.

While other chapters review the evidence of DBS in these and other disorders, and suggest algorithms for stimulation and troubleshooting, this chapter will focus on the neurosurgical aspect of DBS, from surgical planning to implant and postoperative care, in addition to surgical complications of the procedure.

INTRODUCTION

When functional neurosurgery procedures were first introduced in the 1940's and 1950's, they were carried out largely on empirical basis. Over time, the rationale for performing functional neurosurgical interventions has become clearer.

Several factors have contributed to progress in functional neurosurgery such as effective animal models and the development of precise brain imaging methods that allow for the evaluation of patients and animal models with these disorders.

Refinements in patient selection, improved understanding of the pathophysiology, and increasing accuracy of neurosurgical targets has translated into increased safety, effectiveness, and overall success of deep brain stimulation (DBS).

Surgical Planning

A. Patient Selection for DBS Neurosurgical Interventions

Successful DBS therapy for the treatment of movement disorders is based on the foundation of careful patient selection, in addition to thought-out target selection, precise lead placement, and proficient electrode programing.

General Selection Process

A thorough selection process should be routinely preformed to ensure that only appropriate candidates are considered for DBS surgery. This type of careful selection process would include the following: 1) a detailed neurological examination, 2) neurosurgical evaluation, 3) neuropsychological testing and psychiatric evaluation, 4) neuroimaging, and 5) medical clearance.

Neurological Evaluation

Preoperative evaluation for DBS usually begins with a complete neurological assessment by a neurologist who specializes in the management of movement disorders. This examination is targeted on establishing that a diagnosis amenable to neurosurgical interventions has been made correctly. Furthermore, the physician should review the medical management of the patient to ensure that all reasonable pharmacologic therapies have been attempted prior to discussing neurosurgical treatment options. For example, when a patient with Parkinson's disease (PD) is being considered for DBS, examination of the patient both "off" and "on" medications should be performed. The patients response and degree of benefit from levodopa has well-documented diagnostic and prognostic implications.

The determination of which PD patient is most likely to have a good response to DBS is in part related to how well the patient responds to levodopa administration. Additionally, a pre-operative clinical neurological baseline of the patient is established at this point.

Neurosurgical Evaluation

Once the neurologist has confirmed the correct diagnosis and medical strategies have not provided satisfactory control, the patient should then be referred to a functional neurosurgeon. It is the obligation of the neurosurgeon to assess the risk-benefit ratio of the DBS surgery on an individual basis for every patient.

A neurological examination is again performed and a clinical baseline is established at this time. During this evaluation, the neurosurgeon discusses the surgical options, the surgical procedure, the risks and possible complications from anesthesia and the DBS procedure itself. Preoperative, operative, and postoperative processes are discussed in detail with the patient. Importantly, a review of the patient's expectations from DBS is performed and followed by a discussion of what the realistic goal should be.

During this evaluation, the patient is reminded that further surgery for battery replacements will be necessary approximately every 2 to 8 years depending on the type of battery implanted and the stimulation setting used. If the patient is a good candidate for DBS and decides to proceed to the next step, a tentative date for surgery is scheduled and a referral for medical clearance is made in high-risk individuals.

Finally, in order to minimize the risk of hemorrhage, patients scheduled for DBS surgery should be instructed to discontinue platelet inhibitors (i.e. aspirin, clopidogrel, aspirin/ extended-release dipyridamole), anticoagulants (i.e. warfarin, rivaroxaban, dabigatran, apixaban), vitamin E and other medications that interfere with the normal coagulation process, 1 to 2 weeks prior to surgery.

Neurocognitive and Psychiatric Evaluation

Psychiatrist and neuropsychologist are essential members of a multidisciplinary DBS program. Proper cognitive assessment and psychiatric screening are fundamental steps in a patient selection for DBS. The purpose of this evaluation is to identify patients with dementia, severe deficits in executive function, signs of untreated depression or psychosis, dopaminergic dysregulation syndrome, medication-induced hypomania/mania, and high suicide risk. These conditions can contra-indicate DBS, influence the choice of the target or can worsen after DBS and thus need to be treated before surgery.

Neuroimaging

Preoperative imaging, preferably magnetic resonance imaging (MRI) without contrast, is needed during the process of evaluating patients considering DBS surgery. The MRI is needed to identify any structural lesions or anatomic abnormalities that may interfere with proper DBS targeting, or other pathological processes (i.e. brain tumors, cerebral abscess), which may be contraindication for DBS interventions.

It also plays an important role in helping to determine the most optimal entry points. For example, during the preoperative planning, the gadolinium enhanced T1-weighted MRI is particularly useful in visualizing major vessels that allow for the adjustment of entry points in order to avoid any cortical arteries, as well as any cortical draining veins or venous lakes. Care is also taken to avoid sulci and the ventricular system when planning the entry point and trajectory in order to minimize the risk of hemorrhage, as well as loss of CSF with penetration of the ventricles.

Historically, ventriculography was the gold standard for the identification of the anterior and posterior commissures, but it has been replaced by MRI. The time at which the MRI is acquired for surgical planning purposes, however, differs from center to center. Some centers obtain the MRI on the same day of surgery, while others acquire the MRI the day before surgery. Another option is to obtain the MRI several days prior to surgery and to obtain a computed tomography (CT) on the day of surgery and to merge it with the MRI images using the FrameLink software (Medtronic, Minneapolis, US).

The introduction of 3T MRI scanners has not only further increased the image quality and resolution of brain imaging, it has also allowed for the creation of patient-specific and treatment-specific target models utilizing diffusion tensor imaging (DTI).

Ideally, a 3T MRI with several MRI sequences is used, each with its own information that is collectively incorporated into making the final surgical plan. A T1 weighted image (T1WI) MRI with contrast is useful to delineate and avoid the cortical vessels during the planning for the entry point and the location of the cranial burr holes. Additionally, a T2 weighted image (T2WI) without contrast is particularly useful for visualizing the anatomy of the basal ganglia.

Medical Clearance

Medical clearance is usually the last step prior to proceeding with DBS implant. This evaluation normally includes standard preoperative blood tests and electrocardiography (ECG). A cardiac stress test may be indicated in some cases. General contraindications to surgery should also be explored further. Patients with uncontrolled hypertension, diabetes, coronary artery disease, cardiac pacemakers, liver or kidney failure, intractable seizure disorders or coagulopathies may be poor surgical candidates. During that visit, patients have their medications reviewed again so that any medication which may increase the risk of hemorrhage can be discontinued in a timely fashion.

B. Pre-Operative Planning: Direct vs. Indirect Targeting

Surgical planning includes determining the exact location of the specific DBS target and the best trajectory to reach it. Although several different frameless systems using skull-based fiducials are available, we will focus on our personal experience with the stereotactic head frame system, specifically the Leksell Stereotactic System used with FrameLink (Medtronic, Minneapolis, US), a stereotactic software program that calculates the target coordinates (X, Y and Z) using a tridimensional Cartesian system.

Indirect targeting uses standardized stereotactic atlases and a formula, using the anterior commissure (AC) and posterior commissure (PC) landmarks as references. With indirect targeting, T1WI MRI sequences are used to identify visible anatomical landmarks: the AC and PC location, the distance between AC and PC, the intercommissural line (ICL) or the intercommissural plane (ICP), the midcommissural point (MCP), and the height of the thalamus above the AC-PC plane. In addition to these anatomical landmarks, indirect targeting also utilizes a standard atlas such as the Schaltenbrand atlas, which is reformatted and adjusted to the patient's ICL. Moreover, indirect targeting can utilize the anatomical relationships between the target of choice and the structures other than the AC and PC, such as the wall of the third ventricle or the borders of the red nucleus (RN).

Conversely, direct targeting involves the direct visualization of the target nucleus on T2WI MRI, and thereby a calculation for that particular target coordinate is made utilizing the FrameLink software. Currently no clear advantage has been established for direct versus indirect targeting in regards to the accuracy of targeting.

Although targeting techniques may vary depending on the target, a combination of indirect and direct anatomical targeting strategies are typically compared with each other prior to surgical implantation. For example, when targeting the subthalamic nucleus (STN), we initially begin by implementing indirect targeting by applying the typical anatomical coordinates for STN, which are 11-13 mm lateral to the midline, 4 to 5 mm ventral to the ICP, and 3 to 4 mm posterior to the MCP. Once these coordinates are inserted into the planning software, the target is examined and modified as needed via direct targeting that is utilized by direct visualization of the STN on T2WI sequences. The axial and coronal T2WI sequences are particularly useful in the visualization and delineation of the nucleus against the surrounding white matter structures.

Furthermore, neighboring structures clearly visualized on T2WI may be used for further positioning of the final target point, such as visualizing the RN and its borders when localizing the STN during its targeting.

Similarly, in regards to targeting the globus pallidus internus (GPi), indirect targeting is implemented by using the typical coordinates, which are 19 to 21 mm lateral to the midline, 2 to 3 mm anterior to the MCP, and 4 to 5 mm ventral to the ICP. Once the initial target coordinates have been entered into the surgical planning software, careful windowing of the T2WI sequences allows for direct visualization of the GPi as well as the globus pallidus externa (GPe), which is then used to further refine the target coordinates. Additionally, using the T2WI sequences, the optic tract and the internal capsule can also be visualized. Since the optic tract is located ventral to the GPi, its anatomical relationship can be used as an additional landmark when targeting the GPi [1, 2].

Although the thalamus and its boundaries can easily be visualized using the T2WI sequences, the subdivisions and the individual sub-nuclei within the thalamus cannot be directly visualized with current imaging techniques. Therefore, the ventral intermediate nucleus (Vim) of the thalamus can only be targeted by the implementation of indirect targeting, along with intraoperative electrophysiological mapping and intraoperative testing of the impact of stimulation on the patient's symptoms. The typical coordinates for indirect targeting of the Vim of the thalamus are approximately 11 to 13 mm lateral to the midline, or approximately 10 mm lateral from the wall of the third ventricle at the level of the ICL [3]. In relation to the anterior-posterior axis, the Vim is usually found between $1/6^{th}$ and $1/4^{th}$ of the AC—PC distance rostrally from the PC [3, 4, 5, 6, 7].

In patients with narrow or wide third ventricles, adjustments in the Vim targeting are made by its relationship to the width of the third ventricle. This is traditionally accomplished by implementing Guiot's formula [8] according to which the distance of the Vim from the midline is 11.5 mm + V/2, where 'V' is the width of the third ventricle [5]. It is important to understand that this formula is based on the assumption that the wider the third ventricle is, the more lateral the Vim is located. Moreover, a study by Bardinet et al. has shown that this calculation may result in localizing a target located more laterally than the actual position of the Vim [5]. It is therefore recommended that at least one microelectrode should be placed more medially than the target determined through this formula during microelectrode recording (MER) and intraoperative testing [5].

Once again, after the indirect atlas-based and formula-based targeting is completed, those coordinates are typically analyzed and correlated with direct visualization of the target when applicable. In addition to specific subcortical nuclei, the stereotactic targeting of white-matter tracts such as the dentato-rubo-thalamic tract (DRT) and the medial forebrain bundle (MFB) are increasingly implemented for treatment of essential tremor (ET) and medically refractory depression respectively [7, 9]. This is mainly accomplished by direct targeting of such tracts visualized by the use of tractography using a pre –operatively obtained MRI DTI sequence.

Traditionally, targeting of the Vim nucleus of the thalamus has been used in the surgical treatment of medically refractory tremor. More recently, the DRT white matter tract has emerged as a new target for tremor control [7, 10], and we have had good success in controlling ET by directly targeting the DRT. The DRT is the main fiber bundle that composes the superior cerebellar peduncle (SCP). Fibers mostly originating from the dentate nucleus (DN) enter the contralateral RN and continue to ascend and terminate in both the ventralis oralis posterior nucleus (VOP) and the Vim nucleus of the thalamus. These nuclei then project to the primary motor cortex [7, 9, 11]. Mapping the location of the DRT-fiber tract is performed at our institution using the StealthViz DTI software application (Medtronic, Minneapolis, US) after acquisition of the proper MRI sequences.

As described by Coenen et al., such tractography is accomplished upon identification of a cubic volume of interest (VOI) defining the region of the cerebellar dentate nucleus (DN) on the high-resolution T2WI MRI. The resulting fibers following the superior cerebellar peduncle are included with a second VOI box (end region) around the fibers that reach the precentral gyrus [7, 9]. The subsequent fiber tracts are fused to the T2-weighted and T1-weighted MRI sequences and transferred to the stereotactic planning system FrameLink for direct targeting.

DBS Surgery

A. Patient Positioning and Surgical Exposure

Depending on whether or not the patient's intraoperative feedback in needed, i.e. whether or not brain mapping is done, the 1 surgical implant of the intracranial DBS lead may be performed either under local or general anesthesia. In general, most of the intracranial DBS lead implants are done under local anesthesia in order to perform brain mapping.

Prior to beginning the procedure, cefazolin (or vancomycin, if the patient has a history of allergy to penicillin) is administered to the patient. Depending on the procedure, the entire scalp or the neck, chest, and/or abdomen are clipped of hair, degreased, and then prepared with 2% chlorhexidine gluconate and 70% isopropyl alcohol (ChloraPrep; Enturia, Inc.).

To begin the first stage of DBS surgery, the placement of intracranial electrode leads, the stereotactic head frame is affixed to the skull of the patient via four points of fixation using local anesthetics, two on the forehead above the eyebrows, and two in the suboccipital region. A stealth CT scan of the head with the head frame in place is then obtained.

The CT stealth scan is then merged with the preoperative MRI in order to increase the spatial accuracy inherent to CT imaging and to utilize the benefit of the high image resolution, while minimizing the image distortion that occurs with MRI scans, particularly with the presence of the stereotactic head frame [12, 13, 14]. Although there still exists inherent inaccuracies that occur with the merging of MRI and CT imaging, this merging allows to take advantage of both direct and indirect imaging methods, and simultaneously minimizes the disadvantages of each strategy [15].

Once the patient returns to the operating suite after completion of the head CT, the patient and the head frame are secured to the operating table using a skull fixation device (i.e., Mayfield) along with the appropriate y- and z-coordinates for the specific DBS target. Due to the length of the procedure, the patient's comfort should be optimized. The head and the neck are maintained in a neutral position to ensure an adequate airway, but, overall, the patient is positioned in a reclined, semi-sitting position with the operating bed placed in a slight Trendelenburg position.

In other institutions, the patient is laid flat on the back. The surgical sites are cleaned with 70% isopropyl alcohol prior to marking the two surgical incisions on the skull with a surgical marking pen. First, a curvilinear incision is marked over the coronal suture, ensuring that the incision remains behind the frontal hairline, along with ample space to allow for burr holes to be well behind the surgical incision. The second incision is marked over the left parietal eminence, approximately 2cm behind and 2cm above the pinna.

At this point the patient is prepped and cleaned with a mix of 2% chlorhexidine gluconate and 70% isopropyl alcohol (ChloraPrep; Enturia, Inc.). Then, the patient is draped in the usual sterile fashion, using a transparent drape to separate the surgical sterile field from the non-sterile patient-side. This allows the patient to communicate clearly, and the surgeon to monitor the patient's movements during the procedure.

A generous amount of local anesthetic is injected along both surgical sites. A 10-blade scalpel is used to make the initial skin incisions. A bipolar electrocautery instrument is used to obtain meticulous hemostasis. Rainey hemostatic clips are then placed over the skin edges of the coronal incision, and the scalp is flapped and secured posteriorly.

The entry point through the bone is then identified and marked. The entry point should be at least 3 cm lateral to the midline. This minimizes skiving through the lateral ventricles and reduces the risk of injury to the superior sagittal sinus, its draining veins, or any large venous lake that are found along the midline. The entry point and trajectory would have been determined in advance, with the help of pre-operative MRI as discussed above.

After the entry point has been identified on the skull, 14 mm burr holes are made along the coronal suture using a high-speed drill. It is important to have continuous irrigation and prompt placement of bone wax along the edges of the burr holes in order to avoid an air embolus. For further discussion on the avoidance of complications, please refer to the surgical complication section below. Once the burr holes are completed, the dura-mater is identified and coagulated thoroughly. For cosmetic purposes, further bone is drilled off using a high-speed drill with a 5mm round cutting burr. This makes a trough circumferentially around the burr hole. The DBS anchoring device is then secured over the burr hole. The drilled out trough creates a recess in which the DBS anchoring device and cap, along with the Stimloc system (Medtronic, Minneapolis, US), can sit and discretely remain underneath the scalp.

Once the anchoring device is in place, the dura is opened using an 11-blade in a cruciate fashion. Again the edges of the dura are coagulated using the bipolar electrocautery instrument to ensure meticulous hemostasis and an unimpeded entry point. Care is taken to minimize cerebral spinal fluid (CSF) loss, thus minimizing brain shift. Next, vessels along the cortical surface are identified and avoided. If an unexpected vessel is encountered, the burr hole can be expanded to avoid injury to any major cortical vessels. In order to minimize the risk of hemorrhage, the bipolar electrocautery instrument is used to coagulate a small cortical surface along the entry point before using the 11-blade to pierce through the leptomeninges. This also allows for less brain shift and easier passage of the cannula into the brain parenchyma, as well as minimizes the potential for the development of a subdural hematoma from brain movement and tearing of bridging veins during electrode penetration into the brain parenchyma. Meticulous hemostasis is obtained prior to proceeding to the next step of the procedure. At this point, the x-coordinate is set on the Leksell Stereotactic Arc before mounting it on the head frame. This assures fast and correct positioning when fitting the arc onto the head frame.

B. Microelectrode Recording, Intraoperative Stimulation and Implant

Mapping strategies vary from center to center, but can be broadly categorized into two groups: those who only rely on macrostimulation to elicit clinical effects and side effects, and those who utilize microelectrode recording (MER) prior to macrostimulation.

MER is a neurophysiological technique which detects and amplifies the activity of individual neurons. This is an important technique which incorporates real-time anatomic verification of the target region and identifies its borders. Moreover, when treating movement disorders such as PD, MER can confirm the presence or absence of movement-responsive neurons.

Although there remains some controversy whether MER may cause an increased risk of bleeding, the risk against imperfect placement of the DBS electrode by not utilizing MER must be weighed against the risk of hemorrhage when using MER—particularly, in patients who are older, as well as in patients who are hypertensive [16, 17, 18].

There are several factors that can result in suboptimal targeting, including brain-shift upon trepanation, the inherent distortions and imprecisions of the imaging acquired, the head frame, and the software merger, just to name a few. For this reason, we apply the additional information provided by MER and macrostimulation to further refine final electrode placement and to ensure the best possible outcome. However, whether target refinements by MER in fact lead to improved outcomes, or whether non-MER techniques may be equivalent, has not been fully resolved. We will discuss MER briefly, as it will be discussed in further detail in chapter 5.

Per protocol, we record single-unit action potentials with MERs typically beginning 10mm above the specific DBS target point. Some institutions start recording at 15mm above the target. It is essential to avoid deflection of the electrodes by bone, dura, and even pia, as they are placed and advanced to the target. The microelectrode is advanced to target in a controlled and precise manner using a micro-motor driving system. The amplitude, frequency, and pattern of the action potentials are recorded. MER is useful in order to identify, localize, and outline the shape of the targeted nuclei.

As will be discussed further in the next chapter, MER can be supplemented by microstimulation in the microampere range (up to 90 microamps). After successful localization of the target is confirmed by MER, with or without microstimulation, the permanent DBS electrode lead is implanted. After removal of the MER system, a rigid guiding cannula is placed at the target and the DBS electrode is inserted through this cannula. Sharp instruments and forceps with teeth should not be used in manipulating the DBS electrode and special caution must be taken not to crush or damage the DBS lead. At our institution, we use rubber shodden instruments and bayonets without teeth when manipulating the DBS lead.

Currently, there are two widely used Medtronic DBS lead models: The 3387 model, which is composed of four 1.5mm cylindrical electrodes that are each 1.5mm apart; and the 3389 model, which was designed to minimize the intercontact interval to 0.5mm in comparison to the 1.5mm intercontact interval found in the 3387 model. In the 3389 model, by reducing the intercontact interval, the overall span of the electrode contacts is also reduced from 10.5mm, as is found in the 3387 model, to 7.5mm. In general, we use the 3387 model in all our patients. In regards to STN targeting, it is still uncertain whether the theoretical target is actually within the STN or just above. Thus, the longer 1.5mm interval provided by the 3387 model, allows for the ability to stimulate a greater region outside of the theoretical target, and, additionally, the longer length of the contact distribution permits greater ability for programing compensation in a suboptimally placed DBS electrode. Other institutions use the 3389 model in the STN because of its small size, and the 3387 model in the GPi and Vim.

Once the DBS electrode is in place intra-cranially, it is tested intra-operatively to assess benefits and side effects at that location before finalizing and closing. There are 2 ways to perform macrostimulation through the DBS lead: using a bipolar or a monopolar configuration, and these are not mutually exclusive.

When using a bipolar configuration, the Medtronic model 3625 handheld pulse-generator is attached to the DBS lead higher end. Stimulation is performed usually at a high frequency (>130 Hz) and over the widest range of contacts on the lead (ventral most contact 0-, dorsal most contact 3+). We usually begin at 1V and, in a stepwise fashion, gradually increase in increments of either 0.5V or 1V up to a maximum of typically 5-10 volts, depending on the structure targeted during surgery. Typically, in STN targeting, limiting adverse effects from current spreading to the internal capsule, such as dysarthria or facial contractions, occur above 6 volts.

If the threshold of adverse effects is lower than expected in this situation, this indicates that the DBS electrode is positioned too laterally and should be repositioned at least 2 mm medially [1]. Furthermore with STN targeting, intermittent paresthesias are expected when the testing voltage is increased and signify a more posterior location of the electrode. Unless the paresthesias do not spontaneously resolve, this is not considered a contraindication for final DBS implantation at that particular target [3]. The maximum testing voltage used varies from patient to patient because it is the adverse effect felt by the patient or seen clinically that ultimately set the limit. It is important to note that the patient may experience a "shock-like" sensation over the contralateral side of the body if the voltage is increased too quickly. However, this is less likely to occur if the voltage is gradually increased. Typically for STN targeting, up to 4 volts are generally tolerated without adverse effects [3]. In contrast, when targeting GPi, slightly higher thresholds to adverse effects should be expected [3]: for example, dysarthria, facial pulling, and/or transient visual phenomena typically occur anywhere from 6 to 12 volts [10].

Overall, if adverse effects occur at lower voltages than expected, then testing with closer contacts (1-, 2+), and thereby theoretically testing a smaller volume of activated tissue [19, 20, 21], should be done. If the threshold is still low, lead repositioning should be considered.

In the monopolar configuration, a Medtronic model 8840 handheld pulse-generator, similar (but no identical) to the one used for postoperative programming in clinic, is connected to the DBS lead higher end with a screening cable model 3550-67: the cathode is linked to the contact used and the anode is linked to the frame or the scalp. Stimulation is performed usually at a frequency of 130HZ to 185Hz, and at a pulse width of 60 microsecs, although a higher pulse width can be used in the GPi. The most ventral contact (contact 0) is tested first. The amplitude is increased in a similar fashion than in the bipolar configuration, with benefits on the abnormal movement and side effects by spreading of the current to adjacent structures being assessed at each step. Effects and side effects typically occur at lower thresholds in the monopolar configuration, because of the bigger field created by that configuration at the same amplitude, compared to the bipolar configuration. Once limiting side effects such as muscle contraction, gaze deviation or dysarthria are observed, the amplitude is brought down to zero and another contact is tested. To change the active contact, the surgeon needs to manually move the cable connecting the programmer to the higher end of the lead and link it to the appropriate contact. If results are satisfactory in contact 0 with a low threshold to improvement and high threshold (typically above 4V) to side effect, then contact 2 can be tested next.

Otherwise, it might be necessary to test contact 1 first. In the STN, stimulation at contact 0 is the most likely to cause side effects by spreading of the current to the internal capsule, so more dorsal contacts need to be tested before planning to reposition the lead, as the threshold to capsular side effects might be higher and thus acceptable with a more dorsal stimulation. All 4 contacts are rarely tested in the operating room, as testing 2 or 3 contacts is usually enough to grossly assess efficacy and safety of the location of the lead.

Once the DBS electrode is in the final position, special care is taken to ensure that it does not move, as it can migrate in the vertical plane Therefore, the exit point of the DBS electrode is marked and kept in position, using rubber shodden hemostats during removal of the cannula and the electrode stylet. After the DBS electrode is "clipped" to the Stimloc anchor, the cap is carefully placed and secured.

A temporary protective cap is placed over the proximal lead end which is tunneled to the parietal scalp and secured under the galea just posterior and superior to the pinna of the ear. This end will be accessed during the programmer implant, which the second stage of the surgery, and is typically scheduled 2 weeks after the lead's implant.

Intraoperative imaging is essential for confirming final lead location. At most centers, an intra-operative lateral x-ray/fluoroscopy or computed tomography image (via Medtronic's O-Arm system or intraoperative CT) is obtained to confirm lead target placement, depth, and to rule out any lead migration that may have occurred during the process of securing the lead. At our center, we obtain an intraoperative computed tomogram using the O-arm just prior to the conclusion of the procedure and merge it with the pre-operative imaging in order to confirm the final target and trajectory. If displacement of the lead is detected, we immediately reposition the lead to the proper target location, re-secure the lead, and obtain an additional intraoperative stealth head CT to confirm the new position of the lead.

Once the lead position is deemed satisfactory, irrigation with povidone-iodine solution diluted to near 1% concentration is performed at each incision site, and is followed by the addition of 1 gram of vancomycin powder over the inserted hardware and within the surgical incisions. The surgical incisions are then closed with 3-0 resorbable sutures in the galea, usually followed by skin staples in order to minimize any potential damage to the DBS electrodes during the suture process.

Functional neurological improvement of the patient may be seen during MER and/or macrostimulation. Any improvement observed during this time is usually considered a good indicator of the patient's ultimate clinical outcome.

However, patient's abnormal movements, occasionally improve by the mere implant of the DBS lead without any stimulation. This effect is called the "microlesion effect." Typically, the symptom improvement is temporary and usually only lasts for up to 4 weeks. However a longer-lasting microlesion effect on tremor control can be seen when targeting the Vim nucleus of the thalamus. The presence of the microlesion effect is believed to be a positive prognostic indicator.

C. Post-Surgical Care

As mentioned above, it is our protocol to obtain a postoperative CT of the head to ensure the absence of any intracerebral hemorrhage or extra-axial hemorrhage, and verify the final DBS lead position.

The preoperative MRI and the postoperative head CT are merged using stereotactic planning software in order to confirm the anatomical target around each electrode contact. Moreover, the pre- and postoperative image merger allows for the evaluation of the accuracy of the procedure by comparing the planned trajectory and target with the final DBS electrode position. At our institution, the patient is monitored in the neuro-intermediate care unit (NIMU) post operatively for one day, and all appropriate home medications are restarted. After completion of the postoperative protocol of IV antibiotics for 24-hours (cefazolin, or vancomycin if the patient has a history of allergy to penicillin), oral cephalexin (or ciprofloxacin/clindamycin if the patient has a history of allergy to penicillin) is routinely administered to all patients for 7 days after the procedure as prophylactic therapy.

Additionally, in order to avoid postoperative seizures, our protocol consists of loading the patient with an anticonvulsant, such as levetiracetam. If the patient remains seizure free, the anticonvulsant is discontinued upon discharge, usually the day after the procedure. If the patient has a seizure, the anticonvulsant is continued after discharge for several months.

D. Pulse Generator Implant

Two weeks after the intracranial lead implants, the stage I procedure, the patient returns for an outpatient procedure during which the implantable pulse generator (IPG) and the lead extensions are placed subcutaneously—otherwise known as stage II procedure.

During this procedure, the patient is placed under general anesthesia and the parietal incision is reopened to externalize the leads' distal ends. The protective caps, which were placed during the initial procedure, are removed from the distal ends of the leads which are then connected and secured to the lead extensions that are tunneled subcutaneously to reach the site of the pulse generator. While there is variation from center to center, we use one dual-channel IPG, instead of two single-channels, for several reasons. First, the need and time for repositioning, re-preparing, and re-draping are eliminated with the use of one dual-channel IPG. Additionally, the surgical time is decreased when only one surgical incision is made, and only one subcutaneous tunneling pass for the lead extensions is needed.

Currently, Medtronic is the only US supplier of FDA approved DBS devices, and provides three different models of pulse generators from the new Activa family: a single-channel primary cell (non-rechargeable) Activa SC, a dual-channel primary cell (non-rechargeable) Activa PC, and a dual-channel rechargeable cell Activa RC.

All IPGs have their advantages and disadvantages, but the Activa class is more reliable than its predecessors, the Soletra and Kinetra. The PC model is larger and is more rectangular in shape compared to the RC and SC, which are similar in shape and size, but with rounder edges that contour to a subcutaneous pocket. At times, such sharp dimensionality of the PC can make it more prone to erosion in frail, thin-skinned patients [22, 23].

One major disadvantage of the dual-channel IPGs is that if an infection develops, both DBS leads are placed at risk if the generator must be explanted. At our institution, we mostly use either the Activa PC or RC. Whether the Activa PC or RC version is implanted is a decision that is made by the patient. For example, individuals who do not wish to take time to recharge their IPG, would be better suited with the Activa PC. However, the lifespan for each IPG must be kept in mind.

In general, the Activa PC lasts between 3-5 years, and therefore will require more frequent surgical exchanges than the RC version, which can last as long as 9-years, but requires recharging sessions. The pulse generator is commonly placed over the superiolateral quadrant of the left chest, about 3 cm inferior to the clavicle, in the subcutaneous space, above the fascia of the pectoralis muscle. It can be placed underneath the fascia in thin patients. In thin women or young patients who want better cosmetic results, a subcostal placement of the pulse generator might be preferred. Implant of the pulse generator usually requires a 5-cm linear subclavicular or subcostal incision, that will constitute the superior margin of the subcutaneous pocket for the IPG.

Again, the incisions are closed with 3-0 resorbable sutures in either the galea or deep subcutaneous tissue, followed by either skin staples or 3-0 running monofilament nylon sutures. Prior to closure, irrigation with a povidone-iodine solution diluted to near a 1% concentration is performed at each incision, followed by the addition of 1 gram of vancomycin powder on to the newly implanted hardware and within all surgical incisions.

After the stage II procedure, the patient is discharged on the same day with 7 days of oral antibiotics. It is important to note that the role of prophylactic antibiotics has not been clearly established in the literature. Please refer to the section on infections below. The patient follows up in clinic 2 weeks later for wound check and suture removal.

Surgical Complications of DBS Implant

A. Infections (Scalp, Neck, or Pocket Infections)

Wound complications are uncommon following DBS surgery. Nevertheless, certain key technical steps can be performed in each procedure to minimize this still troublesome risk.

As DBS techniques evolve and become more available, wound complications (including infections) related to the implanted hardware will inevitably also rise, as well as their need to be treated. The risk of infectious complications from DBS is reviewed in a number of reports in the literature, and varies from 0% to more than 15% [22, 24].

However, interpretation of these data is difficult because the definition of infection is variable and is further complicated by small size series, restricted perioperative analysis, and limited discussion of cranial wound management. Few reports detail the comprehensive incidence and management of all postoperative wound complications that are self-limited, in addition to those requiring a return to surgery, without excluding noninfectious wound dehiscence and/or erosions over a long follow-up period [22, 24].

The use of copious amounts of diluted povidone-iodine irrigation at a 1% concentration for both stage I and stage II procedures prior to closure, must be underscored. Povidone-iodine has bactericidal activity against a wide spectrum of pathogens, including methicillin-resistant Staphylococcus aureus (MRSA), and is maximally effective against MRSA in a dilution of 1:25 to 1:200 (0.5–4% betadine). This has been shown to be superior to saline irrigation alone [22, 24]. Indeed, the use of povidone-iodine has potentially contributed to minimizing our patient infections, possibly due to its bactericidal activity. Other groups have experienced success in reducing their own patient infection rates using other antibacterial applications prior to wound closure; and no there is no data to suggest one agent over the other.

The routine postoperative administration of oral staphylococcal prophylaxis via cephalexin (or ciprofloxacin/clindamycin in patients with penicillin allergy) for 7 days following each procedure could also potentially contribute to our low infection rate, but this cannot be adequately proven nor supported [22, 24]. There is only anecdotal evidence to support the extended use of perioperative antibiotics after implantation of devices into the CNS. The use of systemic antibiotic prophylaxis for more than 24 hours after ventriculoperitoneal shunting is uncertain, as concluded by a recent meta-analysis [22, 24]. What has been demonstrated, aside from evidence suggesting decreased postoperative infection with antibiotic impregnated devices (such as catheters during shunting) and frequent glove changing, is that reducing operative time is directly associated with reduced infection risk during implantation procedures [22, 24]. At out institution, the procedural time from incision to closure is routinely under 2 hours for a stage I bilateral lead placement, and around 30 minutes for a stage II procedure. It is important to minimize handling of the implant, reduce operating room traffic, give attention to meticulous surgical tissue manipulation, and to work with an experienced team [22, 24].

Given that the number of DBS hardware implants will continue to increase, and new applications for this procedure appear on the horizon, we must determine how to prevent, as well as manage, such complications if and when they arise.

Infections at the burr hole and the IPG site tend to present soon after surgery. However, more distal infections, such as at the connector sites, may be related to skin erosion and their presentation is more variable [22, 24]. Superficial infections, mainly cellulitis of the surgical wound, are usually treated conservatively with IV or oral antibiotics, as well as close clinical monitoring.

Deep infections involving loculated and purulent collections around the implanted hardware usually require surgical washout along with removal of the hardware in active infections. Conversely, if no skin erosion is present, antibiotic therapy without removal of the hardware can be attempted with a low threshold to implement surgical intervention for washout and removal of the hardware.

Moreover, given the high likelihood of hardware co-contamination, with infections of the IPG site, removal of the IPG as well as the lead extension cables should be considered. A period of 4-6 weeks of antibiotherapy followed by 2-4 weeks of observation off antibiotics, is recommended prior to re-implantation of any new hardware, assuming complete resolution and no recurrence of the infection [22, 24].

B. Vascular Complications

The most serious complication from DBS lead placement is a symptomatic vascular accident. Fortunately, in a large retrospective review of 728 patients who underwent 1333 DBS lead implants by a single neurosurgeon between 2002 and 2010, symptomatic vascular complications were noted to be overall uncommon for both intracerebral hemorrhages (ICHs) (1.1%) and infarctions (0.4%). Interestingly, 7 of the 8 symptomatic ICHs reported occurred when targeting the STN, but this could be a selection bias as over half of the DBS implants were targeting the STN [24].

More commonly, a small amount of intraventricular hemorrhage (IVH) was noted in either the atrium of the occipital horns of the lateral ventricles in 28 patients (3.8%). Only three of these patients (0.4%) were symptomatic with transient confusion post operatively [24].

C. Other Adverse Events

In this same study, the most common intraoperative adverse events of DBS implant were vasovagal responses (0.8%), hypotension (0.3%), and seizures (0.3%) [24].

Vasovagal responses were described as episodes of coughing and blood pressure changes shortly following the placement of the burr holes. This may represent the clinical manifestation of an air embolism. Patients who undergo DBS implant are at risk for developing air emboli because they are in a semi-sitting position, with the head above the heart, and are spontaneously breathing, which generates negative venous pressures upon inspiration. During the time of the burr hole placement, the neurosurgeon should anticipate the episode of air emboli and take the proper measures to prevent its occurrence.

In order to best minimize the risk of air emboli, timely and meticulous waxing of the bone edges of the burr holes, copious and continuous irrigation of the surgical field, and maintaining clear communication with the anesthesiology team are all essential.

The most common side effects in the immediate postoperative period in this study were headaches (4.2%) and confusion, either with (0.5%) or without (1.0%) agitation [24]. Fortunately, those side effects were mostly transient and resolved without intervention [24]. Long-term adverse events (occurring greater than 2 weeks post operatively) principally consisted of wound complications and hardware complications.

Among wound complications, infection was the most common, occurring in a total of 23 cases (3.1%), 10 (1.4%) of which were self-limited, and 13 (1.7%) of which required a return to surgery for debridement and/or device removal (Table). Erosions and dehiscence occurred in 2 patients (0.3%), each requiring surgical debridement only [24].

Table 1. Summary of adverse effects after DBS device implantation

Event	No. of Patients (%)
intraoperative	
asymptomatic IVH	25 (3.4)
symptomatic ICH	8 (1.1)
asymptomatic ICH	4 (0.5)
acute perilesional edema	2 (0.3)
cortical/subcortical ischemic infarction	3 (0.4)
vasovagal response	6 (0.8)
hypotension	2 (0.3)
confusion	2 (0.3)
anxiety	5 (0.7)
seizure	2 (0.3)
arrhythmia	1 (0.1)
aborted procedure	7 (1.0)

Event	No. of Patients (%)
perioperative (<2 wks)	
headache	31 (4.2)
Hemiparesis w or w/o decreased LOC	13 (1.7)
confusion	7 (1.0)
confusion/agitation	4 (0.5)
respiratory distress	3 (0.4)
seizure	3 (0.4)
Hallucinations	3 (0.4)
somnolence	1 (0.1)
Fall	1 (0.1)
long-term postoperative (>2 wks)	
wound complications	
wound infection–self limited	10 (1.4)
wound infections	
requiring system removal	7 (1.0)
requiring lead removal only	1 (0.1)
requiring IPG/extension removal only	3 (0.4)
requiring debridement only	2 (0.3)
skin erosion–device removal	2 (0.3)
wound dehiscence–debridement only	2 (0.3)
hardware complications	
lead fracture–lead revision	7 (1.0)
lead malposition–lead revision	9 (1.2)
lead migration–lead redirection w/o removal	4 (0.5)
lead malfunction/high impedance–lead revision	2 (0.3)
flipped IPG–revision	4 (0.5)
malpositioned/uncomfortable IPG–revision	4 (0.5)
IPG malfunction/high impedance–replace	1 (0.1)
lead extension malfunction/high impedance–replace	1 (0.1)
lead extension fracture–replace	3 (0.4)
satisfaction-related complications	
loss of system efficacy over time–lead revision	19 (2.6)
decreased efficacy over time–no revision desired	10 (1.4)
results not as desired–no revision desired	7 (1.0)
complete system removal w/o replacement	5 (0.7)
lead extension incision uncomfortable	8 (1.1)
IPG site uncomfortable/hematoma–no revision	3 (0.4)

LOC: loss of consciousness.

All hardware-related complications required a re-operation. Lead malposition (9 cases (1.2%)) or migration (4 cases (0.5%)), were the most common hardware complications, leading to revision at an average of 1.3 years after initial implantation (range 0.25–6 years) [24]. Lead fractures (7 cases (1.0%)) and lead extension fractures (3 cases (0.4%)) were also found to be common hardware complications, followed by component malfunction (4 cases (0.5%)) as identified by high impedance in the system, resulting in either lead revisions (2 cases (0.3%)), or lead extension or IPG revisions (1 case each (0.1%)) which occurred at an average of 4.4 years after the initial operation (range 0.5–8.7 years). Four patients (0.5%) had an IPG that flipped, or an uncomfortable or malpositioned IPG, all of them required repositioning of the IPG [24]. If the total number of hardware complications (n = 29), infections (n = 13), and erosions (n = 2) requiring reoperation were combined, the total number of long-term device-related complications requiring repeat surgery was be 44 (6%) (Table) [24].

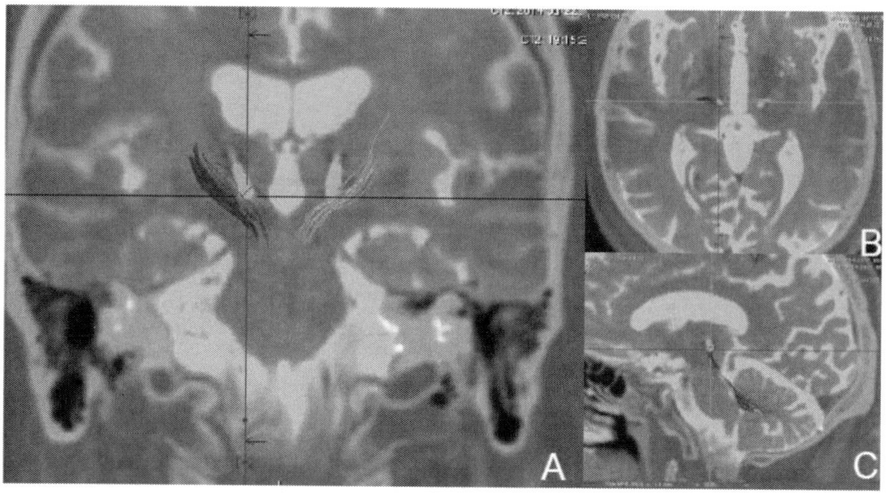

Figure 1. Illustration of use of MR diffusion tensor imaging to map the dentate-rubro-thalamic (DRT) tract for direct targeting in an patient with ET. Tractography performed from source images using seed VOI at dentate gyrus, end VOI at precentral gyrus. (A,B,C) Superposition of post-op CT showing final lead placement onto tracts drawn for planning, showing final location of lead that was tested intraoperatively to obtain good tremor control.

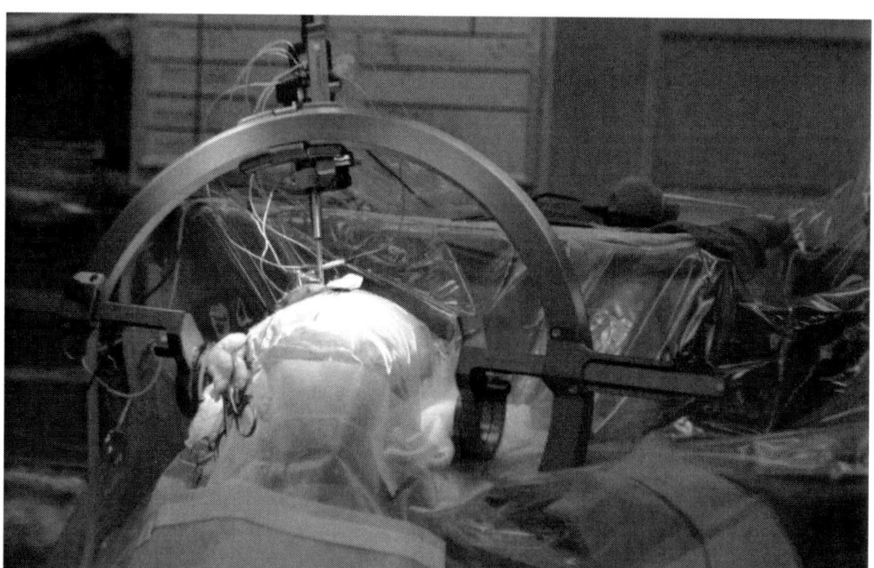

Figure 2. Intraoperative picture showing draping of patient, Leksell frame placement, and microelectrode drive descending multiple microelectrodes in parallel trajectories.

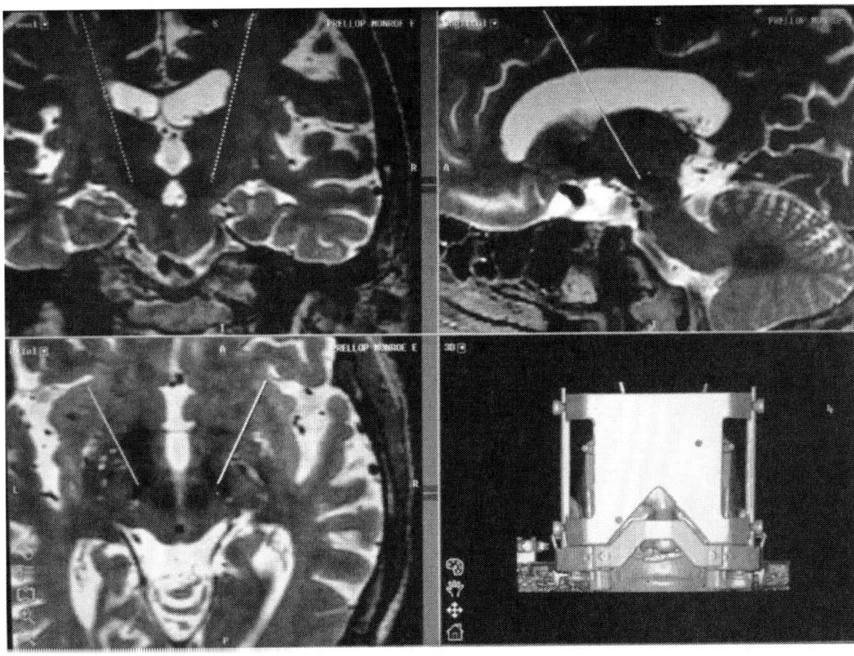

Figure 3. Depiction of intended trajectories targeting the STN, planned on Framelink software using the Stealth System (Medtronic, Minneapolis). Here, a 3T T2 MRI is merged with a stereotactic CT with frame for registration. A combination of indirect targeting (using coordinates) and direct targeting (using MRI) was employed.

CONCLUSION

DBS implant is a process requiring a multi-disciplinary team, careful planning, thorough surgical technique and proper post-operative care. These allow for optimal results with adequate lead location for symptoms control, while minimizing short and long term surgical complications.

REFERENCES

[1] Starr, P. A., Turner, R. S., Rau, G., Lindsey, N., Heath, S., Volz, M., Ostrem, J. L., Marks, W. J. Jr. Microelectrode-guided implantation of deep brain stimulators into the globus pallidus internus for dystonia: techniques, electrode locations, and outcomes. *J. Neurosurg*. 2006;104:488-501.

[2] Starr, P. A. Placement of deep brain stimulators into the subthalamic nucleus or Globus pallidus internus: technical approach. *Stereotact. Funct. Neurosurg*. 2002;79):118-145.

[3] Machado, A., Rezai, A. R., Kopell, B. H., Gross, R. E., Sharan, A. D., Benabid, A. L. Deep brain stimulation for Parkinson's disease: surgical technique and perioperative management. *Mov. Disord*. 2006;21 Suppl. 14:S247-258.

[4] Anthofer, J., Steib, K., Fellner, C., Lange, M., Brawanski, A., Schlaier, J. The variability of atlas-based targets in relation to surrounding major fibre tracts in thalamic deep brain stimulation. *Acta Neurochir.* (Wien). 2014;156:1497-1504.

[5] Bardinet, E., Belaid, H., Grabli, D., Welter, M. L., Vidal, S. F., Galanaud, D., Derrey, S., Dormont, D., Cornu, P., Yelnik, J., Karachi, C. Thalamic stimulation for tremor: can target determination be improved? *Mov. Disord.* 2011;26:307-312.

[6] Schlaier, J. 1., Anthofer, J., Steib, K., Fellner, C., Rothenfusser, E., Brawanski, A., Lange, M. Deep brain stimulation for essential tremor: targeting the dentato-rubro-thalamic tract? *Neuromodulation.* 2015;18:105-112.

[7] Coenen, V. A., Allert, N., Mädler, B. A role of diffusion tensor imaging fiber tracking in deep brain stimulation surgery: DBS of the dentato-rubro-thalamic tract (drt) for the treatment of therapy-refractory tremor. *Acta Neurochir.* (Wien). 2011;153:1579-1585.

[8] Dormont, D., Cornu, P., Pidoux, B., Bonnet, A. M., Biondi, A., Oppenheim, C., Hasboun, D., Damier, P., Cuchet, E., Philippon, J., Agid, Y., Marsault, C. Chronic thalamic stimulation with three-dimensional MR stereotactic guidance. *AJNR Am. J. Neuroradiol.* 1997;18:1093-1107.

[9] Coenen, V. A., Panksepp, J., Hurwitz, T. A., Urbach, H., Mädler, B. Human medial forebrain bundle (MFB) and anterior thalamic radiation (ATR): imaging of two major subcortical pathways and the dynamic balance of opposite affects in understanding depression. *J. Neuropsychiatry Clin. Neurosci.* 2012;24:223-236.

[10] Hamel, W., Herzog, J., Kopper, F., Pinsker, M., Weinert, D., Müller, D., Krack, P., Deuschl, G., Mehdorn, H. M. Deep brain stimulation in the subthalamic area is more effective than nucleus ventralis intermedius stimulation for bilateral intention tremor. *Acta Neurochir.* (Wien). 2007;149:749-758.

[11] Carpenter, M. B. *Core Text of Neuroanatomy.* Williams and Wilkins Eds., 1991.

[12] Rezai, A. R., Kopell, B. H., Gross, R. E., Vitek, J. L., Sharan, A. D., Limousin, P., Benabid, A. L. Deep brain stimulation for Parkinson's disease: surgical issues. *Mov. Disord.* 2006;21 Suppl. 14:S197-218.

[13] Walton, L., Hampshire, A., Forster, D. M., Kemeny, A. A. A phantom study to assess the accuracy of stereotactic localization, using T1-weighted magnetic resonance imaging with the Leksell stereotactic system. *Neurosurgery.* 1996;38:170-176.

[14] Walton, L., Hampshire, A., Forster, D. M., Kemeny, A. A. Stereotactic localization with magnetic resonance imaging: a phantom study to compare the accuracy obtained using two-dimensional and three-dimensional data acquisitions. *Neurosurgery.* 1997; 41:131-137.

[15] Duffner, F., Schiffbauer, H., Breit, S., Friese, S., Freudenstein, D. Relevance of image fusion for target point determination in functional neurosurgery. *Acta Neurochir.* (Wien). 2002;144:445-451.

[16] Palur, R. S., Berk, C., Schulzer, M., Honey, C. R. A metaanalysis comparing the results of pallidotomy performed using microelectrode recording or macroelectrode stimulation. *J. Neurosurg.* 2002;96:1058-1062.

[17] Gorgulho, A., De Salles, A. A., Frighetto, L., Behnke, E. Incidence of hemorrhage associated with electrophysiological studies performed using macroelectrodes and microelectrodes in functional neurosurgery. *J. Neurosurg.* 2005;102:888-896.

[18] Ben-Haim, S., Asaad, W. F., Gale, J. T., Eskandar, E. N. Risk factors for hemorrhage during microelectrode-guided deep brain stimulation and the introduction of an improved microelectrode design. *Neurosurgery*. 2009;64:754-762.

[19] Mädler, B., Coenen, V. A. Explaining clinical effects of deep brain stimulation through simplified target-specific modeling of the volume of activated tissue. *AJNR Am. J. Neuroradiol*. 2012;33:1072-1080.

[20] Butson, C. R., McIntyre, C. C. Tissue and electrode capacitance reduce neural activation volumes during deep brain stimulation. *Clin. Neurophysiol.* 2005;116:2490-2500.

[21] Butson, C. R., McIntyre, C. C. Role of electrode design on the volume of tissue activated during deep brain stimulation. *J. Neural Eng*. 2006;3:1-8.

[22] Fenoy, A. J., Simpson, R. K. Jr. Management of device-related wound complications in deep brain stimulation surgery. *J. Neurosurg*. 2012;116:1324-1332.

[23] Son, B. C., Han, S. H., Choi, Y. S., Kim, H. S., Kim, M. C., Yang, S. H., Lee, S. W. Transaxillary subpectoral implantation of implantable pulse generator for deep brain stimulation. *Neuromodulation*. 2012;15:260-266.

[24] Fenoy, A. J., Simpson, R. K. Jr. Risks of common complications in deep brain stimulation surgery: management and avoidance. *J. Neurosurg*. 2014;120:132-139.

In: Deep Brain Stimulation
Editor: Raja Mehanna

ISBN: 978-1-63483-282-3

Chapter 5

INTRAOPERATIVE MICROELECTRODE RECORDING FOR PARKINSON'S DISEASE, ESSENTIAL TREMOR AND DYSTONIA

Scott E. Cooper MD, PhD*

Department of Neurology, Center for Neurological Restoration, Cleveland Clinic, Cleveland, OH, US

ABSTRACT

Microelectrode recording, the use of a microelectrode during DBS surgery, to record and stimulate, helps guide intraoperative decisions about DBS electrode location. The first part of this chapter reviews pros and cons of the technique, relevant basics of biophysics and stereotaxis, equipment and general techniques for recording, stimulating, and testing responsiveness of neuronal activity. The second part of the chapter discusses MER with respect to individual DBS targets. Thalamus (for tremor, and less often Parkinson's Disease), subthalamic nucleus (for Parkinson's disease, and less often dystonia) and globus pallidus (for dystonia, and less often Parkinson's disease) are reviewed, including typical electrophysiological findings confirming DBS electrode target, atypical findings suggesting a need for target adjustment, and information to be gleaned from multiple microelectrode tracks.

INTRODUCTION

Definition of MER

In this chapter, we take the term "microelectrode recording (MER)" to cover a broad range of electrophysiological techniques which use a microelectrode to determine, confirm, or refine the target for implanting a deep brain stimulation (DBS) macroelectrode.

---

* Scott E. Cooper MD, PhD. Present address: Department of Neurology, University of Minnesota, Minneapolis, MN, US.

This definition includes microstimulation, making "microelectrode *recording*" something of a misnomer; we prefer the term "microelectrode mapping" or "microelectrophysiology," but "MER" is more widespread. There are almost as many variants of MER as there are centers using MER techniques, and, in what follows, we have tried to cover a range of techniques. However we focus on the techniques with which we have the most personal experience; for other perspectives, the reader is referred to [1-3].

Is MER Useful?

The first point to be addressed in any discussion of MER is whether it should be done at all. For the past two decades, a broad, but by no means universal consensus has existed that MER is useful, or even necessary for DBS surgery. For an introduction to the contrary view, the reader is referred to the article from Zrzino et al. [4], its accompanying editorial and response. Here, we will summarize briefly the disadvantages of MER before moving on to its advantages, thereafter commenting on how future developments in neuroimaging may alter the balance between MER advantages and disadvantages.

Disadvantages of MER

Increased Surgery Duration

All else being equal, MER prolongs the surgery, and, as a general heuristic, increased surgical duration increases complication rates if for no other reason than the increased risk of infection. In the particular case of DBS, increased surgical time increases pneumocephalus (see below) which may increase postoperative confusion [5] and may contribute to lead misplacement. Moreover, operating room time is an expensive resource, efficient use of which requires minimizing procedure times.

Risk of Hemorrhage

While surgical planning of the electrode's path can avoid blood vessels large enough to be seen on MRI, smaller vessels are encountered with low, but nonzero probability, and hemorrhage may result.

Presumably if one or more microelectrode penetrations are made in addition to the DBS (macro-) electrode penetration, then the risk of this is increased. Increased relative risk of hemorrhage related to MER (use vs. non-use, or number of microelectrode penetrations) has been reported by some [6-8] but not others [9-12] or only in a high-risk subgroup [e.g. 13].

Other reports emphasize a low absolute risk of hemorrhage when MER is used [14-17]. Taking the available data together with common sense it seems likely there is some relation between MER and risk of symptomatic hemorrhage, but the effect size may be small.

Requirement for Awake Patient

MER is done in awake, and, generally, unsedated patients. This is, to say the least, inconvenient for both surgeon and patient, and requires considerable attention by OR staff to the patient's comfort and emotional state. There are several reasons for this requirement. First, some parts of MER (e.g. detecting microstimulation-evoked paresthesias) are only possible if the patient can report on subjective sensations.

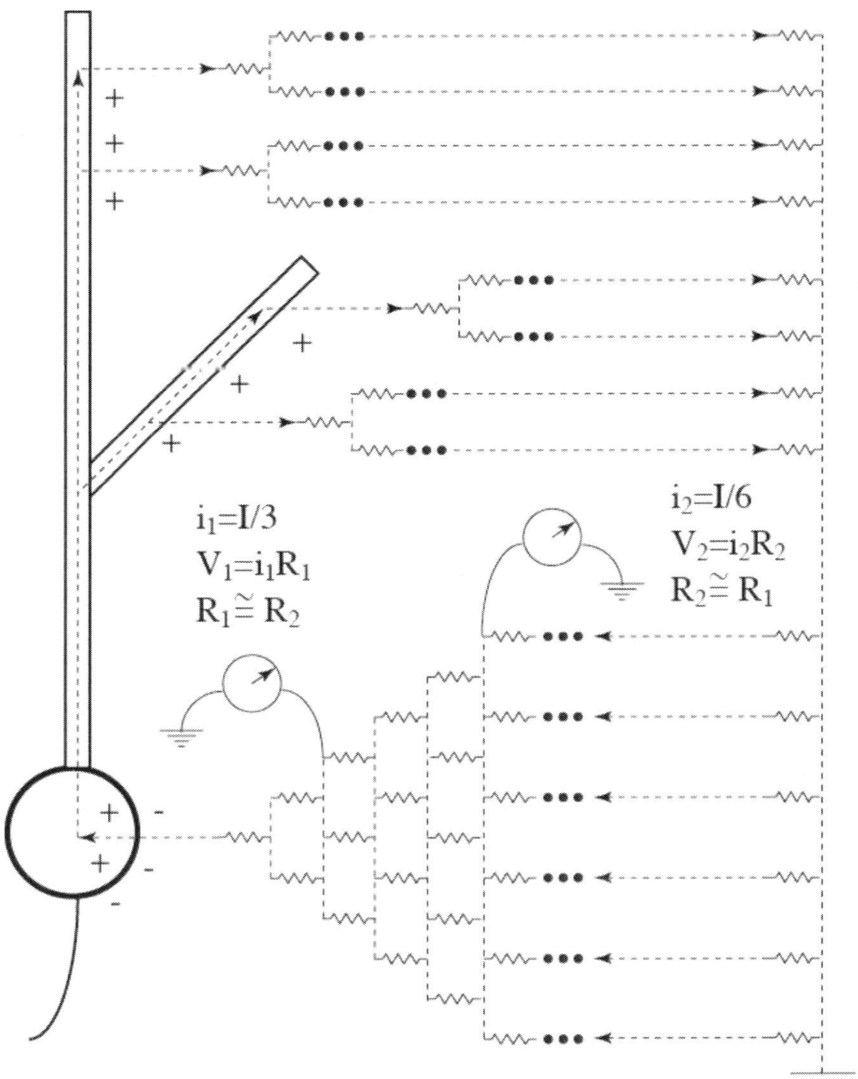

During an action potential, current flows inward across the membrane, and the same total current must complete a circuit to arrive back at its source. Far away from the neuron, that current is distributed over many resistive elements; close to the neuron, the same current is distributed over only a few. By Ohm's law, the voltage is proportional to current, hence, voltage associatedwith an action potential is larger when measured by an electrode closer to the neuron.

Figure 1. Highly simplified, schematic illustration of how current flows through the extracellular space during an action potential.

Others, such as testing for orolingual receptive fields, are not practical in a patient who is intubated and unable to make voluntary tongue movements. Moreover, neuromuscular blockade, which is routine with general anesthesia, thwarts any attempt at detecting muscle contraction evoked by stimulation of internal capsule.

Finally, anesthesia or even sedation may alter the firing pattern of neurons [18], interfering with MER. It is reported [19] that dexmedetomidine sedation does not impair MER, but this has not been our experience: in subthalamic nucleus, firing patterns were still recognizable, but far fewer neurons were detected by the electrode than in unsedated patients, making boundaries of the nucleus harder to determine accurately.

Nonetheless, we have found light dexmedetomidine sedation invaluable as an alternative when patients are unable to tolerate a fully awake state during DBS surgery.

ADVANTAGES OF MER

Precision

One advantage of MER is its contribution to greater precision for DBS implantation. Motion of the electrode along its own length is controlled to an accuracy of microns, and the distance needed to move, before losing the signal from one neuron, and picking up the signal from another, is about 250 to 500 microns, that is, one quarter- to one half-millimeter. This defines the accuracy with which MER can locate landmarks such as, e.g. the borders of the subthalamic nucleus. This far exceeds the precision of 3 Tesla clinical MRI.

However the above needs to be qualified in several respects. First, precision is not the same as accuracy [20]. Assessing the accuracy of MER localization would require either a gold standard, or at least a systematic investigation of reproducibility. Second, sub-millimetric precision is only obtained along the electrode axis (i.e. approximately dorsoventral).

Mapping on other axes (mediolateral, anteroposterior) requires removing the electrode from the brain, moving it, and then reinserting it into the brain. Such movement is, for practical purposes, never less than 1 mm, which sets a limit on precision (Most stereotactic systems won't permit a smaller movement; even when that is possible, the tendency of the electrode to follow the path of least resistance may result in it following the old track, if it is moved less than 1 mm, either because the electrode deviates, or because the brain does). MER thus has its greatest accuracy along the axis of the electrode, but targeting errors along that axis can to some degree be compensated for by selecting different contacts along the DBS electrode.

Finally, it may legitimately be asked if sub-millimetric precision affects clinical outcomes. This question is difficult to answer from the published literature, but Figure 2 in [21] shows large differences in motor outcome with electrode targeting errors on the order of one millimeter. Our own opinion is that there is no lower limit below which improvements in accuracy have no effect on clinical outcome (although there will certainly be limits to the statistical power of any study which assesses the relation between accuracy and outcome), and we try for the greatest accuracy practically achievable.

Compensation for Brain Shift

The brain, being of a gelatinous consistency, and being located at the top of the body, above the heart, tends, all things being equal, to flow downward toward the foramen magnum. For that to occur, something would have to fill the space that appeared between the top of the brain and the inner surface of the skull. This doesn't happen, because the skull is (normally) sealed, and the entry/exit of fluids such as blood and CSF is (normally) tightly regulated.

The brain is, so to speak, pulled up in the skull by suction in the subdural potential space just as the lungs are pulled outward in inspiration by suction in the pleural potential space.

When neurosurgeons breach the skull and incise the dura, they create pneumocephalus (analogous to pneumothorax), and the brain begins to sag downward. The movement is not enough to cause herniation, but it does mean that neuroanatomical structures are now in a slightly different location relative to the skull than when the preoperative CT or MRI was done [22-25].

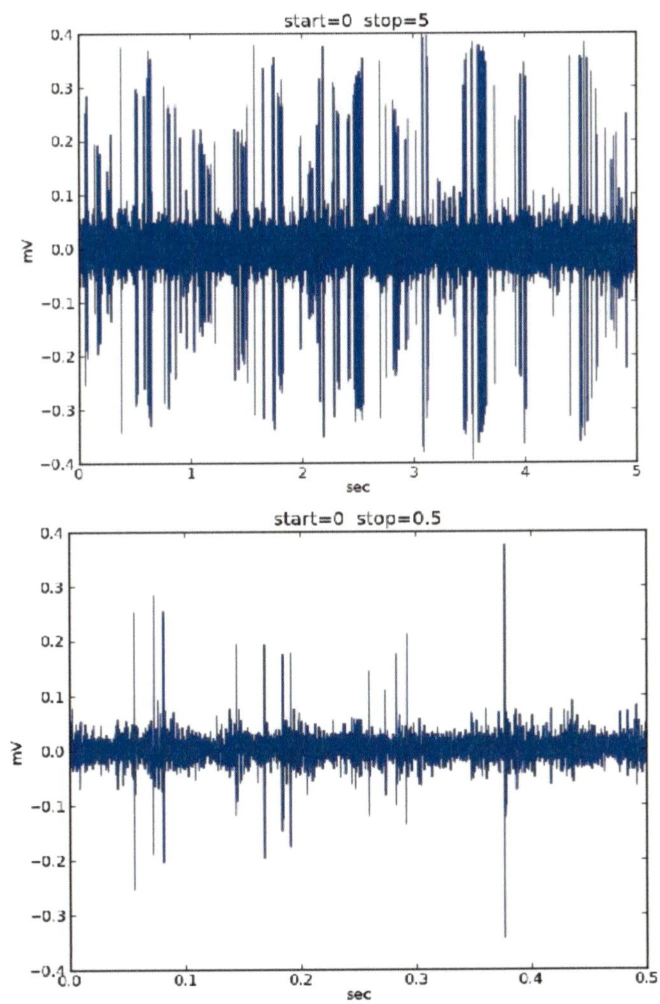

Figure 2. (Continued).

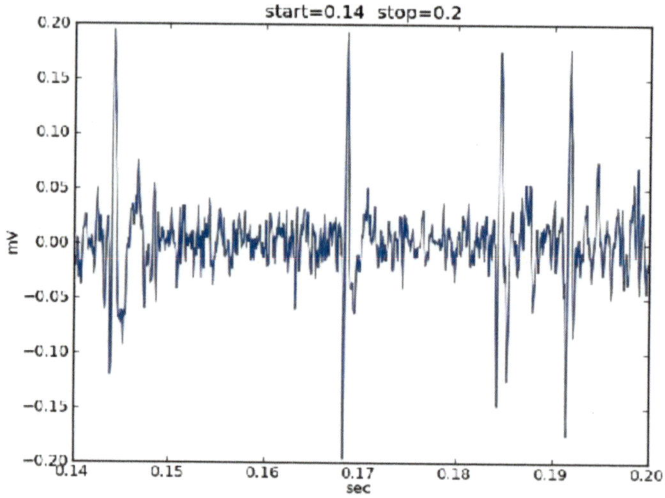

Spontaneous activity recorded from the subthalamic nucleus, at (from top to bottom) progressively faster oscilloscope "sweep speeds" (compare X axes). In Figure 1a, many action potential spikes per second, with amplitudes ranging from about 0.15 to 0.4 mV, are clearly distinguished from background noise with amplitude about 0.05 mV. Even though the sweep speed is too slow to distinguish spike waveforms, the wide variation in spike amplitudes suggests that that the spikes are not all from one neuron, i.e. this is grey matter, and the neuronal density is high. Figure 1c, with fast sweep speed (expanded X axis) highlights 4 spikes; the first two are probably from the same neuron, while the second two likely represent activity of a second neuron also adjacent to the microelectrode tip. Note that, whereas both pairs of spikes have a fast (narrow) initial negative phase, followed by a fast initial positive phase, in the first two spikes this is followed by a slow negative, then a slow positive phase, while, in the second pair, it is followed by a fast negative phase only. Specialized spike-sorting software can perform this sort of comparison more accurately than "by-eye" comparisons.

Figure 2. Spontaneous activity recorded from the subthalamic nucleus.

Since the stereotactic frame maintains a constant relationship to the skull, such "brain shift" introduces targeting error. Historically, one of the chief advantages of MER is that it determines target location after the skull is opened, i.e. the target location after brain shift begins to occur. However, this advantage has been somewhat eroded by the introduction of intraoperative MRI scanners capable of imaging the brain in the operating room after the dura has been breached [26]. This is a new technology which is still proving itself clinically and is not yet widely available, but offers an alternative to MER at least in patients unwilling or unable to undergo awake surgery.

Functional vs. Anatomical Mapping

Another advantage of MER is that it is a physiological rather than an anatomical technique. The target of a DBS electrode is chosen by physiological criteria. For example (see below) the target for subthalamic nucleus stimulation is not merely the subthalamic nucleus per se -- which is an anatomical structure with boundaries visible on MRI, or on cresyl violet stained microtome tissue sections -- but the somatomotor region, where neurons process information related to limb movement. This physiologically defined region looks the same as the rest of the subthalamic nucleus on MRI or even stained microtome tissue sections. It can only be recognized by "eavesdropping" on neuronal activity by electrophysiology (e.g. MER) techniques. The same situation applies to globus pallidus, while in thalamus the difficulty is almost as great (here, light microscopy reveals cytoarchitectonic boundaries between regions -- i.e. different thalamic nuclei – but these are not visible on clinical (3 Tesla) MRI).

However, this advantage has been somewhat eroded by recent developments in MRI. There is really no such thing as a purely physiological regional difference; differences in the information processed by e.g. the somatomotor region reflect differences in which neuroanatomical structures project to that region, and the new MRI technique of diffusion tractography allows such projections to be seen [27].

Application of this technique to DBS targets is still in its infancy, but foreseeably it will grow in importance in the future. Another new MRI technology, high field strength, 7 Tesla MRI, is capable of showing the cytoarchitectonic boundaries between thalamic nuclei. However, higher field strength may introduce more geometrical distortion [28]. In any case, 7 Tesla scanners are rare, and likely to remain so for years to come, but here, too, the boundary between physiology and anatomy is becoming blurred.

REVIEW OF BASIC BIOPHYSICS

Microelectrode Recording

Most readers will be familiar with the concept of action potential (AP) generation and propagation along a neuron. An AP is an extremely localized, extremely brief change in electrical potential ("depolarization"), and consequent flow of electrical (ionic) current, into the neuron across the neuronal membrane.

Intracellular recording is not feasible in neurosurgical patients, so we detect APs from the flow of current in the extracellular medium near the depolarized neuronal membrane. This works because the current which flows into the neuron across the depolarized membrane must complete a circuit, flowing back out of the neuron through another part of the membrane (generally the dendrites), through the extracellular medium, and back to its source at the depolarized patch of membrane.

As we follow the flow of current through this circuit, the total amount of current remains constant but, at a large distance from the neuron, it is spread out through a large volume of extracellular tissue, while close to the neuron it is concentrated in a small volume near the membrane through which it flows. Consider a small volume element of extracellular tissue, through which current flows. Far from the neuron, current through that element is small, because the total current is distributed through many volume elements. The share of current through an element closer to the neuron is larger, because total current is more concentrated in fewer volume elements.

By Ohm's law, electrical potential (voltage) across a volume element is proportional to current, so the voltage signal from an AP is larger when measured closer to the neuron [Figure 1]. This leads to our first practical fact about MER: the signal we measure is dominated by action potentials close to the recording electrode.

In practice, microelectrodes used for MER have about 10 microns of electrically conductive surface at their tips (giving a resistance in the hundreds of kiloohms) and record AP within a few hundred microns of the exposed electrode tip. The spatial precision of MER is on the order of a few tenths of a millimeter.

If the MER voltage is plotted versus time (e.g. by an oscilloscope), nearby APs appear as transient deflection from a stable baseline, or "spikes." The deflection may be either positive or negative: since, during an action potential, current flows back out of the neuron through the dendrites, the neuron can, in theory, be viewed as a dipole with a current sink in the soma, and a current source in the dendritic tree; the electrode will record a positive or negative spike depending on which is closer. In practice the action potential waveform recorded extracellularly proves to be more complex than a simple monophasic positive or negative spike because it reflects multiple factors, including the timing of current entry into and exit from different parts of the neuron, as well as the shape of the neuron and the location of the electrode relative to it. Consequently, when examined closely the spike usually has a complex waveform, crossing repeatedly from positive to negative and back. Little clinically useful information can be derived from the waveform, however the waveform remains constant while the electrode isn't moved, therefore, two spikes with different waveforms recorded from the same stationary electrode necessarily come from two different neurons [Figure 2].

The size of the spike will depend on the total amount of current flowing, which depends on the total membrane area involved in the AP. This leads to another important practical fact about MER: spikes recorded from microelectrodes reflect almost exclusively APs occurring in neuronal somata and not axons. This means that many spikes will be recorded when the tip of the electrode is in grey matter, near the soma or proximal dendrites of spiking neurons, and very few when it is in white matter. [Of note, APs in axons are detected if the electrode tip is adjacent to an active axon, which happens only rarely. Axonal APs are recognizable by narrow spike duration (<1 msec), and a tendency to disappear if the electrode is moved even slightly, in contrast to somatic APs, which have broader, often polyphasic spikes, and persist over 10s or hundreds of microns of electrode movement]. The grey-white distinction is the most basic discrimination that can be made with MER.

By connecting the amplifier output to an audio speaker, spikes can be heard, as well as seen, and the experienced electrophysiologist can recognize "by ear" characteristic patterns of activity distinguishing different grey-matter nuclei.

Microstimulation

As noted previously, the term "microelectrode recording (MER)" is a misnomer, because valuable information is often also obtained by using the microelectrode for microstimulation. In our opinion, if a microelectrode is used at all, then microstimulation should also be done, because it yields additional information complementary to the recording of spikes. Whereas in microelectrode recording, an AP causes current flow through the extracellular space, leading to a potential, which we measure with an electrode, in microstimulation the reverse happens: the electrode induces a current in extracellular space, which causes an electrical potential that leads to an AP. As in MER, all of this occurs relatively close to the electrode tip (probably within 1 mm or less).

The results depend on the electrode tip location: for example, stimulation of somatosensory thalamic nucleus will produce paresthesias, stimulation of optic tract, phosphenes, stimulation of the posterior limb of internal capsule muscle contractions. Unlike MER, which "sees" only neuronal somata, microstimulation affects axons at least as much as soma (in fact, probably more [29-31]). Therefore, microstimulation complements MER, when the electrophysiologist is concerned to judge the location of the electrode relative to a white-matter structure, such as the internal capsule.

The goal of microstimulation is to induce a flow of current, inducing a potential gradient sufficient to depolarize some neurons to their threshold for action potential initiation. The pulse of current is biphasic: first in one (negative) direction, then in the other (positive) direction, so that the integral of current over time is zero.

In other words, there is no net movement of electrical charge, and at the end of a pulse, everything is the same as before, except that some neurons have fired APs. This requires that the process which carries current across the electrode tissue interface must be fully reversible; in fact, there are multiple mechanisms, and some are not reversible.

Such "irreversible Faradic" mechanisms do electrochemical work on -- i.e. damage to -- the electrode or surrounding tissue when current exceeds the capacity of reversible mechanisms [32]. This imposes a practical limit on the amplitude of stimulation. The tiny microelectrode is fragile and has low capacitance, making it vulnerable to such effects. The practical consequence is that microstimulation current must be limited to avoid damaging the microelectrode. In practice, we observe a limit of 90 microamperes, which in our experience is enough to cause a drop of several hundred kiloohms in measured electrode impedance, but without impairing electrode performance.

Review of Basic Stereotaxis

Coregistration of Differing Frames of Reference

Stereotaxis is a large topic, and we provide here only a brief overview sufficient to make a few points of practical importance to the electrophysiologist. The essence of stereotaxis is to rely on external or internal fiduciary points to target a structure which is typically deep inside the brain -- hence not directly visible. The target is a point defined in some coordinate system, usually some version of the familiar 3-dimensional Cartesian X,Y,Z system [Figure 3].

By convention, stereotactic X,Y, and Z are aligned as closely as possible with the anatomical mediolateral, anteroposterior, and dorsoventral axes. The origin point (i.e. the point with coordinates 0,0,0) is not, however, necessarily the same.

For example, brain atlases [33] typically use an internal landmark – the midcommissural point located midway between anterior commissure (AC) and the posterior commissure (PC), whereas the origin point of the Leksell stereotactic frame is located outside the patient's head.

Thus a 1 mm movement on the frame's X axis corresponds closely to 1mm mediolateral movement in the atlas, but the numerical coordinates representing a particular anatomical structure in frame coordinates will differ by a constant offset from the coordinates of the same structure in the atlas.

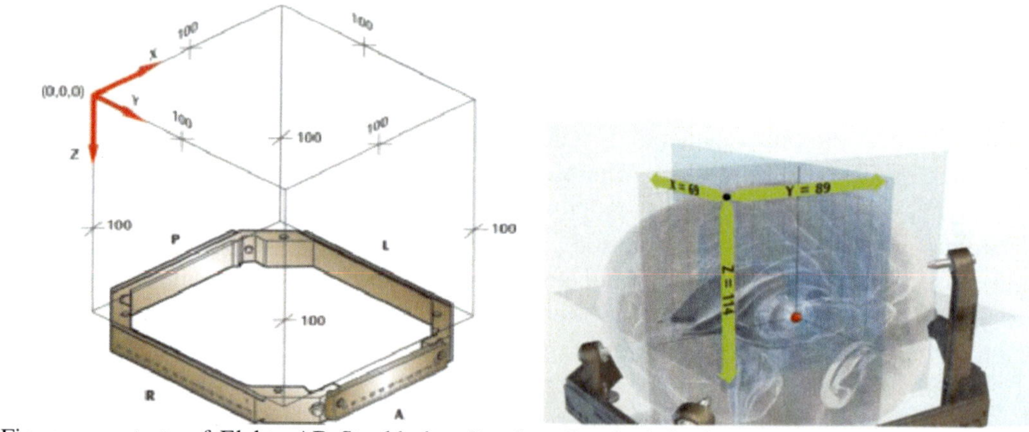

Figures courtesy of Elekta AB Stockholm, Sweden. On the left, the stereotactic axes defined by the frame. On the right, the frame and axes in relation to the brain.

Figure 3. Stereotaxis.

Targeting Workflow

Surgical planning begins by identifying the anterior and posterior commissures in three-dimensional images, typically a preoperative volumetric brain MRI. The midcommissural point is then established, and targeting can proceed by either the indirect or the direct method (or a combination of both).

Indirect vs. Direct Targeting

Indirect targeting relies on coordinates derived from atlases that indicate the location of subcortical structures in a typical, cadaveric brain. Distances between the subcortical structures and either the posterior commissure or midcommissural point in the cadaver brain indirectly indicate the location of the same structures in the patient's brain. In direct targeting the target is visualized in the patient's own brain (i.e. MRI). For structures like subthalamic nucleus and globus pallidus which are visible in routinely available MR sequences, direct and indirect methods can be combined. However, thalamic nuclei cannot be delineated with standard clinical 3 tesla MRI and so indirect methods alone are used, usually the Guiot method [34]. In this method, the upper extremity region of the Vim nucleus of the thalamus is estimated to be 1/4th of the length of the AC-PC line from the posterior commissure and 10-11 mm lateral to the wall of the third ventricle.

Coregistration of Anatomical with Stereotactic Space

The electrode cannot be positioned relative to the midcommissural point. It can only be positioned relative to the stereotactic frame. Therefore, once the chosen target's coordinates are known relative to the midcommisural point, its coordinates relative to the frame ("stereotactic coordinates") must be established.

This is done by attaching the frame to the skull, attaching markers ("fiducials") to known points on the frame, and then obtaining a volumetric (no gaps) image (CT or MRI) which includes in one image both the fiducials and known points in the brain (including anterior and posterior commissures). The relation of stereotactic to anatomical coordinates is now known, giving the target's stereotactic coordinates.

In fact, the surgeon now has a complete map from the brain image to stereotactic coordinates: not only the target, but also e.g. ventricles and blood vessels may be located in stereotactic coordinates, so that the electrode trajectory can be planned to avoid them.

Two-Step Coregistration

Sometimes two brain images are used for coregistration: an MRI of the brain without frame fiducials, and a CT of the head, with frame fiducials. The CT and MRI share a rich set of anatomical landmarks, including skull and ventricles, by which they may be coregistered (usually by automated software).

This establishes a fixed spatial relationship between fiducials and known points in the brain, including anterior and posterior commissures, as required.

Angle of the Electrode to the Anatomical Axes

The electrode passes through cerebral cortex and other overlying structures to reach its target. The track it follows is planned to avoid structures such as primary motor cortex, sulci, and blood vessels. Satisfying these constraints, while still arriving at the planned stereotactic target, usually requires an electrode track that does not coincide with any of the three stereotactic planes, i.e. it makes neither a 0 degree nor a 90 degree angle with any of the three stereotactic axes.

Determining these angles is not simple; in the Leksell stereotactic system, for example, the surgeon sets an "arc" and a "ring" angle; the arc angle corresponds to the coronal angle of the electrode, i.e. an angle measured in the sagittal plane; the ring angle, however, is measured in a plane which depends on the arc angle. Computing the electrode angle relative to anatomical axes requires at minimum trigonometry in 3 dimensions if not linear algebra as well. With frameless stereotactic systems, the problem is even more complex. The position of the electrode along its track (its "depth") is read directly off the microdrive. If the angles of approach are approximately vertical, this can be thought of as approximately the anatomical Z (superior – inferior) axis.

However, the angles are often far from vertical and no correlation between the Z axis and the electrode track should be assumed. Put more mathematically, we have two Cartesian coordinate systems: the first, X,Y,Z is the anatomical (mediolateral, anteroposterior, dorsoventral) stereotactic frame, while the second X',Y',Z' is related to the first by a rotation (the angle of the electrode), with Z' being the axis of the electrode track. Motion limited to the Z' axis results in motion along all three of X,Y, and Z axes.

XY Stages

These distinctions become important if one has made a microelectrode track at some particular X and Y coordinates and now plans to make another track, or to place the DBS electrode at different X and or Y coordinates. In this case, it is important to distinguish between two different systems for altering the stereotactic coordinates of an electrode track.

The first system uses an "XY stage," which is a horizontal platform at right angles to the electrode track (the electrode is "normal to" the plane of the XY stage). All tracks are normal to this plane, and the XY stage allows the electrode to be moved not only on the Z' axis (by the microdrive) but on the X' and Y' axes orthogonal to it. The stage may allow continuous variation of X' and Y', or, more commonly, it provides a pre-defined grid of X' and Y' coordinates. For exactly the same reason that motion on the Z' axis produces motion on all three of X, Y, and Z axes, motion on the X' or Y' axis using the XY stage in theory produces motion on all three of X,Y, and Z axes. In practice, the XY stage is rotated about the Z' axis so that the Y' - Z' plane is parasaggital; in this configuration, motion on Y' produces only motion on Y and Z, while motion on X' produces only motion on X and Z. This simplifies things, but it is still true that when using an XY stage, changing either X' or Y' means that the same electrode depth on two different electrode tracks **does not** correspond to the same Z (dorsoventral) stereotactic location [Figure 4].

Exactly how much the Z coordinate changes depends on the angle of the electrode track to the anatomical axes. The second system changes the track location using the stereotactic frame itself; that is, the stereotactic target itself is changed each time the electrode track is moved. In this case, X and Y motion is really along the X and Y axes -- not X' and Y' axes. The same electrode depth on two different tracks *does* correspond to the same Z (dorsoventral) stereotactic coordinate.

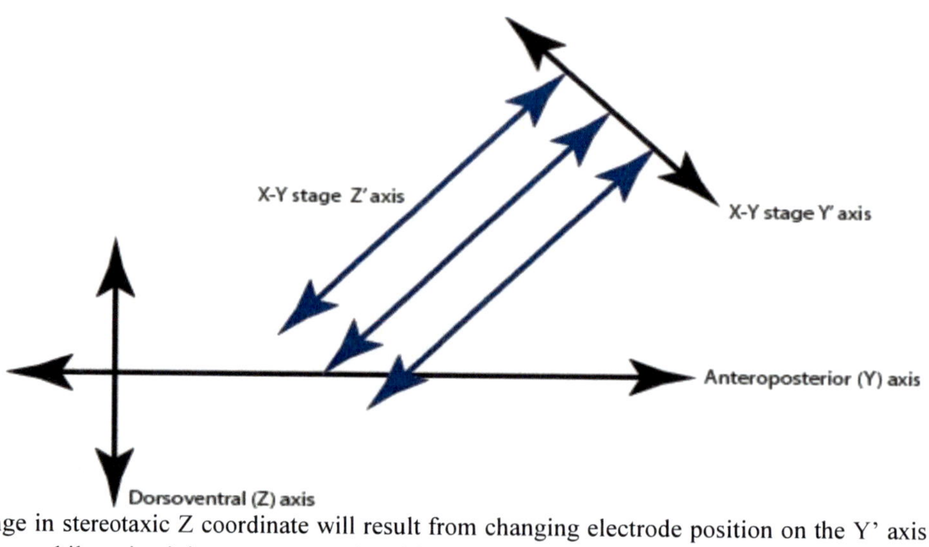

A change in stereotaxic Z coordinate will result from changing electrode position on the Y' axis of the stage while maintaining a constant microdrive depth (Z').

Figure 4. Y' and Z' axes defined by the X-Y stage in relation to the stereotactic Y and Z axes.

MER EQUIPMENT

In the early days of MER, electrophysiologists assembled their own "rigs" from components (often designed and marketed for other purposes).

Nowadays, complete MER systems are available off the shelf from multiple manufacturers. These differ in physical configuration and in various ancillary features, but all have the same core components.

Microdrive

The microdrive is essentially a device for converting large movements into small ones, very accurately. The large movements are made by the operator's hand (or by a motor controlled by the operator) and these are geared down by the microdrive so that the electrode can be moved in increments of microns. The electrode moves on only one axis: parallel to its own length, since, obviously, motion in any other direction while in the brain would have a cutting action. The microdrive is necessarily attached to the stereotactic frame on the patient's head; most systems allow it to be controlled remotely by an operator outside the sterile field. The connection from the operator's control to the microdrive may be hydraulic or electrical. In the hydraulic case (rarely seen these days) the operator manipulates a master cylinder, which is connected by an oil-filled tube to the slave cylinder mounted on the stereotactic frame. The electrical method mounts a DC stepper motor on the microdrive, connected by an electrical cable to controlling electronics outside the sterile field. The latter system is far more convenient, although the jerky motion of the motor, together with the electrical pulses required to operate it, create signal artifact, so that it is often necessary to alternate moving the electrode with listening to / looking at the signal, rather than moving and looking/listening simultaneously.

Electrode

Microelectrodes for extracellular recording consist of thin (a few hundred microns) stiff metal wires, sharpened at their tips, and insulated except at the tip. Microelectrodes used for MER have about 10 microns of uninsulated surface at their tips giving a resistance in the hundreds of kiloohms. Manufacturers use various proprietary processes to control tip size and electrical characteristics of the electrode; for example, plating powdered platinum ("platinum black") onto the tip reduces its resistance by increasing its tip area at a sub-micron scale, without enlarging the tip at the relatively coarser micron scale. Microelectrode tips are extremely delicate: accidental contact with anything stiffer than brain parenchyma will not only spoil it electrically, but will typically bends it into a microscopic hook which will cause tissue damage on insertion and (especially) withdrawal. It is wise to inspect the electrode tip under a bright light before inserting into the brain. At most, though not all centers, the electrode is inserted into the brain through a thin metal tube ("cannula") which penetrates through the meninges and some distance into the brain parenchyma. The cannula remains in place, and, using the microdrive, the tip of the electrode is advanced out of the cannula into brain. At this point a useable signal is obtained.

Like any voltage, the electrical potential measured at the electrode tip must be measured relative to the potential in some other location, i.e. a reference electrode is required. In MER, this needs to be larger than the microelectrode tip so that it will average activity from many neurons to give a reference signal which does not itself contain any individual spikes.

Apart from that, it should ideally pick up all the same extraneous ("noise") signals encountered by the electrode tip, since the measurement of tip potential relative to reference potential will, in that case, contain none of the noise ("common mode rejection"). Therefore, the reference electrode should be close to the electrode tip. The cannula through which the electrode is inserted can be used as the reference electrode, if electrically conductive, as it usually is. Some electrode designs include a second exposed contact higher up the electrode shank with an area intermediate between the tip and reference electrode, from which averaged activity of multiple neurons within a limited volume of tissue ("local field potentials" LFPs) may be recorded. LFPs may also be recorded from the microelectrode tip, by using signal processing techniques to remove spikes from the signal, or from the DBS electrode itself. Some research [35] suggests that power spectra of LFPs may help locate optimal DBS electrode location.

Amplifier

The amplifier occupies a central, critical role, but its internals are the province of the electrical engineers who design it. Its role is to transform the tiny voltage fluctuations at the microelectrode into larger, but perfectly proportional voltage fluctuations at its output that are more readily handled by visual displays, audio monitors etc. An amplifier may consist of multiple stages, with the output of one stage connected to the input of another. In some MER systems, care is taken to put the first amplifier stage as close as possible to the electrode ("head stage"). This reduces the length of the cables connecting electrode to amplifier, which reduces its propensity to act as an antenna, picking up stray electromagnetic signals, the electrophysiologist's bête noire. Almost every piece of electrical equipment in the operating room generates them, including florescent lights. Of course, there is still a long cable connecting the head stage to the rest of the electronics, located in a rack or cabinet outside the sterile field. However, this cable is less vulnerable to noise because of the signal processing done by the headstage.

Filters

Any signal (mathematical esoterica excepted) is a sum of simple sinusoids; complicated waveforms are built up of sinusoids at many different frequencies, each with an appropriate amplitude and phase; the set of amplitudes, phases, and frequencies of the sinusoids constituting an arbitrary signal can actually be calculated (its Fourier transform). Signals which change slowly and smoothly over time contain only low frequency sinusoids. Signals which contain abrupt transitions -- such as MER spikes -- contain high frequencies as well. MER systems include a band pass filter which effectively decomposes the microelectrode signal into its component sinusoids, suppresses those below (low-pass cut-off) and above (high-pass cut-off) specified frequencies, then reconstitutes the signal from the altered components. This is actually accomplished by a considerably more efficient process, but the result is the same. The voltage which the amplifier picks up from the electrode contains a mixture of signal (the spikes) and noise (a mixture of unwanted signals, including aggregate activity in distant neurons, artifacts of electrode motion, electromagnetic interference from other electrical equipment in the operating room) and the job of the filter is to attenuate the noise, while preserving the signal. The electrophysiologist will sometimes need to adjust the filter settings from their defaults, but spikes are generally recognizable as spikes over a fairly wide range of filter settings, so, if spikes are expected, but not observed, the problem is probably not with the filter settings.

Oscilloscope

The oscilloscope draws a visual picture of the microelectrode signal. The oscilloscope "beam" (nowadays simulated digitally) sweeps horizontally across the screen at constant "sweep speed" and is deflected vertically by changes in measured voltage i.e. APs.

The sweep speed is adjustable; a value of around 10 cm/sec works well for this purpose: at that speed, a spike looks like a vertical tick-mark drawn against a horizontal baseline. Increasing the sweep speed allows the electrophysiologist to see the spike waveform which, as noted above, reveals whether the spikes being recorded are from one or several neurons.

Simply increasing the sweep speed works rather poorly however, because the spike waveform will appear at random intervals at random locations on the screen. MER systems provide a triggered fast sweep feature to solve this problem: a fast sweep is triggered when the signal rises above a user-specified threshold, so that the spike waveform appears still at irregular intervals, but now always in the same location: it is then much easier to judge by eye whether the waveform is constant or variable.

Audio Monitor

The audio monitor allows the MER signal to be heard as a sound, rather than seen as a picture. This is extremely valuable: in our experience it is much easier to distinguish among different patterns of activity, notice changes, and detect receptive fields using the ear than the eye.

Pulse Generator

When microstimulating, the amplifier is disconnected from the electrode, and a separate set of electronics is connected to it which delivers controlled electrical pulses. Microstimulation is done with current controlled (more loosely, "constant current") pulses i.e. the stimulator supplies whatever voltage is required to ensure that the specified current flows during stimulation. This gives more consistent results than constant voltage stimulation in which the stimulator applies a specified voltage to the microelectrode, and the amount of current is determined by resistance of tissue between the microelectrode and reference electrodes, and also, in particular by the resistance of the electrode-tissue interface, which varies over time, and also varies in response to stimulation. The local potential gradient at the neuron responding to stimulation is determined by the current flowing across the volume element occupied by that neuron which is usually a fixed, but unknown fraction of the total current.

With constant voltage stimulation, the total current will vary with the electrode-tissue resistance; as a result the current, and local potential gradient, experienced by the neuron will be variable, and less faithfully follow the stimulus waveform. As a result, thresholds for stimulation effects will be inconsistent. With constant current stimulation, the total current is constant, and thresholds are in general more consistent.

Several parameters of stimulation may be varied. Individual pulse durations are typically about 200 microseconds, and this can generally be left constant. Pulses are repeated with a frequency of typically about 300 Hz (historically, a third of a kilohertz; the more precise value of 333 Hz satisfies tradition, but has no other virtue) and this, also, rarely if ever needs to be adjusted. The pulses continue for a period of time (train duration) which may be either preset (0.5 to 1.0 seconds is typical) or the stimulator can be configured so that pulses continue for as long as the electrophysiologist keeps a finger on the button: we favor fixed train durations for greater consistency in determining thresholds. Pulse amplitude is the only parameter which the electrophysiologist will vary routinely.

Impedance Tester

Most readers will be familiar with concepts of electrical voltage, current, and resistance: current (I) is a flow of electrons or anything else with a charge (e.g. ions in solution); voltage (V) is the force which drives the flow, and resistance (R) is a property of the medium through which current flows, and defines how much voltage is required for a given current, by Ohm's law V=IR. When current and voltage are time-varying, concepts of capacitance and inductance come into play, and R is replaced by a more general quantity, impedance, which is a complex number i.e. one containing both a real and an imaginary part ("imaginary" in the sense that it is a multiple of the square root of negative one). This is an electrical engineer's understanding of impedance, and strictly speaking, it varies with frequency, i.e. if the impedance of an electrical circuit is measured with sinusoidally varying voltage and current, it will be different for different frequencies of the sinusoid. Loosely speaking, however, impedance can be thought of as equivalent to resistance.

MER systems include an "impedance tester" which does not actually measure "impedance" in the electrical engineering sense. MER impedance testers deliver a (not necessarily sinusoidally) varying voltage at a standard frequency and measure the resulting current. Information about phase shift is discarded giving a real number with no imaginary part. The amplitude and frequency are low enough to avoid any biological effect of what is otherwise, effectively microstimulation. While this may not satisfy a purist's definition of impedance, it is nonetheless extremely useful: by testing the electrode's impedance, the electrophysiologist can detect faulty or damaged electrodes, and can also monitor the changes to the electrode tip induced by microstimulation.

Electrode impedance should be checked as soon as the electrode enters the brain, (if not before: out-of brain testing can be done by dipping the tip in saline solution in continuity with the reference lead of the tester). If the measured impedance exceeds the manufacturer's specifications, the electrode may be defective. Microelectrodes used in MER for DBS surgery have impedances in the 200-800 kiloohm range. Impedances above 1 megohm tend to pick up more noise, and fewer spikes. Lower impedances suggest a manufacturing defect or damage to the electrode during sterilization or other handling.

Initial impedances in the 1.0-1.5 megohm range, however, can often be brought into the desired range by microstimulating, and such electrodes tend to perform well thereafter.

Approach to Recording and Stimulating

Approach to Recording

General Principles

Using the microdrive, the electrode is advanced point first into the brain, slowly (about one mm per minute is typical) characterizing electrical activity along the way, until the electrophysiologist builds up a one-dimensional map of the territory explored (an electrode "track"). This is then co-registered with a two- or three-dimensional brain atlas, either formally (for example by overlaying acetate drawings on a printed stereotactic atlas), or more informally, via the clinical judgment of the electrophysiologist and surgeon.

Discrepancies, if any, with the expected atlas location may lead to a change in target location for the DBS electrode; conversely, if the results of MER are as expected, this provides confirmation of the initial target. The MER map is one-dimensional because the electrode can only be moved along its own length while in the brain, but a two- or three-dimensional map can be built up by making multiple electrode penetrations, either one at a time or simultaneously [Figures 5 and 6].

Pros and Cons of Serial vs. Simultaneous Tracks

The disadvantage of multiple microelectrode tracks is that it presumably increases the risk of accidentally encountering a small blood vessel and causing hemorrhage. Multiple microelectrode tracks can be made serially, i.e. one at a time, or they can be made simultaneously. A disadvantage of serial tracks, compared to simultaneous tracks is increased time; not only do serial tracks prolong the surgery, they also allow more time for brain shift to occur: as a result the true location of the target may change from the time the initial penetrations are made, to the time the DBS electrode is implanted.

A disadvantage of simultaneous tracks compared to serial tracks is that simultaneous tracks require a pre-determined number of electrodes in a pre-determined spatial relationship. In contrast, with serial tracks the number and location of each penetration can be chosen based on the results of preceding penetrations and also each penetration can be independently planned to avoid any blood vessels large enough to be seen on MRI. Another advantage of serial tracks is that the electrophysiologist can give full attention to a single microelectrode, rather than dividing it among several.

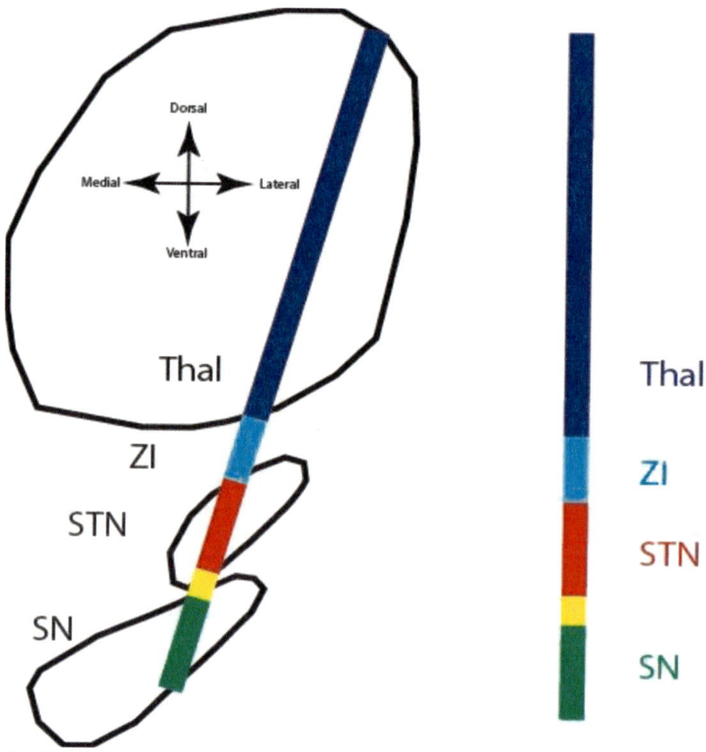

Example of how MER yields a one-dimensional brain map. Left: The electrode track (in color) is overlayed on a conventional (two-dimensional) brain map (in black). Thal: Thalamus; STN: subthalamic nucleus are shown as well as SN: substantia nigra and ZI: Zona incerta, a region of low neuronal density between thalamus and subthalamic nucleus. Right: the same electrode track, in isolation, to emphasize the one-dimensional nature of the map.

Figure 5. One dimensional MER map of subthalamic nucleus.

Spontaneous Activity

Cell Density

The most basic distinction MER can make is between regions of high and low neuronal density. By "neuron" we really mean neuronal soma, since, as noted earlier, to be detectable as spikes in the microelectrode signal, action potentials must occur in neuronal somata close to the tip. Neuronal density may be appreciated in two ways: First, in regions of high cell density, the electrode records spikes from more than one neuron simultaneously (in clinical electromyography, what would be called an "interference pattern"). This state of affairs is recognizable because spikes from different neurons will have different waveforms; as noted above, the spike waveform from any one neuron should not vary, as long as the electrode is not moved (two exceptions to this rule, both easily recognized, are injury discharges, and cardioballistic firing, discussed below). Modern MER systems have features (e.g. threshold-triggered fast oscilloscope sweeps and template matching) for distinguishing spikes with differing waveforms, but in practice it is usually enough to look at the standard display and note that spike heights vary. The second manifestation of high neuronal density is that neurons are encountered frequently as the electrode is moved. In a region of low cell density, one records spikes, which fade away as the electrode is advanced, moving away from the neurons; it may move hundreds or thousands of microns along its track before it approaches new neurons and spikes are again detected.

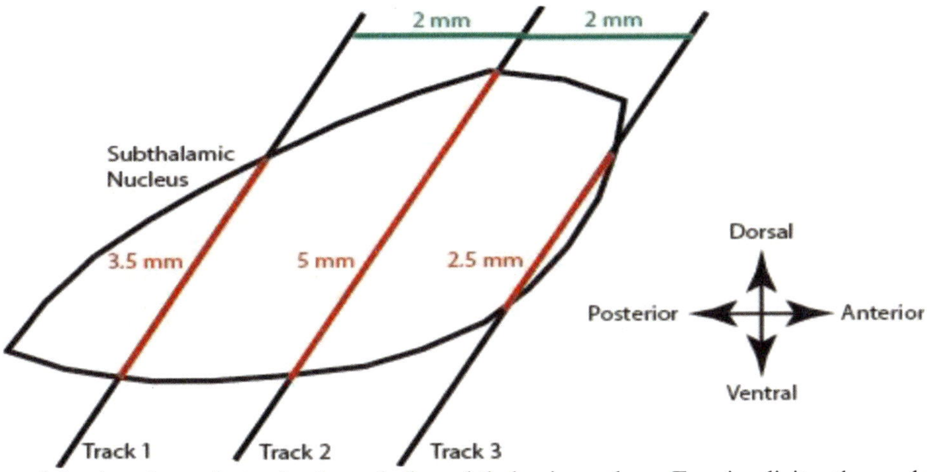

Diagram of 3 microelectrode tracks through the subthalamic nucleus. For simplicity, the nucleus and the tracks are shown strictly parasagital. The portion of each track within the nucleus is shown in red, together with its length. The red segment is longest for Track 2, which passes nearest the center of the nucleus, Overlaying the three tracks, with their known spacing, on the outline of the nucleus (e.g. from a sterotactic atlas) yields more information than considering a single track in isolation.

Figure 6. Mapping subthalamic nucleus with multiple microelectrode tracks.

In a region of high neuronal density "new" spikes fade in as "old" spikes fade out and there are no stretches of the track without spikes. Distinguishing the old from the new spikes is again facilitated by differences in waveform, although here the audio monitor is more useful than the oscilloscope display: the electrophysiologist is like a person walking through a crowded room full of people talking; voices fade out and fade in as one moves away from and closer to different people, but it is actually not difficult to tell the voices apart: this is something most human beings are naturally good at [We are indebted to Dr. Erwin Montgomery for the crowded-room simile]. Usually, these two measures of neuronal density covary, but occasionally not: for example, in substantia nigra pars reticulata (SNr), often cell density is high by the second measure, but not by the first, and this is occasionally useful in locating the boundary between SNr and subthalamic nucleus (STN).

Temporal Pattern

Individual nuclei can be distinguished from each other by the temporal pattern of spikes recorded there. Recognizing these patterns is to some extent like recognizing the voice of a friend or acquaintance, and can only be learned with experience. However, this should build on a systematic approach to classifying neuronal activity patterns. The first, and most basic classification is regular vs. irregular firing pattern. Regular firing, in which spikes come at a constant, unvarying rate, is actually rather uncommon and distinctive: regular firing at 60-80 Hz is characteristic of substantia nigra, while "border cells" encountered at the boundary between Globus Pallidus pars externa and pars interna (GPe and GPi) also fire very regularly at lower frequency of 20-30 Hz. Some neurons fire irregularly, but with a fairly constant average firing rate; this pattern is one of the least distinctive, and is seen in the majority of thalamic neurons. Some neurons fire very regularly but only for brief periods: some thalamic neurons (thalamic bursting neurons), for example, are silent, except for brief (about 10-20 msec) bursts of perfectly regular, very high frequency spikes, 2-10 spikes per burst (similar to "complex repetitive discharge" in clinical electromyography) and this pattern is quite distinctive. Similarly, some neurons in globus pallidus pars externa (GPe) exhibit brief (< 100 msec) bursts of high-frequency spikes against a background of low-frequency firing (low frequency burst neurons). The majority of GPe neurons, however, exhibit the inverse pattern: brief cessation of spiking interrupting a high frequency background (high frequency pause neurons). Some thalamic, and many subthalamic nucleus (STN) neurons modulate their firing rate smoothly in phase with the patient's tremor (if any; similar modulation is sometimes observed in the absence of visible tremor). However, the commonest form of STN neuron activity is an "irregular bursting" pattern in which firing rate varies from moment to moment in a random and unpredictable fashion.

In all these cases, spiking modulates in pattern or frequency of spikes, but not in spike shape or amplitude: the latter occurs only as an artifact, either of motion of the neuron relative to the electrode, or of injury to the neuron. In cardioballistic modulation, spikes appear to be modulated in synch with the patient's heartbeat, due to pulsatile tissue movement towards and away from the electrode. Spike amplitudes then vary sinusoidally. In injury discharges, the electrode passes so close to a neuron that the neuronal membrane is torn, and the membrane potential is lost: depolariziation results in a very high (hundreds of Hz) firing frequency; both the frequency and the amplitude diminish over several seconds as ionic gradients equilibrate, producing a characteristic diminuendo (similar to the myotonic discharge encountered in clinical electromyography, and commonly described as a "dive-bomber" sound).

"Irritable" Activity

Finally, thalamic and striatal neurons exhibit a distinctive form of "transient" or "irritable" activity in which the inciting stimulus is not activation of a receptive field, but motion of the electrode: each time the electrode is moved, it records a flurry of spikes, which decrease in frequency, and finally cease as the electrode sits motionless for a few tens of seconds.

Receptive Fields

General Principles

Many regions explored with the microelectrode may be recognized by the way spike rates respond to some form of provocation, generally stimulation of a receptive field. A receptive field is characterized by a sensory modality and a location (for example, if we say that a particular neuron has a tactile receptive field located at the tip of the right thumb, we mean that neuron increases its spiking frequency when the tip of the right thumb is touched).

Testing for receptive fields is a specialized form of neurological exam, and, as with the general neurological exam, the goal, which is to test comprehensively, and at the same time efficiently, is achieved only with practice.

The basic procedure is to deliver the stimulus -- e.g. move a joint, or touch a patch of skin -- while listening to the audio monitor for an increase in spike rate which consistently coincides with the stimulus. Receptive fields are almost always contralateral to the electrode, so only one half the body need be tested.

In nuclei where spike rates fluctuate a great deal spontaneously, it can be difficult to tell whether these variations are random or related to the joint movements (this is particularly true of STN, in fact, almost characteristic of it). In this situation, take plenty of time to get a sense of the baseline fluctuations, before delivering the stimulus; it may also help to wait for a lull in firing, or to deliver the stimulus in some recognizable pattern, e.g. three times in rapid succession, then pause, then three times again.

It helps to have a well-practiced routine, but this works best if modified flexibly. For example, efficiency is increased by testing first for the location or modality judged most likely at any given point along the electrode track, and only testing for others if no field is found on the first attempt. Also, at times, one can avoid wasting time on distinctions which do not matter. For example, it is generally more important to distinguish the location of a proprioceptive field when the target is in thalamus than when it is the subthalamic nucleus. When testing for receptive fields, the electrode is often picking up spikes from more than one neuron in the vicinity of its tip; in that case, there may be only one neuron which responds to the stimulus, and one should focus attention one at a time on each (akin to picking out individual voices from the hubbub of a crowded room).

Proprioceptive Receptive Fields

In neurons with proprioceptive receptive fields, spike rate responds to movement of a limb or other body part. Proprioceptive fields are the most common and important type, in MER, since DBS is most often done for treatment of movement disorders, and in this type of surgery, the electrophysiologist is generally exploring regions related to movement. To test for proprioceptive fields, passively move the patients' joints. The neuronal response is greater with larger, faster movements, so the movement should be as large and as brisk as possible. Be aware of any joint pathology which might limit range of motion, and watch the patients face, at least the first few times with each joint, to be sure there is no discomfort. Systematically test distal and proximal joints testing each joint in both flexion and extension. For example: fingers, thumb, wrist, elbow, shoulder (flexion/extension and ab-/ad-duction), or ankle, knee, hip (flexion/extension and internal/external rotation)). Orolingual fields are common and therefore important to test, but these structures are difficult to move passively: we ask the patient to actively protract and retract the tongue (the tongue can be moved passively by grasping it with a gauze pad, but this is rarely useful).

To move the arms and legs, it may be necessary to disencumber the patient, somewhat, from bedclothes, pneumatic calf compressors, IV lines, noninvasive blood pressure cuffs, pulse oximeters, and the like. We also recommend securing the Foley catheter so as not to put traction on it when passively moving the hip. Once a single receptive field is found, it is usually unnecessary to look for others, before advancing the electrode; therefore it is usually most efficient to test higher- before lower-yield locations, hence, orolingual and upper extremity before lower extremity, and distal before proximal.

Most neurons with proprioceptive fields are activated by passive movements, but neurons in the anterior ventral lateral (basal ganglia - receiving) thalamic nuclei (Voa, Vop: ventralis oralis pars anterior and posterior) respond better to voluntary (active) movements than to passive ones: but this distinction is rarely worth making. A more important distinction is between passive-proprioceptive neurons responding to joint movement per se (presumably to Golgi tendon organs) vs. those which respond to muscle spindles. This type of neuron has high localizing value, because it is found only at the border between cerebellar-receiving (Vim: ventral-intermediate) and dorsal column - receiving (Vc: ventral caudal) ventral lateral thalamic nuclei. Spindle-responsive neurons can be recognized by gently pinching the muscle belly transversely, so that the spindles are stimulated without moving the joint.

Tactile Receptive Fields

In neurons with tactile fields, spike rate responds to touching the skin. These units are encountered when mapping thalamus, but not STN or GPi. They are encountered in the dorsal column -receiving nuclei of the thalamus (Vc: ventral-caudal; also known as VPL/VPM: ventral posterior lateral/medial). They are exquisitely sensitive to the lightest of touch -- for most, a wisp of cotton, or the corner of a gauze pad is enough -- and highly selective as to the location of stimulation: usually, a patch of skin no more than 10mm in diameter, and nowhere else. This is what is known as the location of the receptive field. A subset of neurons with tactile fields requires a slightly stronger stimulus -- just enough to dimple the skin, slightly -- and have fields located on the finger pads: these units are found right on the border between Vim and Vc [Figure 7].

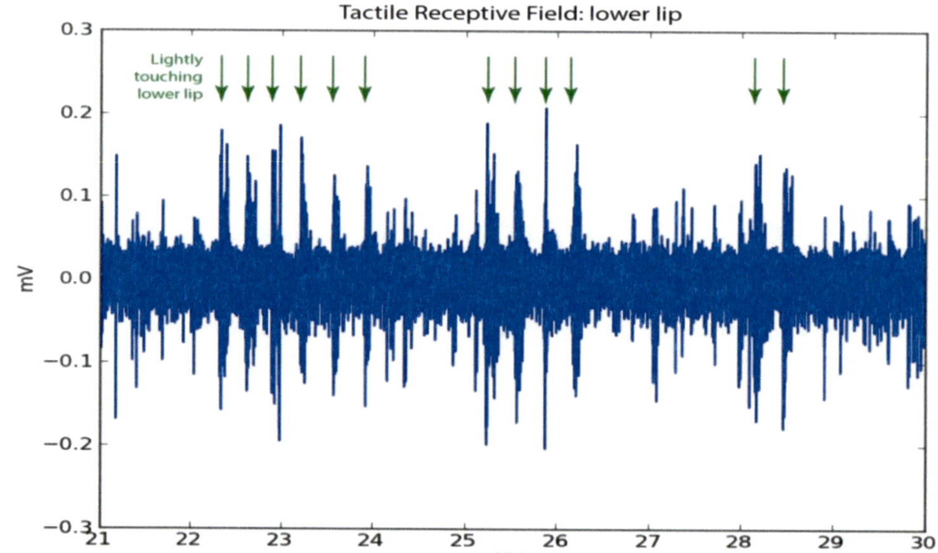

Spikes evoked in ventral caudal (Vc) thalamic nucleus, by lightly touching a tactile receptive field, in this case, on the patient's contralateral lower lip.

Figure 7. Tactile unit in Vc.

The key to finding tactile fields is to screen for them efficiently, then, if screening is positive, refine the search until the field's location is known. Sweep the hand over as much of the patient's lower extremity, upper extremity, and face as are accessible. Tactile fields on the tongue, inside the mouth, and sometimes the lips as well are far more easily screened for by asking the patient to protrude / retract the tongue than by trying to touch all these surfaces oneself. As this advice suggests, tactile fields are easily mistaken for proprioceptive ones, because moving a body part may result in rubbing the skin, e.g. tongue against lips, or arm against bedclothes.

Therefore, on identification of a putative proprioceptive field, the affected body part should be screened for tactile fields: e.g. by sweeping the hand over the arm leg, or face, or stroking the tongue, lips, and buccal mucosa with a cotton-tipped applicator.

Once a tactile field is found, it should be possible to locate the exact location of the receptive field, generally very small and well-demarcated. This is not always possible -- sometimes a field is simply inaccessible (e.g. posterior pharynx) -- but without it, one cannot be sure the field is really tactile.

Visual Receptive Fields

Neuronal activity responding to visual stimulation is encountered immediately ventral to the GPi when the microelectrode approaches or enters the optic tract. Of course, this is a pure white matter structure, so no spikes are observed. However, the electrode records the summed activity of innumerable axonal action potentials, individually too small to observe, and this sounds, on the audio monitor, like a hiss, or a rushing wind. A bright light flashed briefly in either eye will evoke an audible increase in this sound. Finding the location of such a visual field on the retina would require more sophisticated equipment than a penlight, and is not useful in GPi DBS surgeries.

Approach to Microstimulating

General Principles

Microstimulation pulses are biphasic, as noted above, to insure no net movement of electrical charge ("charge balance"). A typical pulse duration is 200 microseconds. Single pulses are not useful; clinically detectable effects require a series of repeating pulses at, typically, 330 Hz, for period of time ("train duration") of 0.5 to 1 sec. In searching for microstimulation effects, amplitude should start low (5-10 microamps) and move up (we use steps of 10-20), in order to avoid startling the patient with an overly intense effect due to suprathreshold stimulation. Amplitude should increase until either an effect is observed, or a limit is reached at which faradic processes become significant, as indicated by stimulation-induced changes in electrode impedance (we limit stimulation to 90 microamps, which generally drops the impedance by a few hundred kiloohms the first time, and has no further effect after that). Once an effect is detected, amplitude should be varied in smaller increments, in order to define a threshold (the minimum amplitude at which the effect occurs). This can be done to any degree of accuracy, but 10 microamperes accuracy is usually sufficient for clinical purposes. The patient should also be asked after each stimulus train whether he or she felt anything.

Internal Capsule

The internal capsule (IC) is the structure most often encountered in microstimulation, since it envelops the anterior, lateral and inferior STN, the posterior GPi, and (of less practical importance) the medial GPi and the lateral thalamus. Also, and unlike other commonly stimulated structures, microstimulation of the IC produces effects -- muscle twitching --

which can be objectively detected. Strictly speaking, muscle twitching is evoked from corticospinal (and corticobulbar) fibers which occupy only a portion of the IC, but in practice, that is the part typically encountered. In looking for IC stimulation effects one should devote the most attention to the body parts where an effect is likely to be seen, i.e. those most overrepresented in the pyramidal system "motor homunculus": the foot, hand, face and tongue. The tongue is not only highly overrepresented, it is also nearly "naked" exposed muscle, making tiny muscle twitches easy to detect (just as, in the ordinary neurological exam, the tongue is a prime location for detecting fasciculations).

All these locations can be efficiently scrutinized as follows: the examiner holds the patient's hand loosely, while looking at the patient's face. The patient opens his mouth, while the tongue and pharynx are illuminated with a penlight. A hand twitch is felt, rather than seen by the examiner; face or tongue movements are detected visually, and a third party is delegated to watch the patient's toes (if no technician or resident is available, the anesthesiologist or circulator may be willing).

In this way, one can be thorough, without loss of efficiency. As noted above, the patient should be asked whether stimulation produced any subjective sensation; sometimes, patients will report this in the absence of visible movement, and in that case, the effect is either a paresthesia, or a very subtle muscle contraction perceptible to the patient but not detectable by the examiner. In the latter case, increasing stimulus amplitude by a few 10s of microamps should bring out a clear twitch in the body part where the patient reports the sensation.

Medial Lemniscus, Vc

Paresthesias are the second most commonly encountered microstimulation effect, and result from activation of fibers in the medial lemniscus, or their terminals and postsynaptic targets in the thalamus. They are a wholly subjective phenomenon, so some skill is required from the electrophysiologist to distinguish real from imagined sensations (we leave to philosophers the difficulties posed by the concept of an imaginary sensation).

Awake neurosurgery is an anxiogenic, distracting, and fatiguing experience, moreover, patients lack experience of distinguishing stimulation effects from various itches, aches, dry mouth, etc. Increasing stimulation amplitude often helps with this: once a clear, strong paresthesia has occurred, the patient will provide more reliable reports thereafter. Another useful tactic is "placebo" stimulation i.e. clicking the button to deliver a stimulus, but with the amplitude set at zero.

Intracranial Oculomotor Nerve (CN III)

Oculomotor effects are uncommon, but highly localizing: They usually result from current spread to fibers of the intracranial oculomotor nerve. Although shown in some atlases as paramedian, they actually "bow" laterally as they travel from dorsal to ventral midbrain and so may be encountered even several millimeters lateral to the midline. Nonetheless, they are only ever encountered when an electrode track directed at STN is more medial than intended; in this situation, microstimulation evokes a twitch of the globe of the *ipsi* lateral eye -- this is easy to overlook since the electrophysiologist will be focusing attention on the contralateral face (and on facial musculature, rather than the eye proper). A second kind of eye movement may be evoked from the portion of the anterior capsule which lies anterior to the STN. Such movements are generally conjugate (bilateral, and the same in both eyes) and horizontal; moreover, they are far less common with microstimulation than when stimulating with the DBS electrode. They presumably result from activation of projections from the frontal eye field to mesencephalon.

Optic Tract

The optic tract is encountered as a cell-free zone beneath the GPi, and stimulation here produces phosphenes. Operating room lights should be dimmed and the patient asked to fixate a spot on the ceiling while stimulation is delivered, and report any flashing or sparkling (which is likely to be restricted to a small portion of the visual field). The same procedure can then be repeated with the lights full-on, looking for a transient focal visual distortion or scotoma affecting the patient's view of the ceiling.

STRATEGY AND TACTICS FOR SPECIFIC TARGETS

General Principles

In MER, one either 1) directs the microelectrode track at the planned target of the DBS electrode, or 2) directs the microelectrode at some other structure which is to be avoided, with the plan of placing the DBS electrode some distance away from that structure. The goal of MER is either 1) to confirm the initial stereotactic target (or, in a minority of cases, detect an anomaly which requires further microelectrode penetrations and/or adjustment of the target) or 2) refine the initial target by prompting small adjustments (generally in the 0.5 to 2.0 mm range) to the initial target. In practice, these approaches are often combined, with proportions varying according to target nucleus and even individual patient characteristics.

SUBTHALAMIC NUCLEUS

Target and Constraints

Although compact and histopathologically homogeneous, the subthalamic nucleus is subdivided into somatomotor, limbic, and associative zones, based on connectivity (especially with cerebral cortex) and presumed function. DBS for PD motor symptoms targets the somatomotor region located dorsolaterally; clinical and laboratory evidence indicates that stimulating outside this zone leads to unwanted cognitive or emotional side effects [36-39]. The somatomotor STN is recognized electrophysiologically by the presence of proprioceptive receptive fields. However, the STN is bordered laterally by the internal capsule; therefore, the electrode cannot be positioned in the extreme dorsolateral corner of the STN, lest spread of electrical current to the IC cause involuntary muscle contractions.

The electrode's final position is thus a compromise between countervailing imperatives to position it more laterally, but to avoid the laterally situated IC. At our institution we try to place the tip of the DBS electrode 3-4 mm medial to the STN's (estimated) lateral border in the same Y-Z plane, on or near a track which passes through at least 5 mm of STN, where proprioceptive fields were observed, and where no IC microstimulation effects were observed at least 2-3 mm ventral to the STN.

Canonical Track

At our institution, for STN surgeries, MER begins 15 mm "above" the stereotactic target which is set at the ventral border of the STN (By "above" we mean that advancing the electrode 15 mm along its track will bring it to the target). Consequently, the first neurons from which spikes are recorded are thalamic. Because the electrode is angled away from the Z axis, in both coronal and parasagital planes, it may traverse several mm of internal capsule before it enters the thalamus and spikes are recorded (Occasionally, the angle is so great that the electrode passes directly from IC to STN, bypassing thalamus).

Thalamic activity recorded along the first 6-8 mm or so of the track establishes a baseline relative to which the electrophysiologist detects changes indicating entry into the STN. Most thalamic neurons encountered dorsal to STN in the ventral lateral tier fire in an irregular pattern, not in itself very distinctive, but "irritable" firing (transient increase in spike rate with moving the electrode) and occasional thalamic-bursting neurons, if present, help with recognizing them.

Further along the track, "below" the thalamus is a zone of low cell density designated "zona incerta" (ZI), which contains the Fields of Forel (white matter structures) and the nucleus of the zona incerta, which contains neuronal somata, but at such low density that only a few scattered spikes, if any, are observed. Such ZI cells have characteristics similar to thalamic neurons. Since the hallmark of ZI is a drop in neuronal density, its dorsal border is hard to discern when neuronal density in the thalamus is also low, as is often the case.

Just before entry of the microelectrode into the STN, "background" noise picked up by the electrode will often increase; this is normally followed within a few hundred microns by well-isolated spikes in an irregularly bursting pattern. Typically, the transition from "quiet" spike-free recording to a "noisy" one crowded with spikes from multiple neurons is dramatic and easily recognized, but the border of the STN is not always so abrupt; changes in background noise, and firing characteristics of individual neurons should be noted with especial care at this point in the track, as this information may be critical later on.

Once the microelectrode has entered the STN, the next task is to test for proprioceptive receptive fields, as described above. This should be done with especial thoroughness for the first few mm of STN encountered along the track, since it is here, in the dorsolateral part of the nucleus, that somatomotor neurons are most likely to be encountered. Our practice is to establish a clear proprioceptive field for 2-3 neurons and not to test additional neurons along the track.

The next landmark to be sought is the ventral border ("bottom") of the STN. Typically, this is recognized when MER signal becomes abruptly quieter, with few or no spikes. A narrow (less than one mm) white matter zone is then followed by the substantia nigra pars reticulata (SNr) with its characteristic high frequency regular firing pattern completely unlike that of the STN. Another difference between STN and SNr is that, in SNr, neurons are more widely dispersed, so that one does not record spikes form multiple neurons in the same electrode location as one usually does in STN.

Unfortunately, a clear-cut a transition between STN and SNr is more the exception than the rule. "Quiet" zones may come and go inside the STN before the ventral border is encounterd. Cell density may be lower than average in ventral STN, or higher than average in SNr.

Firing patterns often transition gradually from irregular bursting to high frequency regular, with ventral STN neurons that sound a bit like SNr, and dorsal SNr neurons that sound somewhat like STN. Nonetheless, by the time the electrode track is finished, the electrophysiologist should be prepared to designate a definite point as the ventral border of STN, in order to calculate the total "length" of the STN measured along the electrode track (i.e. how many mm along the track from the dorsal to the ventral border). On a canonical track, this will be 5-6 mm; 4 mm may be acceptable if the electrode angle is close to the vertical (Z) axis but anything less should raise suspicions that the track did not pass through the centroid of the STN. The most efficient way to do microstimulation is to begin once the electrode has reached its most ventral point. We ordinarily continue the track 2-4 mm below the ventral border of the STN, and microstimulate there, then move back up the track stimulating at additional points along the way, including at least one or two within the STN.

The usefulness of microstimulating below the ventral border of the STN is that it provides information about the mediolateral location of the track. Because the IC curves in the coronal plane from a position lateral to the STN to one ventral to it, it will be encountered at progressively more ventral points with progressively more medial electrode tracks [Figure 8].

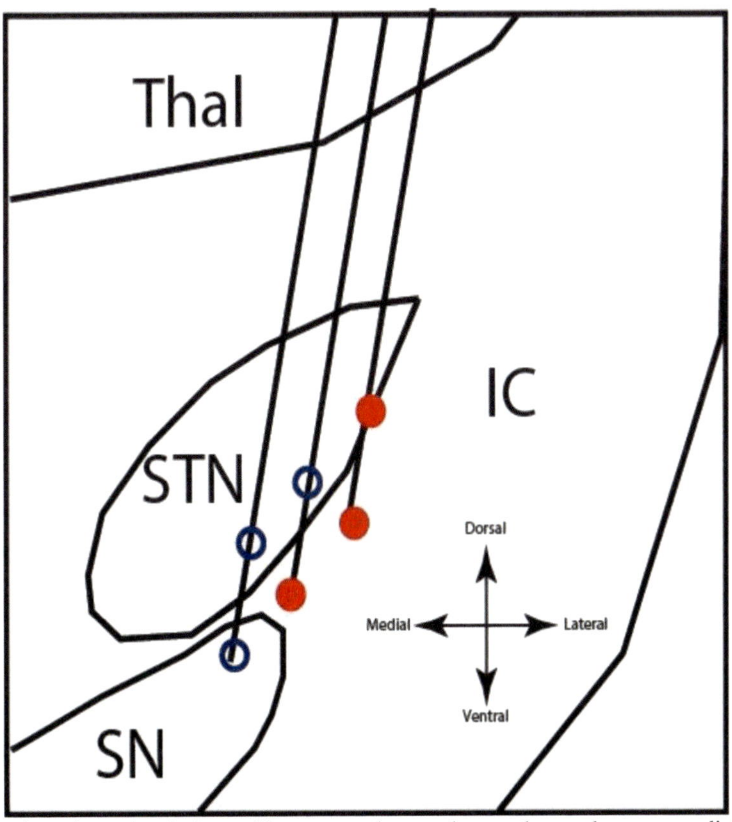

No internal capsule microstimulation effects are observed anywhere along a medial track. Internal capsule microstimulation effects are observed everywhere along a lateral track. Along an intermediate track, no capsular microstimulation effects are seen within the subthalamic nucleus, but capsular microstimulation effects are seen below the ventral border of the nucleus.

Figure 8. microstimulation in subthalamic nucleus.

If microstimulation 3 mm past the ventral border of the STN produces no microstimulation effects, this provides some reassurance that the electrode track is not so close to the IC mediolaterally that implanting the DBS electrode on that track is likely to result in side effects from activation of IC axons.

Interpretation of Non-Canonical Tracks

Such a "canonical" track can be taken as confirming the stereotactic target. A non-canonical track should prompt the electrophysiologist and the surgeon to consider whether that target might be improved upon. The strongest indication that a track deviates from the centroid of the STN is if the length of the STN along the track was less than 4-5 mm.

Other details of the track may then indicate whether deviation in the lateral, medial, anterior, or posterior direction. Lateral deviation is suggested by the presence of IC microstimulation effects either within the STN, or (a weaker indicator) within 3 mm past its ventral border. Medial deviation is suggested by oculomotor microstimulation effects, but these are rarer, and so, less useful; medial tracks are also characterized by a lack of somatosensory receptive fields, and by a generally lower STN neuronal density.

Anterior and posterior tracks are harder to recognize, though on a very posterior track, microstimulation may evoke paresthesias, and an anterior one may give a comparatively long distance of STN along the track, but with extremely low neuronal density, and ambiguous dorsal and ventral borders. Both lateral and anterior tracks will give unusually wide gaps between thalamus and STN (>3-4 mm) and between STN and SNr (>1mm).

A robust thalamus with high cell density makes it unlikely the track is either anterior or lateral; the converse (low density thalamus implying lateral or anterior track) is a weaker indicator, since a perfectly satisfactory track may bypass the thalamus entirely, passing directly from IC into STN, due to the angle of the electrode in the brain.

Additional Tracks

A single microelectrode track provides exquisitely precise information along the axis of the electrode, and some information about the X and Y axes may be extracted as well. However, precise X and Y information requires additional electrode tracks. Additional tracks may be done either routinely, or on an as-needed basis.

Our practice is shifting from doing additional tracks routinely, to doing them in cases where the initial track was not canonical. Additional tracks may have as their goal either to find a better match for the ideal "canonical" track, or to find the edges of the STN, in order to position the DBS electrode a set distance away from them.

At our institution, additional penetrations generally include at least one lateral to the initial target, and often one anterior to it as well; the goal is to position the DBS electrode 3-4 mm medial to the lateral edge of the STN, and 3-4 mm posterior to its anterior edge; the posterior and medial edges are harder to find, and we do not ordinarily attempt that.

An electrode track which passes through the STN close to its edge will traverse a short length of STN, and neuronal density will generally be low -- often so low that it is hard to tell if the track passed through the nucleus or not.

Depending on whether the additional track seems to have passed cleanly through the nucleus, or merely grazed it, or passed entirely outside it, the DBS electrode may be placed nearer, or further from the track.

Multiple Simultaneous Electrode Tracks

When making multiple simultaneous electrode penetrations, the electrophysiologist is attending to multiple signals, and the information derived from each is correspondingly more limited. At our institution, we delineate the dorsal and ventral border of the STN on each track, and choose whichever of the pre-planned tracks had the greatest length of STN as the location of the DBS electrode, with, perhaps, some adjustment for neuronal density, somatosensory receptive fields, and/or microstimulation effects.

VIM THALAMIC NUCLEUS

Target and Constraints

The thalamus is divided into many nuclei; only a few, located in the ventral lateral tier, are relevant to movement disorders DBS surgery. From anterior to posterior these nuclei relay inputs from basal ganglia (GPi, SNr), from cerebellum (dentate, interpositus) and from the dorsal column nuclei of the spinal cord (gracile, cuneate) to cortical regions concerned with motor planning, motor execution, and somatosensory perception.

Nomenclature of the thalamic nuclei is confusing and stereotactic surgery usually uses the system of Hassler [40] in which the cerebellar- and dorsal column- receiving nuclei are designated ventral intermediate (Vim, the target nucleus for treating tremor) and ventral caudal (Vc) respectively. The nuclei are histopathologically distinguisable with classical light microscopy, but not in vivo using 3-Tesla MRI. MER, however, is exquisitely sensitive to the boundary between Vim and Vc and may be used to identify that landmark. Since the target nucleus, Vim is only about 3-4 mm in anteroposterior extent, and since the electrode runs from anterodorsal to posteroventral, the DBS lead should be placed near the posterior border of the nucleus. However, Vim is bordered posteriorly by Vc, therefore the electrode cannot be positioned at the extreme posterior border of Vim lest spread of electrical current to Vc cause intense, uncomfortable paresthesias.

The electrode's final position is thus a compromise between countervailing imperatives to position it more posteriorly, but to avoid the posteriorly situated Vc. At our institution, we try to place the DBS electrode tip about 3 mm anterior (Y) to the estimated Vim-Vc bounday in an X-Y (horizontal) plane approximating the ventral border of the thalamus, and at a mediolateral (X) position where MER receptive fields are predominantly in the upper limb. MER in the thalamus is less concerned with grey-white transitions, and much more concerned with receptive fields, than is MER in the STN.

Canonical Track

The initial microelectrode track is intended to locate Vc, hence, is posterior to the expected final location of the DBS electrode; the stereotactic target is set at the ventral border of the thalamus. MER at our institution begins 15 mm above that target, in the dorsal tier of thalamic nuclei. Receptive field testing begins when the electrode reaches the ventral tier, which may sometimes be recognized by an increase in neuronal density; if not, we begin testing about 10 mm above the stereotactic target.

Proprioceptive receptive fields indicate that the electrode is in Vim; as it moves posteriorly, it passes into Vc, which is recognized by the presence of tactile receptive fields. In fact, it is frequently possible to track the progression from proprioceptive fields, to spindle fields (responsive to joint motion but also to pinch of muscle bellies), to deep-tactile fields (responsive to touching skin enough to dimple it slightly), to ordinary tactile fields (responsive to the lightest of touches) [Figure 9].

The spindle and deep-touch zones occupy less than a millimeter along the track, making them valuable landmarks for the Vim-Vc border. As the electrode continues along its track, it passes out of the thalamus ventrally: this is indicated by decrease in neuronal density, but in Vc, the transition is not abrupt or clear, and spikes may continue to be observed even ventral to thalamus (disappearance of tactile receptive fields is a more reliable indication that the electrode has passed out of the thalamus). An electrode track which passes through 2-4 mm of Vc is probably leaving the thalamus about 1-2 mm posterior to the Vim-Vc border, i.e. about 4 mm posterior to a suitable DBS electrode location.

Receptive fields (both proprioceptive and tactile) on an altogether typical track will be predominantly in the upper extremity. In both Vim and Vc, receptive fields are arranged, from medial to lateral, in the order Face-Arm-Leg.

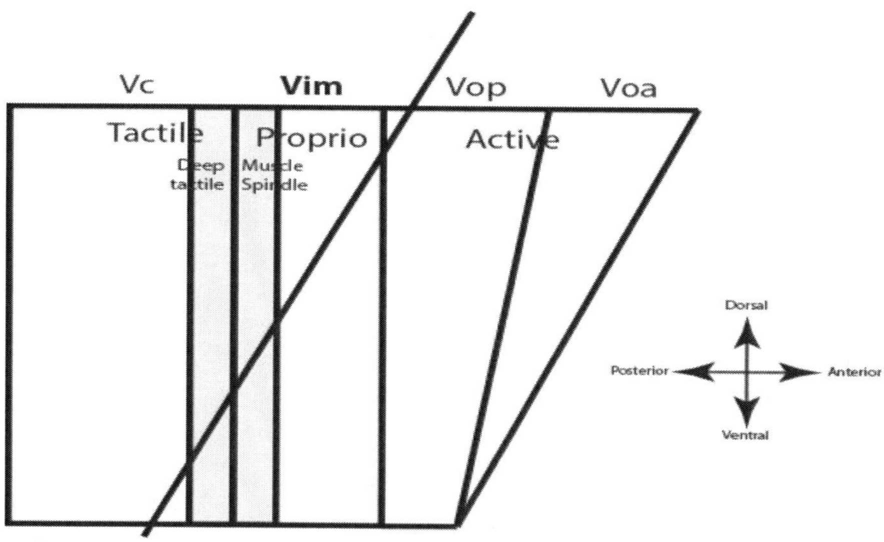

Schematic of the ventrolateral thalamic nuclei showing the types of receptive field to be found in each, and the order in which they are encountered on a typical microelectrode track with target in ventral Vc.

Figure 9. Schematic sagittal view of thalamus.

However, when viewed in a coronal plane, the three zones have the shape of a letter C with the open part of the letter facing the midline [Figure 10]. Thus, along an electrode track, one typically encounters fragments of the sequence "Leg - Arm - Face - Arm - Leg" (rarely the entire sequence) and must characterize the track by its predominant somatotopy.

Microstimulation in the vicinity of Vc almost always yields paresthesias, typically at very low threshold (often less than 10 microamperes). Caution is required to avoid startling the patient. Thresholds along an electrode track often follow a J-shaped curve, with low thresholds below the thalamus, lower thresholds in Vc, and higher thresholds further up the track in Vim. Paresthesia thresholds on a posterior penetration are most useful as confirmation that the track was in Vc, or, on tracks without tactile receptive fields as an indication of proximity to Vc. They have some value for establishing somatotopy, but less than receptive fields, because microstimulation activates fibers of passage (axons en route to other parts of the nucleus [29].

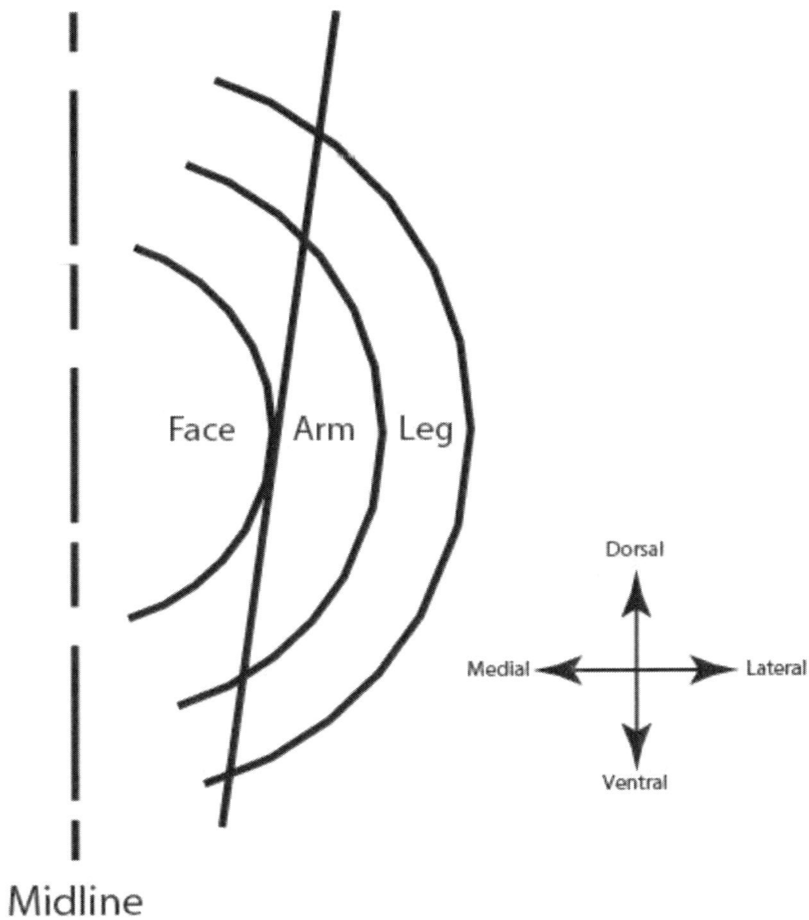

Face, arm, and leg regions of both Vc and Vim have a C-shaped configuration in the coronal plane. A typical microelectrode track will encounter predominantly neurons with upper extremity receptive fields, but may encounter lower extremity fields above and/or below the arm region, and may even encounter a few facial receptive fields as well. If, however leg (face) fields predominate, then the track may be lateral (medial) to the optimal DBS electrode location.

Figure 10. Schematic coronal view of thalamus.

Interpretation of Non-Canonical Tracks

A track which fails to encounter Vc (i.e. no tactile receptive fields) should raise a strong suspicion that the track was more anterior than intended, by a sufficient margin to require revising the planned location of the DBS electrode. If the track encounters 4 or more mm of Vc, this may indicate that it was more posterior than intended.

If receptive fields are predominantly facial, then the DBS electrode location should have a more lateral position, to avoid facial paresthesias and effects on speech as side effects of stimulation; receptive fields that are predominantly in the lower extremity may indicate that the DBS electrode location should be more medial.

The location of the ventral border of the thalamus is typically not confidently established by a track in Vc: not only is the ventral border of thalamus ill-defined posteriorly, but also, it is located up to 2 mm more ventral, in Vc, than it is anteriorly in Vim.

Nonetheless, if positioning the DBS electrode based on a single microelectrode penetration in Vc, we determine the Z coordinate from the estimated ventral thalamic border on the MER track; this conservative strategy may put the tip of the DBS electrode ventral to the thalamus, but if necessary this can be compensated by using higher contacts. Arguably, it is even advantageous to stimulate cerebellothalamic fiber ventral to thalamus [41, 42].

Additional Tracks

If Vc is not encountered, than another electrode track should be done, about 2 mm posterior to the first. If Vc is encountered at the firs penetration, another penetration 2 mm anterior to the first can be made, either just in cases where Vc occupied more than 3-4 mm along the first track, or routinely (in which case, the two penetrations may be consecutive or simultaneous). Ideally, this second penetration will not encounter Vc, in which case, the location of the Vim-Vc border has been "bracketed" to an accuracy of ±1mm. If Vc is encountered again this raises a strong suspicion that the stereotactic target is more posterior than planned, and the target for the DBS electrode may need to be revised. A third microelectrode penetration should be made 2 mm anterior to the second. Predominantly facial receptive fields indicate the need for a lateral adjustment of the final DBS electrode position, but a small one (0.5 to 1mm); similarly, mostly leg fields indicate a medial adjustment should be made. However, somatotopy moves about 1 mm medially for every 5 mm anteriorly the electrode moves; this means that, if facial receptive fields are encountered in Vc, and the DBS electrode is positioned 4 mm anterior to that, at the same mediolateral position, then the DBS electrode is probably in upper extremity zone, as intended.

Generally, the DBS electrode is implanted anterior to the microelectrode penetrations; occasionally, it is useful to make electrode penetration at that location. This serves primarily to identify the ventral border of the thalamus (which is usually better demarcated anteriorly) and to confirm somatotopy (but this is usually less well-demarcated anteriorly). If such a track is done, then microstimulation evoked paresthesias should be seen only at high currents (70-90 microamps) if at all, otherwise the DBS electrode target may be too posterior, leading to troublesome paresthesias as a side effect of stimulation. On the other hand, the somatotopy of such paresthesias is probably somewhat predictive of what will occur with a DBS electrode in that location.

Globus Pallidus Pars Interna

Target and Constraints

GPi is the least common of the three targets discussed here, because it is (perhaps undeservedly [43, 44]) less popular than STN as a target for treating Parkinson's disease. Although GPi is (perhaps undeservedly [45]) the preferred target for treating dystonia, dystonia is a less common indication for DBS surgery.

Furthermore, MER is more often omitted in GPi surgeries. There are several reasons for this. First, the surgeries are usually done in cases of generalized dystonia, which may interfere with putting, or keeping the patient in a stereotactic frame. Second, many patients undergoing such surgery are children, hence judged unable to remain cooperative through a prolonged awake surgery. Finally, the GPi is a larger structure than STN, and less hedged in by other structures to be avoided, therefore, it is widely felt, more tolerant of small inaccuracies in electrode placement which might result from the omission of MER.

As in STN, the target is the somatomotor region of the GPi, located in its most postero-ventro-lateral portion, and is recognized electrophysiologically by the presence of proprioceptive receptive fields. GPi is bordered posteriorly by internal capsule, therefore, the electrode cannot be positioned in the extreme posteroventrolateral corner of the GPi, lest spread of electrical current to the IC cause involuntary muscle contractions. The electrode's final position is thus a compromise between countervailing imperatives to position it more posteriorly, but to avoid the posteriorly situated IC. In GPi, unlike STN, one cannot conclude, just because the electrode track passed through several mm of the nucleus, that the target is necessarily correct; the track can be too anterior, and still traverse several mm of GPi. One must rely on the absence of proprioceptive fields, and also on additional microelectrode tracks, to detect this situation. In contrast, the number of mm of GPi traversed by the electrode track is an excellent clue to position on the mediolateral axis, because the GPi in coronal section is shaped like a wedge of pie, with the point towards the midline. However, this relies on distinguishing GPe from GPi, which, while comparatively straightforward in Parkinson's disease is difficult in dystonia.

The optic tract lies ventral to GPi, and stimulation here will cause phosphenes, or, worse, mechanical disruption of the track by the electrode tip might cause a scotoma. Therefore, (unlike STN and Vim) one is not altogether free to 'hedge ones bets' by implanting the tip of the DBS electrode a little more ventral than necessary and compensating during programming by using more proximal electrode contacts.

Canonical Track

The stereotactic target is at the ventral edge of posterolateral GPi. If recording starts 15 mm above that target, the first units recorded will be in striatum; cell density is low, and activity is typically 'irritable' as in thalamus. If it is the caudate, rather than the putamen which is traversed, the electrode passes through internal capsule before entering GPe. Although IC is a white matter structure, occasional spikes may still be detected here because of the "cords" of neurons joining caudate to putamen across the IC.

As noted above, GPe neurons exhibit one of two firing patterns, which are more or less inverses of each other: In high frequency pause activity continuous high frequency spiking is irregularly interrupted by brief (a few hundred milliseconds) pauses. In low frequency burst activity, which is rarer, a background of low frequency spiking is irregularly interrupted by brief (a few hundred milliseconds) bursts of high frequency firing rates. It is critical to detect the transition from this activity pattern to GPi activity, which has a more undifferentiated irregularly bursting character similar to STN (and also usually a higher density of neurons). Usually they are separated by a thin white matter lamina. The transition may also be marked by a "border neuron." These units, found in a thin shell surrounding GPi, have large-amplitude, isolated spikes, usually more than 1msec in duration (which gives them a distinctive sound on the audio monitor) at moderate and very regular frequency. Because the shell is so thin, it is rare to encounter more than one or two border neurons, and quite common to encounter none at all. Border neurons may also be encountered at the ventral border of the GPi. Misleadingly, they may be encountered in the interior of GPi, in a thin white matter lamina present posteriorly, which divides it incompletely into dorsal and ventral portions. The ventral border of GPi is more easily recognized by the drop in neuronal density as the electrode leaves the nucleus, and by visual phenomena (visual evoked potentials, and microstimulation induced phosphenes) as the electrode approaches the optic tract.

Microstimulation is also done more dorsally with the goal of detecting IC effects (muscle contractions) [Figure 11]. Along a typical track through the thickest part of somatomotor GPi, the distance from first encountering GPi to leaving the nucleus will be 6-8 mm (longer distance with more lateral tracks, or electrode angle further from vertical). Proprioceptive fields will be detected in GPi, the optic track may be encountered ventrally, and IC microstimulation effects will not be encountered dorsally.

Interpretation of Non-Canonical Tracks

A track which is too anterior will not encounter GPi neurons with proprioceptive receptive fields (upper extremity fields imply a slightly more posterior and lateral track than lower extremity fields). A track which is too posterior will have internal capsule microstimulation effects evoked from within GPe and GPi; in this case, the track will probably traverse less than 7mm of GPi. A track which is too medial will also have less than 7mm of GPi, and may or may not have capsule microstimulation effects: a track with less than 7mm of GPi and no microstimulation effects is probably either too medial, or too lateral; too lateral is the more likely possibility if the GPi was virtually absent. If optic track is encountered, then the track is probably not too lateral.

Additional Tracks

Additional microelectrode tracks are particularly useful with the GPi target. If the first track encounters 6-7 mm of GPi, we make another track about 3 mm posterior to that, looking for evidence that the second track is approaching IC. Ideally, that track encounters about 4 mm or less of GPi, with IC microstimulation effects. If not, we make a third track 2-3 mm posterior to the second.

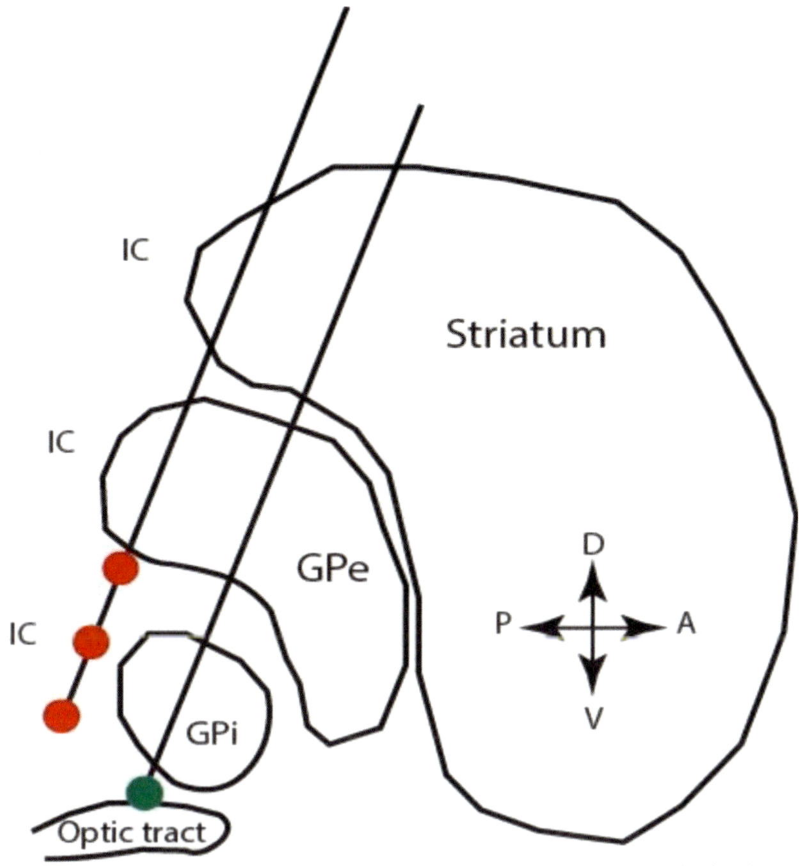

The first penetration encounters first the striatum, then GPe, passes through the internal medullary lamina to reach the GPi, then, passing out of the GPi ventrally, reaches the optic tract, where microstimulation evokes phosphenes (green dot). The second penetration, posterior to the first, encounters GPe, but for most of its length is in, or near internal capsule, where microstimulation evokes muscle contractions (red dots).

Figure 11. Globus Pallidus mapping.

Once a track is found which is judged to be close to the IC, the planned anteroposterior location of the DBS electrode is set to be about 4.5 mm anterior to that (a greater distance is allowed between DBS electrode and IC than for the STN target in anticipation of higher DBS amplitudes with GPi). The planned dorsoventral location of the DBS electrode is the ventral border of GPi as established on the first track (or the closest track to the final DBS electrode location). An additional track can be done to establish mediolateral position: our procedure is as follows: We compare the 2 or 3 tracks done so far with a stereotactic atlas, looking for a best match in the parasagital plane.

From there, we estimate how far laterally we have to move, relative to the initial penetrations, to be just at the lateral border of the GPi, and make a penetration at that location (and at the previously chosen anteroposterior coordinate). That track should encounter GPe, but barely any GPi (it may actually reenter GPe below GPi). The mediolateral position of the DBS electrode is set 2.5 mm medial to the estimated lateral border of GPi.

Conclusion

MER can contribute a considerable amount of information to intraoperative decisions about DBS electrode location. The amount of information, hence the value of the MER, depends on details of technique (e.g. whether microstimulation is used, whether one, or several microelectrode tracks are used) and on the knowledge and skill of the electrophysiologist, both regarding basic principles and with respect to the electrophysiological characteristics of the individual surgical targets.

Acknowledgments

For helpful comments on the manuscript,
Kenneth B. Baker PhD, University of Minnesota
Matthew D. Johnson PhD, University of Minnesota
Andre G. Machado MD, PhD, Cleveland Clinic
Jerrold L. Vitek MD, PhD, University of Minnesota

References

[1] Israel, Z. and Burchiel, K. J. 2004. *Microelectrode Recording in Movement Disorder Surgery*. New York: Thieme.
[2] Bakay, R. 2009. *Movement Disorders Surgery: The Essentials*. New York: Thieme.
[3] Montgomery, E. B. 2014. *Intraoperative Neurophysiological Monitoring for Deep Brain Stimulation*. New York: Oxford.
[4] Zrzino, L., Foltynie, T., Limousin, P., and Hariz, M. I. 2012. Reducing hemorrhagic complications in functional neurosurgery: a large case series and systematic literature review. *J. Neurosurg*. 116:84-94.
[5] Gologorsky, Y., Ben-Haim, S., Moshier, E. L., Bodbold, J., Tagliati, M., Weisz, D., and Alterman, R. L. 2011. Transgressing the ventricular wall during subthalamic deep brain stimulation increases the risk of adverse neurological sequelae. *Neurosurgery* 69:294-299.
[6] Xiaowu, H., Xiufeng, J., Xiaoping, Z., Bin, H., Laixing, W., Yiqun, C., Jinchuan, L., Aiguo, J., Jianmin, L. 2009. Risks of intracranial hemorrhage in patients with Parkinson's disease receiving deep btrain stimuation and ablation. *Parkinsonism and Related Disorders* 16:96-100.
[7] Higuchi, Y. and Iacono, R. P. 2003. Surgical Complications in patients with Parkinson's disease after posteroventral pallidotomy. *Neurosurgery* 52:558-571.
[8] The Deep Brain Stimulation For Parkinson's Disease Study Group 2001. Deep brain stimulation of the subthalamic nucleus or the pars interna of the globus pallidus in Parkinson's disease. *New England Journal of Medicine* 345:956-963.
[9] Piacentino, M., Zambon, G., Pilleri, M., and Bartolomei, L. 2013. Comparison of the incidence of intracranial hemorrhage in two different planning techniques for

stereotactic electrode placement in the deep brain stimulation. *J. Neurological Science* 57:63-67.

[10] Elias, W. J., Sansur, C. A. and Frysinger, R. C. 2009. Sulcal and ventricular trajectories in stereotactic surgery. *J. Neurosurgery* 110:201-207.

[11] Seijo, F. J., Alvarez-Vega, M. A., Gutierrez, J. C., Fdez-Glez, F., Lozano, B. 2007. Complications in subthalamic nucleus stimulation surgery for treatment of Parkinson's disease: review of 272 procedures. *Acta Neurochirurgica* (Wien) 149:867-876.

[12] Ben-Haim, S., Asaad, W. F., Gale, J. T., and Eskandar, E. N. 2009. Risk factors for hemorrhage during icroelectrode-guided deep brain stimulation and the introduction of an improved microelectrode design. *Neurosurgery* 64:754-763.

[13] Gorgulho, A., De Salles, A. A. F., Frighetto, L., and Behnke, E. 2005. Incidence of hemorrhage associated with electrophysiological studies performed using macroelectrodes and microelectrodes in functional neurosurgery. *J. Neurosurg.* 102: 888-896.

[14] Alterman, R. L., Sterio, D., Beric, A., and Kelly, P. J. 1999. Microelectrode recording during posteroventral pallidotomy: Impact on target selection and complications. *Neurosurgery* 442:315-321.

[15] Binder, D. K., Rau, G. M. and Starr, P. A. 2005. Risk factors for hemorrhage during microelectrode-guided deep brain stimulator implantation for movement disorders. *Neurosurgery* 56:722-732.

[16] Chang, W. S., Kim, H. Y., Kim, J. P., Park, Y. S., Chung, S. S., Chang, J. W. 2011. Bilateral subthalamic deep brain stimulation using single track microelectrode recording. *Acta Neurochirurgica* 153:1087-1095.

[17] Zeiler, F. A., Wilkinson, M. and Krcek, J. P. 2013 Subthalamic nucleus deep brain stimulation: An invaluable role for MER. *Can. J. Neurol. Sci.* 40:572:575.

[18] Hutchison, W. D., Lang, A. E., Dostrovsky, J. O., and Lozano, A. M. 2003. Pallidal neuronal activity: implications for models of dystonia. *Annals of Neurology* 53:480-488.

[19] Rozet, I. 3008. Anesthesia for functional neurosurgery: the role of dexmedetomidine. *Current Opinion in Anaesthesiology* 21:537-543.

[20] Eisenhart, C. 1969. Realistic evaluation of the precision and accuracy of instrument calibration systems. In: *Precision Measurement and Calibration*, H. Ku ed. Selected NBS Papers on Statistical Concepts and Procedures Volume 1 Series editor HL Mason. Washington: US Government Printing Office.

[21] Anheim, M., Batir, A., Fraix, V., Silem, M., Chabardes, S., Seigneuret, E., Krak, P., Benabid, A.-L., and Pollak, P. 2008. Improvement in Parkinson disease by subthalamic nucleus stimulation based on electrode placement. *Archives of Neurology* 65:612-616.

[22] Sillay, K. A., Ross, C., Brady, M., Alexander, A., Gupta, N., Adluru, G., Miranpuri, G. S., and Williams, J. C. 2013. Perioperative brain shift and deep brain stimulating electrode deformation analysis: implications for rigid and non-rigid devices. *Annals of Biomedical Engineering* 41:293-304.

[23] Petersen, E. A., Holl, E. M., Martinez-Torres, I., Foltynie, T., Limousin, P., Hariz, M. I., Zrinzo, L. 2010. Minimizing brain shift in stereotactic functional neurosurgery. *Operative Neurosurgery* 67S1:213-221.

[24] van den Munckhof, P., Contarino, M. F., Bour, L. J., Speelman, J. D., de Bie, R. M. A., and Schuurman, P. R. 2010. Postoperative curving and upward displacement of deep brain stimulation electrodes caused by brain shift. *Neurosurgery* 67:49-54.

[25] Halpern, C. H., Danish, S. F., Baltuch, G. H., and Jaggi, J. L. 2008. Brain shift during deep brain stimulation surgery for Parkinson's disease. *Stereotactic and Functional Neurosurgery* 86:37-43.

[26] Larson, P. S., Starr, P. A., Bates, G., Tansey, L., Richardson, M., and Martin, A. J. 2012. An optimized system for interventional MRI guided stereotactic surgery: preliminary evaluation of targeting accuracy. *Neurosurgery* 70(S1):95-103.

[27] Lambert, C., Zrinzo, L., Nagy, Z., Lutti Antoine, Hariz, M., Foltynie, T., Draganski, B., Ashburner, J., and Frackowiak, R. 2012. Confirmation fo functional zones within the human subthalamic nucleus: Patterns of connectivity and sub-parcellation using diffusion weighted imaging. *NeuroImage* 60:83-94.

[28] Duchin, Y., Abosch, A., Yacoub, E., Sapiro, G., and Harel, N. 2012. Feasibility of using ultra-high field (7-T) MRI for clinical surgical targeting. *PLoS-1* 7:e37328.

[29] Grill, W. M., Simmons, A. M., Cooper, S. E., Miocinovic, S., Montgomery, E. B., Baker, K. B., Rezai, A. R. 2005. Temporal excitation properties of paresthesias evoked by thalamic microstimulation. *Clinical Neurophysiology* 116:1227-1234.

[30] Miocinovic, S. and Grill, W. M. 2004. Sensitivity of temporal excitation properties to the neuronal element activated by extracellular stimulation. *J. Neuroscience Methods* 132:91-99.

[31] McIntyre, C. C., Grill, W. M., Sherman, D. L., and Thakor, N. V. 2004. Cellular effects of deep brain stimulation: Model-based analysis of activation and inhibition. *J. Neurophysiology* 91:1457-1469.

[32] Merril, D. R., Bikson, M. and Jefferys, J. G. R. 2005. Electrical stimulation of excitable tissue: design of efficacious and safe protocols. *J. Neuroscience Methods* 141:171-198.

[33] Morel, A. 2007. *Stereotactic Atlas of the Human Thalamus and Basal Ganglia*. New York: Informa.

[34] Kelly, P. J., Derome, P. and Guiot, G. 1978. Thalamic spatial variability and the surgical results of lesions placed with neurophysiologic control. *Surgical Neurology* 9: 307-315.

[35] Ince, N. F., Gupte, A., Wichmann, T., Ashe, J., Henry, T., Bebler, M., Eberly, L., Abosch, A. 2010. Selection of optimal programming contacts based on local field potential recordings from subthalamic nucleus in patients with Parkinson's disease. *Neurosurgery* 67:390-397.

[36] Bejjani, B.-P., Damier, P., Arnulf, I., Thivard, L., Bonnet, A.-M., Dormont, D., Cornu, P., Pidoux, B., Samson, Y., and Agid, Y. 1999 Transient acute depression induced by high frequency deep brain stimulation. *New England Journal of Medicine* 340:1476-1480.

[37] Krak, P., Kumar, R., Ardouin, C., Limousin, P., McVicker, J. M., Benabid, A.-L., and Pollak, P. 2001. Mirthful laughter induced by subthalamic nucleus stimulation. *Movement Disorders* 16:867-875.

[38] Ulla, M., Thobois, S., Llorca, P.-M., Derost, P., Lemaire, J.-J., Chereau-Boudet, I., de Chazeron, I., Schmitt, A., Ballanger, B., Broussolle, E., and Durif, F. 2011. Contact dependent reproducible hypomania induced by deep brain stimulation in Parkinson's

disease: clinical anatomical and functional imaging study. *J. Neurology, Neurosurgery, and Psychiatry* 82:607-614.

[39] Frankemolle, A. M. M., Wu, J., Noecker, A. M., Voelcker-Rehage, C., Ho, J. C., Vitek, J. L., McIntyre, and Alberts, J. L. 2009. Reversing cognitive-moto impairments in Parkinson's disease patients using a modelling approach to deep brain programming.

[40] Ilinsky, I. A. and Kultas-Ilinisky, K. 2002. Motor thalamic circuits in primates with emphasis on the area targeted in treatment of movement disorders. *Movement Disorders* 17(S3):S9-S14.

[41] Murata, J.-I., Kitagawa, M., Uesugi, H., Saito, H., Iwasaki, Y., Kikuchi, S., Tashiro, K., and Sawamura, Y. 2003 Electrical stimulation of the posterior subthalamic area for the treatment of intractable proximal tremor. *J. Neurosurgery* 99:708-715.

[42] Plaha, P., Khan, S., and Gill, S. S. 2008. Bilateral stimulation of the caudal zona incerta nucleus for tremor control. *J. Neurology, Neurosurgery, and Psychiatry* 79:504-513.

[43] Follett, K. A., Weaver, F. M., Stern, M., Hur, K., Harris, C. L., Luo, P., Marks, W. J. J., Rothlind, J., Sagher, O., Moy, C., Pahwa, R., Burchiel, K., Hogarth, P., Lai, E. C., Duda, J. E., Holloway, K., Samii, A., Horn, S., Bronstein, J. M., Stoner, G., Starr, P. A., Simpson, R., Baltuch, G., De Salles, A., Huang, G. D., and Reda, D. J. 2010. Pallidal versus subthalamic deep-brain stimulation for Parkinson's disease. *New England Journal of Medicine* 362:2077-2091.

[44] Weaver, F. M., Follett, K. A., Stern, M., Luo, P., Harris, C. L., Hur, K., Marks, W. J. J., Rothlind, J., Sagher, O., Moy, C., Pahwa, R., Burchiel, K., Hogarth, P., Lai, E. C., Duda, J. E., Holloway, K., Samii, A., Horn, S., Bronstein, J. M., Stoner, G., Starr, P. A., Simpson, R., Baltuch, G., De Salles, A., Huang, G. D., and Reda, D. J. 2012. Randomized trial of deep brain stimulation for Parkinson disease: thirty-six-month outcomes. *Neurology* 79:55-65.

[45] Ostrem, J. L., Markun, L. C., Glass, G. A., Racine, C. A., Volz, M. M., Heath, S. L., de Hemptinne, C., and Starr, P. A. 2014. Effect of frequency on subthalamic nucleus deep brain stimulation in primary dystonia. *Parkinsonism and Related Disorders* 20:432-438.

In: Deep Brain Stimulation
Editor: Raja Mehanna

ISBN: 978-1-63483-282-3

Chapter 6

DEEP BRAIN STIMULATION FOR PARKINSON'S DISEASE

Raja Mehanna, MD
University of Texas Health Care Science Center at Houston;
Houston; Texas

ABSTRACT

For the last 50 years, levodopa has been the cornerstone of Parkinson's disease (PD) management. However, a majority of patients develop motor complications a few years after therapy onset. Deep brain stimulation (DBS) has been approved by the FDA as an adjunctive treatment in PD, especially aimed at controlling these complications. In this chapter, we review the available evidence supporting the use of DBS in PD, including its potential impact on cognition and behavior. We then discuss the modality of patient screening and selection as well as target selection for DBS. We conclude with a suggested strategy for programming, with a special mention of stimulation induced balance and speech difficulty.

INTRODUCTION

Parkinson's disease (PD) is a neurodegenerative disorder characterized by the clinical tetrad of motor dysfunction, including tremor, rigidity, akinesia (or bradykinesia) and postural instability (TRAP). It has a prevalence of 1 to 2% above the age of 60 years [1] and typically develops between the ages of 55 and 65 years. The tremor typically starts asymmetrically and is present at rest, usually involving hands, legs, jaw, lips, but sparing the head. Pathologically, PD is classified as a synucleinopathy, associated predominantly with the loss of dopaminergic neurons in the substantia nigra, but other brainstem neurons have been found to degenerate in PD, possibly contributing to not only motor but also non-motor impairment [2]. Indeed, PD is now considered to be a complex syndrome, and is no longer regarded as a pure motor system disorder [3]. For example, neurobehavioral abnormalities are frequent in advanced PD and include depression, dementia, bradyphrenia, apathy, fearfulness, anxiety, emotional lability, social withdrawal, visual–spatial impairment, sleep disturbance and psychosis. Autonomic involvement leads to constipation, bladder and sphincter dysfunction and orthostatic hypotension. Dermatological problems such as seborrhea, sensory problems such as pain and tingling, and special sense disorders such as hyposmia and vestibular dysfunction are also well described [3].

Five years after initiation of therapy, a majority of patients develop medication related motor complications, namely levodopa induced dyskinesias (LID) and motor fluctuations. LID are choreic, stereotypic, and dystonic movements affecting any part of the body [2] and occurring either at peak dose or when the medication is kicking in or wearing off (dyskinesia-improvement-dyskinesia effect). Motor fluctuations occur when the duration of each medication dose is too short and the symptoms of PD recur sooner that initially. This weaning off of the medication effect can occur suddenly and unexpectedly, leaving the patient with markedly decreased mobility and/or severe tremor [4, 5]. Deep brain stimulation (DBS) has been developed primarily to address these treatment related motor complications and therapeutic failures.

The estimated annual health care cost of PD ranges from $2,000 to more than $20,000 per patient [6], with an estimated global economic burden of $4.63 billion [7], the greatest part of which being represented by nursing homes and personal care-giving [8-10] which are much higher in the later stage PD [11].

To better understand the hypothesized mechanism of action of DBS in PD, we will first briefly review the motor circuitry of the basal ganglia. These have been covered in detail in chapter 2. Different motor and non-motor cortical areas project primarily to the striatum which has two major projections: the direct pathway to the globus pallidus pars interna (GPi) and the indirect projection to the GPi via the globus pallidus pars externa and the subthalamic nucleus (STN). The GPi serves as the major output nucleus, which connects back to the cortex via the thalamus. Modulated by the substantia nigra pars compacta, the indirect pathway exerts surround inhibition and thus facilitates an excitatory drive to muscles responsible for a given movement and suppresses unwanted motor activity not relevant to the primary movement. Thus, PD is thought to result from overactivation of the indirect pathway leading to an increased output from the GPi and a decrease in spontaneous movement [12]. This model of the basal ganglia and its connections is, of course, an oversimplification of a complex network that, when disrupted, can result in a range of motor abnormalities [13]. For example, a hyperdirect pathway, projecting directly from the cortex to the STN, and from there to the GPi has recently been added to this model [14].

The loss of dopaminergic neurons in the substantia nigra, the main functional characteristic of PD, affects the circuit described above and leads to the cardinal motor symptoms of PD. While the exact mechanism of this process is unknown, animal research as well as human recordings have provided functional and biochemical evidence that bradykinesia in PD results from excessive activity in the STN and the GPi [3, 5-17]. This leads to an exaggerated beta (10-30Hz) synchronization within and between structures in the basal ganglia circuitry [3] that could also contribute to rigidity and akinesia [18, 19].

The pathophysiology of rest tremor in PD is less clear and probably more complicated. The existence of a unique pacemaker driving the tremor in the thalamus or the GPi has been suggested and then rejected [3]. This symptom most likely results from a dysfunction of both the striato-pallidal-thalamocortical and the cerebello-dentato-thalamocortical circuits [20], with hyperactivity and hypersynchronization between central oscillators [21]. However, contrary to bradykinesia, tremor does not seem to be dependent on beta oscillatory synchronization [22, 23].

DBS acts through delivering an electrical current in a specific target area of the brain. This current can be modulated through modification of voltage, frequency and duration of each electrical pulse delivered. The delivered energy creates an electrical field of variable size and shape according to the parameters used for stimulation. Although initially believed to stimulate the target, thus the name of the whole process, it seems that DBS actually excites the neuronal fibers, but inhibits the neural cells [24, 25]. In fact, GPi DBS decreases the GPi mean firing rate back to a normal range in animal models as well as PD patients [26], and high frequency DBS has a similar effect as dopamine replacement therapies, and promotes faster (about 70 Hz) non-hypersynchronous activity in the basal ganglia, correlated with clinical improvement [27-30]. This might be achieved through stimulation of bypassing inhibitory pathways, synaptic inhibition, depolarizing blockade, synaptic depression, and simulation-induced disruption of pathological network activity [26, 31]. Overall, this leads to modifications of the firing rate and pattern of neurons [32] in the basal ganglia, as well as local release of neurotransmitters such as glutamate and adenosine [33-35]. In addition, it seems that DBS also increases blood flow and stimulates neurogenesis [36].

Over the last few years, functional imaging, specifically functional magnetic resonance imaging (fMRI), positron emission tomography (PET) and single-photon emission computed tomography (SPECT), has been used in an attempt to clarify the mechanism of action of DBS. In fMRI, blood-oxygen-level-dependent (BOLD) signals are acquired, and oxygenated blood marks areas of neural stimulation or inhibition [37-40]. On the other hand, PET and SPECT allow for imaging of multiple activity markers, such as blood flow, glucose and oxygen metabolism [40, 41] . While fMRI is less powerful than nuclear medicine techniques, it provides a much better spatial and temporal resolution.

Because of the suspected inhibitory DBS effects in electrophysiological studies, reduced STN blood flow or glucose metabolism would have been expected on functional imaging. However, the opposite has been found to be true in an overwhelming majority of imaging studies to date [42-49]. In addition, BOLD activation in the area surrounding the electrode has been reported [48, 49], despite the electrode imaging artifact preventing direct observation of the STN around the electrode. This discrepancy between apparent STN inhibition in single-cell studies and activation in imaging studies might be explained by a few hypotheses [50]. First, electrophysiological recordings identify short neuronal modulation (in the order of milliseconds) while neuroimaging methods may reflect the summed activity changes over seconds to minutes. Second, non-neuronal contributions to the change in blood flow and/or glucose metabolism cannot be excluded, and could confound the results of neuroimaging. Finally, it is possible that PET and fMRI actually detect the increased activity in the axons, rather than in the cell bodies. Complicating matters further, some imaging studies after STN DBS have showed increased activity in the GPi [47, 48, 51] while others reported decreased activity in that nucleus [42, 52].

In summary, it is still unclear how exactly DBS affects the firing rate and pattern of neurons and how these changes actually modify the symptoms of Parkinson's disease. DBS is presently more of an empirically proven treatment in search of physiological explanation [53].

Table 1. Randomized controlled trial comparing DBS to optimal medical management

Author,year	Number of patients	Follow up	Target	Results (primary outcome)
Deuschl et al., 2006[54]	156	6 months	BL STN	-Quality of life better with DBS-Motor symptoms better with DBS.
Weaver et al., 2009[55]	255	6 months	BL STN or GPi	Dyskinesia- free ON time 4.6 hours longer with DBS
Williams et al., 2010[56]	366	12 months	BL STN or GPi	-Quality of life better with DBS

Legend: BL: bilateral; STN: subthalamic nucleus; GPi: Globus pallidum pars interna; DBS: deep brain stimulation.

Reproduced form Mehanna et al. [53] with permission from the authors

A. Review of Evidence for DBS in the Treatment of PD

Benefits

The effect of DBS on the cardinal symptoms of PD have been established in three randomized controlled clinical trials (Table 1) [54-56].

The first trial was conducted in Germany and Austria on 156 patients with PD and persistent motor symptoms despite optimal medical therapy [54]. These patients were randomly assigned to DBS of the STN (STN DBS) or optimal medical management. DBS assigned patients had a statistically better quality of life, as measured by the Parkinson's Disease Questionnaire-39 (PDQ-39), as well as motor symptoms control, as measured by the motor part of the Unified Parkinson's Disease Rating Scale (UPDRS, Part III). Another trial conducted in the United States as a double-blinded randomized study and involving 255 patients showed that DBS in either the STN or GPi increased the amount of dyskinesia free ON time at 6 months by 4.6 hours compared to the optimally managed medical group [55]. The statistically significant improvement in quality of life after DBS compared to optimal medical management was reproduced in a third trial on 366 patients followed for 1 year in the United Kingdom [56].

These and other studies have also shown that DBS typically improves "off" time by 4 to 6 hours per day [55, 57, 58], and reduces off symptoms by 60% and medication induced dyskinesias in STN DBS by 60-80% [59].

DBS is thus a reasonable option to consider when medication adjustments do not control disabling symptoms anymore [6, 60, 61]. Animal models of PD have suggested that STN DBS might prevent further neuronal loss and thus have a neuroprotective effect [62-67]. The mechanisms of such effect are unknown, but could include a reduction in excitotoxic induced damage [66]. However, these results have not yet been reproduced in the few human studies evaluating DBS for a neuroprotective effect [68, 69].

On the other hand, Ngoga et al. reported a decrease in mortality and in nursing home admission after STN DBS [70]. This study compared 106 patients who underwent STN DBS to 41 patients who qualified for DBS but declined surgery and continued optimal drug management. All patients had severe PD defined by a Hoehn and Yahr of 3 or 4 in the OFF state, and the two groups were matched for age, gender, ethnicity, duration of disease, rates of preexisting depression and Levodopa equivalent doses of anti-Parkinson's medications taken. Median age in both group was 60 years, median duration of disease at the time that surgery was offered was 11 years in the surgical and 10 years in the medical group ($p=0.413$), and the median duration of follow-up was 7.4 years for surgical and 6.7 years for medical patients. During that time, mortality rate was 17% in the surgical and 41.5% in the medical group ($p=0.004$, Fisher exact test). The decrease in mortality in the DBS group was also seen in a survival analysis performed using Kaplan–Meier survival curves and a Log-Rank test. After correcting for confounding variables, the Hazard Ratio for survival of surgical patients, with respect to medical patient was 0.29 (Confidence Interval 0.13 to 0.64: $p=0.002$). The authors reported that 20% of medically managed patients died from respiratory causes compared to 2% in the surgical group ($p=0.005$). Aspiration pneumonia being the most frequent cause of death in PD [71], a possible explanation to decrease in mortality after STN DBS might be an improvement in deglutition since STN DBS has been reported to improve the oropharyngeal phase of swallowing on videofluorographic swallowing studies [72-76], through improved mobility and reduction in drug related side effects [70]. The nursing home admission rate in that study was 5.7% in the surgical group and 36.6% in the medical group ($p<0.001$, Fisher exact test). After correction for potential confounding factors, the Odds ratio for nursing admission for surgical relative to medical patients was 0.1 (Confidence Interval 0.0 to 0.3; $p<0.001$) [70]. While the authors suggested that DBS can decrease mortality and nursing home admission in PD patients likely through better symptomatic control, it did not demonstrate any impact on the progression of the disease.

Similar to the medical management of PD, DBS is thus a symptomatic treatment and has not been shown to slow the progression of the disease. The duration of the therapeutic benefit has not been clearly established, but modifying the parameters of the stimulation allows the healthcare provider to tailor delivered energy to the patient's symptoms and evolution, and sustained clinical improvement had been reported up to 11 years after implant [77-83]. However, the greatest sources of disability in late-stage PD, including drug-resistant axial motor features, falls and non motor symptoms, especially psychiatric disorders and cognitive decline, are not significantly and consistently modified by DBS [84-86].

In addition to the improvement of motor symptoms, DBS can also improve pain, emotion, akathisia and autonomic function [59, 87-90]. In a series of 41 PD patients treated with STN DBS [91], pain prevalence decreased from 70% to 21% after surgery ($p < 0.001$) with essentially dystonic and musculoskeletal pain responding well to DBS, but not central pain or neuropathic pain. There was no correlation between pain improvement and motor improvement during stimulation. These results were reproduced in another series of 58 STN DBS patients [92], without correlation with motor improvement, depression scores or L-Dopa reduction.

Table 2. Summary of benefits and side effects of DBS in PD

Reported benefits	Reported side effects
Improved QOL	Wound/hardware infection
Decreased OFF time	Intra cranial hemorrhage
Reduced OFF symptoms	Post-operative seizures
Reduced LID	Muscle twitches or tonic contractions
Improved sleep	Paresthesia
Can also improve	Dysphagia
pain	Cognitive impairment
anxiety	Speech impairment
emotion	Visual complaints
akathisia	Mood disorders
autonomic function	Anxiety
working memory	Apathy
psychomotor speed	Impulse control disorders
	Obsessive-compulsive disorder
	Aggression
	Weight gain

Legend: DBS: deep brain stimulation; QOL : quality of life; LID: levodopa induced dyskinesias. Reproduced form Mehanna et al. [53] with permission from the authors.

Additionally, Buhmann et al. reported that STN DBS, but not best medical therapy, improved driving, evaluated with a driving stimulator, back to the level of healthy controls matched for age, despite the fact that patients in the DBS group had more advanced and more prolonged disease than patient with optimal medical therapy [93]. Within the DBS group, driving was also more accurate with stimulation only ON (without medication) than with medication only (without stimulation).

Finally, working memory and psychomotor speed improved in the ON versus OFF stimulation state of bilateral STN DBS in some studies [94]. Open label studies and prospective series also suggest that bilateral as well as unilateral STN DBS improves sleep quality and increases total sleep time, likely by allowing a better control of PD symptoms at night and by a direct effect on sleep architecture (Table 2) [60, 95, 96].

Occasionally, patients might have a suboptimal response to DBS. In a series of 41 such patients, 31 of whom initially diagnosed with PD, Okun et al. reported poor patient screening and selection as the main causes for DBS failure [97]. Other causes included improper electrode location as well as suboptimal DBS programming and medication management. 51% of these patients markedly improved with appropriate management adjustments [97]. Occasionally, patients might require surgical lead repositioning or even the addition of another lead in another brain structure [98]. Troubleshooting DBS failure will be detailed in chapter 10.

While DBS related expenses such as the hardware, surgery, post-surgical programming visits and personal care-giving are relevant [99], STN DBS seems economically more beneficial than optimal medical management through a decrease in drug requirement and cost as well as a reduction in nursing care cost [59, 100-102]. No such data exist for GPi DBS.

Table 3. Controlled studies assessing cognitive change in PD patients after DBS

Author, year	N	F/u (mo)	Lead location	Status of stimulation/ medication at cognitive assessment	Cognitive improvement	Cognitive decline	No change
Castelli et al., 2010 [122]	27	12	STN	ON/ON	None	L	E,A/C, M, L.
Cilia et al., 2007 [113]	20	12	STN	ON/ON	None	L	GC, L, E, A/C
De Gaspari et al., 2006 [118]	12	12	STN	ON/ON	None	L	None
Gironell et al., 2003 [119]	8	6	STN	ON/ON	None	None	L E, A/C, M, V, PS
Hilker et al., 2004 [120]	8	4	STN	ON/-	M	None	GC, E, L, A/C, M, V
Moretti et al., 2003 [129]	9	12	STN	ON/ON	L	L,E	E,L,, A/C, M, V
Morrison et al., 2004 [121]	17	3	STN	ON and OFF/OFF	None	None	L, A/C, M, E, V
Rothlind et al., 2014 [141]	281	6	STN n=84 and GPI n=80	ON/ON	None	A/C, E, GC. See text	A/C, E, GC, L, M
Sáez-Zea et al., 2012 [127]	9	6	STN	ON/ON	None	None	A,M,V,E, L, A/C
Smeding et al., 2006 [126]	99	6	STN	ON/ON	None	L,A/C	L,M,VS, A/C
Whelan et al., 2003 [121]	5	3	STN	ON/ON	L	L	None
Witt et al., 2008 [125]	60	6	STN	ON/ON	None	A/C	GC, E, L, A/C
Witt et al., 2013 [124]	31	6	STN	ON/ON	None	None	GC, A/C, L
York et al., 2009 [114]	23	6	STN	ON/ON	None	M	GC, E, A/C, M, L,V, PS.
Zangaglia et al., 2009 [128]	32	96	STN	ON/ON	None	L	GC, M, E, A/C

Legend: PD: Parkinson's disease; STN: subthalamic nucleus; N: number of patients; mo: months; A/C: Attention/Concentration; E: Executive; GC: Global Cognition; L: language; M: Memory; PS: Psychomotor/Processing speed; V: Visual. [a] : median; [b] : mean

Side Effects

Like all surgeries, DBS implant is not deprived of potential complications (Table 2). The rate of post-operative wound or hardware infection varies from 1.2% to 15.2% in different series [103-105], and most often such incidences require removal of the hardware in addition to an antibiotic course [6, 105]. Intracranial hemorrhage has been reported in 5% of cases, but was symptomatic only in 2.1% of implanted patients and caused a permanent deficit or death in 1.1% [106]. Another larger study on 299 patients after DBS placement reported 1% of intracranial hemorrhage and stroke respectively [58]. Older age and a history of hypertension have been associated with an increased risk of hemorrhage [106]. Post-operative seizures were reported in 2.4% of patients in one review [107], but these do not increase the risk of epilepsy. Prophylactic anticonvulsive therapy before and around surgery is currently unjustified. A transient postoperative confusional state was reported in around 2.4% of the patients [58].

Because the energy delivered to the target can spread to nearby structures and alter their function as well, DBS can induce cognitive and speech impairment, visual complaints, mood disorders including suicidal ideation [108, 109], dysphagia, paresthesia and muscle twitches or tonic contractions. These are most frequently due to a lead positioned too close to the medial STN, optic tract, oculomotor nerve, internal capsule or lemniscal tract. Ideally, these side effects could be reduced or avoided by optimal placement of the lead, with a combined use of anatomic localization and intraoperative microelectrode recording. In addition, using bipolar stimulation settings will create a smaller field with less spreading to adjacent structures, and consequently fewer side effects.

a. Cognitive Side Effects

The most frequent cognitive side effect to DBS seems to be a decrease in verbal fluency; especially when the STN is targeted; [110] although some authors argue this to be a consequence of the implant rather than the stimulation [6]. It is unclear why STN DBS might have a higher rate of cognitive decline and/or depression in some studies. These finding first need to be reproduced; but both current spreading to limbic regions as well as the decreased dose of dopaminergic drugs might be contributory [111].

A recent review of 54 studies totaling 1296 STN DBS patients and 85 GPi DBS patients for cognitive changes after deep brain stimulation in Parkinson's disease [112] reported that only 10 studies included statistical correction for multiple analyzes [113-122] and 13 had a control arm [13, 114, 118-128]. Since most of the information available stems from open label uncontrolled series; a major concern is that a detected cognitive worsening might be secondary to the natural history of PD rather than DBS. It is then worthwhile to take a closer look at the few controlled studies available (Table 3) [112].

No difference was detected between DBS and non DBS PD patients in 6 controlled studies. Gironell et al. [119] reported 8 PD patients who underwent bilateral STN DBS and compared their evolution 6 months after surgery to 8 age and stage-matched PD patients who refused surgery. Evaluations were done ON medication and ON stimulation, and reported worse semantic verbal fluency in the DBS group. However, when corrected for multiple analyzes, this difference was not statistically significant. In addition, no difference was found in the other cognitive tasks assessed. A year later, Morrison et al. [121] compared 17 PD patients who underwent bilateral STN DBS with 11 non surgically treated PD patients. There was no statistically significant difference at 3 months between the 2 groups. In addition, within the DBS group, there was no difference with stimulation ON or OFF at 3 months, or between the stimulation ON at 3 months and the pre-operative assessment. York et al. [114] compared 23 STN DBS patients to 27 medically managed PD patients and reported worse verbal memory in the DBS group at 6 months. Visual memory, all measures of fluency and other cognitive measures were not statistically different between the groups. However, in a follow up to this study, Williams et al. [123] reported on 19 STN patients and 18 medically optimized PD patients 2 years after surgery. While the authors concluded on worsening of some measures of memory, processing and fluency, this was not significant after correction for multiple analyzes. More recently, Sáez-Zea et al. [127] compared the cognitive outcome of 9 bilateral STN DBS patients with 12 non-surgical PD patients 6 months after surgery.

While 4 measures of language and attention, out of the 18 cognitive measures assessed, worsened during that interval, there was no difference between the 2 groups. In addition, a non-statistically significant trend to worse phonemic verbal fluency was observed in the STN-DBS patients but was significantly correlated with reductions in the L -dopa-equivalent daily dose, suggesting that worse fluency observed after STN DBS might in fact be secondary to decrease in the anti-parkinsonian medication. Most recently, Witt el al [124] randomized 62 STN DBS candidates equally to DBS or optimal medical treatment and reported worsening of semantic fluency 6 months after surgery, with no significant change in letter fluency compared to the non-surgical group. However, this difference was not statistically significant after correction for multiple analyzes. Similarly, the other cognitive measures did not differ between the 2 groups.

In contrast, 6 controlled studies suggested worsening of some cognitive measures after DBS, sometimes mitigated by improvement of others. Moretti et al. [129] reported 9 patients with bilateral STN DBS and compared their evolution 12 months after surgery to 9 non-surgically treated PD patients. Assessments were done ON stimulation and ON medications, and reported worsening of some executive function as well as semantic and syllabic fluency, but with an increase in control of linguistic production. The other cognitive measures assessed were not different between the 2 groups. Zangaglia et al. [128] reported worsening of verbal fluency in the STN DBS group (n=32) compared to the medically optimized patient group (n=33) 3 years after surgery. Other cognitive measures were stable over that period of time and did not differ between the 2 groups. Witt et al. [125] compared 60 bilateral STN treated PD patients with 63 STN eligible PD patients who declined surgery ON medications and stimulation 6 months after implant. While this study did not compare cognitive functions to the preoperative baseline, it did nevertheless report statistically worse attention on 2 measures in the STN group, but no difference in the other cognitive measures assessed. Smeding et al. [126] compared 99 STN DBS patients to 39 non DBS patients 6 months after implant in the ON stimulation/ON medication state. They reported a significantly worse decline in fluency and attention/concentration in the STN group. Other cognitive measures were stable over that period of time and did not differ between the 2 groups. Cilia et al. [113] reported statistically significant worsening of category fluency in a group of 20 DBS patients compared to 12 non-surgically treated PD patients 12 months after surgery. Phonemic fluency and other cognitive measures did not differ between the 2 groups. De Gaspari et al. similarly repotted decrease in category fluency in a group of 12 DBS patients compared to 13 non-surgically treated PD patients 12 months after surgery [118]. Last, Castelli et al. compared the change in score between pre-operative baseline and 1 year follow up for each assessed cognitive measure, between 27 STN DBS patients and 31 matched non DBS PD patients [122]. Phonemic fluency was worse in the STN group, while semantic fluency and other cognitive measures were not statistically different between the 2 groups.

Hilker et al., [120] however, compared 8 PD patients ON stimulation 4 months after bilateral STN DBS with 10 healthy matched controls and reported significant improvement in verbal and nonverbal long-term memory, suggesting STN DBS might in fact improve memory circuits compared to non-surgically treated PD patients. The study was not corrected for multiple analyzes and no exact p value was reported. A post hoc correction was not possible and it is unclear if the improvement would have been significant once this correction had been made.

Finally, Whelan et al. [121] compared language between 5 PD patients 3 months after bilateral STN DBS and 16 non surgically treated PD patients. Each of these groups was then compared to another group of 16 healthy aged matched and that difference was again compared between these 2 groups. PD patients were all ON medications and DBS patients had their stimulators ON. When compared to the non-surgically treated PD patients, post DBS patients had improvement on the word test-revised but decline in the accuracy of lexical decisions about words with many meanings and a high degree of relatedness between meanings. It is unclear however, how much these detailed differential results would impact the patients' daily life.

In summary, only half the available controlled studies reported statistically significant worsening on some cognitive measures after bilateral STN DBS. Different subtypes of fluency (semantic, phonemic, category) worsened in some studies but not others. Worsening of attention was also reported in more than one controlled study. On the other hand, 2 controlled studies reported improvement in some cognitive measure after STN DBS.

Available studies on the cognitive impact of DBS on PD patients yielded different and sometimes opposite results. However, when cognitive worsening was detected; it was usually not reported by patients, caregiver or health care providers, suggesting that any change revealed by cognitive tests is subtle [122]. In addition, quality of life is improved after DBS, even when cognitive worsening is detected [130].

Kumar et al. [131] suggested that this could reflect some variability in lead placement inside the target. Comparing postoperative magnetic resonance imaging scans in 8 patients who developed neuropsychological side effects to 30 who did not, Tsai et al. [132] suggested that the neuropsychological effects of chronic STN-DBS were related to an anteriorly located active contact within the ventral STN. York et al. [114] reported that the surgical trajectory through the frontal lobe, in addition to the precise location of the active electrode inside the STN, might also influence the cognitive outcome. Indeed, Witt el al. [124] reported that a trajectory intersecting the caudate nucleus was associated with a higher risk of decline in global cognition and working memory performance. On the other hand, Smith et al. [133] could not find any correlation between decline in verbal fluency and any of age at surgery, number of intraoperative microelectrode penetrations, coordinates of the lead tip or active stimulation site in a series of 28 STN DBS patients.

In addition, the stimulation parameters might also influence the outcome. Wojtecki et al. [134] reported improvement of verbal fluency in 12 PD patients with low frequency (10 Hz) STN DBS compared to no stimulation. Stimulation at 130 Hz had a non-significant trend towards worsening of fluency compared to no stimulation, suggesting a frequency-dependent modulation of cognitive circuits involving the STN. In another study on 20 PD patients treated with bilateral STN DBS, Schoenberg et al. reported that increased amplitude and pulse width of the stimulation were associated with improved cognitive test scores [135].

Trepanier et al. also suspected variations in the characteristics of the patients selected for surgery between different centers (age, preoperative cognitive status, comorbidity with other conditions such as psychiatric disorders) [136]. While advanced age might be considered a risk factor for cognitive worsening, studies showing executive worsening [78, 115, 120, 129, 137, 138] did not have an older population than studies reporting improvement [122,139,140] (mean age of 56.8 vs 58 years).

In a review of the available literature on cognitive changes after STN and GPi DBS in PD patients, we suggested the following: (1) Worsening of one or more cognitive function is rare after DBS in PD patients. Available literature is conflicting, with controlled studies reporting opposite results. (2) When cognitive worsening is detected; it is usually not reported by patients, caregiver or health care providers, suggesting that any change revealed by cognitive tests is subtle. In addition, quality of life is improved after DBS, even when cognitive worsening is detected. (3) Future studies addressing this topic should ideally have a control arm of non-surgically treated PD patients matched for all clinical and demographic variables to control for the natural evolution of the disease. In addition, assessing the DBS group ON and OFF stimulation would provide direct comparisons of the stimulatory effects while controlling for surgical effects, and yield greater power since patients serve as their own controls. (4) More reports on anatomo-clinical correlation of cognitive worsening after DBS would help improve surgical planning to avoid sensitive structures [112].

More recently, in a prospective unblinded randomized controlled study comparing neuropsychological outcome between patients treated with bilateral DBS ON stimulation and ON medication(164 patients, 84 implanted in the STN and 80 in the GPi) and patients treated with optimal medication management ON medication (n=116), Rothlind et al. reported significantly greater mean reductions at 6-month in performance on multiple measures of processing speed and working memory in the combined DBS group, as well as higher rates of decline in neuropsychological test performance in this group [141]. Decline by multiple indicators in two or more cognitive domains was seen in 11% of the DBS patients and 3% of the medically managed patients. This multi-domain cognitive decline was associated with less beneficial change in subjective ratings of everyday functioning and quality of life. However, the authors noted that the majority of individual patients receiving DBS did not display changes on individual measures or combinations of measures that would clearly distinguish them from patients treated with BMT and in fact showed, for most of them, a balance of isolated declines and improvements in test performance similar to the pattern observed in the BMT arm. In other words, worsening of some neuropsychological tests after DBS was observed at a population level, but was unlikely to affect individual patients in the majority of the cases.

b. Behavioral Side Effects

Abnormal behavior, and specifically impulse control disorders such as dopamine dysregulation syndrome in which the patient becomes addicted to dopaminergic drugs, pathological gambling, hyper sexuality, binge eating or compulsive shopping have been reported to worsen or start after STN DBS in some patients, while improving or completely resolving in others [142, 143]. Despite conflicting data in the literature, the presence of impulse control disorders has been traditionally considered a contraindication to STN DBS and in favor of GPi DBS [58, 144]. More recently, Lhommée et al. reported that STN DBS combined with discontinuation of dopamine agonists lead to marked improvement in impulsivity and mood fluctuations in a prospective study of 63 STN DBS patients assessed at baseline then 12 months after surgery [145]. Specifically, 30/30 patients with some form of addictive habit at their preoperative assessment were free from their addiction at 1-year follow-up. On the other hand, one patient with surgical failure experienced new onset of dopaminergic compulsive medication use that was believed to be secondary to failure in dose reduction of dopamine agonists; and 18/30 patients developed apathy at some point during the postoperative year, believed to be secondary to excessive dopamine agonist reduction. In comparison, GPi DBS does not typically allow a significant decrease in dopaminergic drugs

[58, 146], and has also been associated with post-operative behavioral addictions [147]. In addition, STN DBS allowed improvement in ON-period euphoria likely through a decrease in the total dose of dopaminergic drugs as well as improvement in the OFF-period dysphoria likely through a direct positive psychotropic effect of DBS from current diffusion to the non-motor territories of the STN. Lhommée et al. concluded that non only impulsive control disorders should not deter from STN DBS in favor of GPi DBS, but that "hyperdopaminergic behaviors as well as non-motor fluctuations are becoming new indications for STN DBS" [145].

Similarly, Castrioto et al. reported on a series of 20 patients with improvement in the IOWA gambling task in 7/8 patients 3 months after STN DBS, attributed to decrease in dopaminergic medications [148].

However, further studies formally comparing post-operative behavior after STN and GPi DBS are needed.

c. Mood Changes After DBS in PD Patients

Changes in mood and behavior have been reported after DBS. Bejjani et al. first reported one patient with transient acute depression after STN DBS, but the tip of the electrode was actually misplaced in the substantia nigra (SN) [149]. Then, Berney et al. reported on a series of 24 consecutive PD patients followed for up to 6 months after bilateral STN DBS and found significant worsening of mood in 6 patients (25%) despite a marked improvement in motor symptoms that was similar between depressed and non depressed patients [150]. In this series, post-operative MRI confirmed the accurate location of the lead in the STN. However, Krack et al. reported no worsening of depression 5 years after bilateral STN DBS in a series of 42 PD patients [117].

In contrast, Kulisevsky et al. described 3 patients who developed a manic episode after STN DBS [151]. However, post-operative imaging suggested the implant was too deep and actually located in the SN, and the behavioral abnormality resolved with stimulation of more dorsal contacts. In addition, Romito et al. reported 2 patients, out of a series of 30, who developed mania a few days after turning ON their STN DBS [152]. Mania did not resolve with stimulation parameters change or turning the DBS off for a few hours, or with decrease in L dopa, but gradually disappeared spontaneously over a few months. Most recently, Welter et al. reported hypomania in 19/262 STN DBS patients, which was related to a younger age, shorter disease duration, higher levodopa responsiveness, and a ventral contact location [153].

However, in a small series of 9 PD patients, Okun et al. reported mood improvement after GPi or STN DBS compared to no stimulation and attributed negative mood changes to suboptimal placement of the DBS lead, either ventral or dorsal to the optimal location [154].

On the other hand, in a series of 322 unilateral DBS procedures (195 STN, 71 Vim, and 56 Gpi, Burdick et al. reported an increase in anger score on the visual analogue mood scale after STN or GPi DBS for Parkinson's disease [155]. There was no difference between the 2 targets, and the anger score changes seemed associated to the number of microelectrode pass and not affected by the stimulation status (ON or OFF), suggesting this was an effect of lead implant rather than stimulation. The change was also more evident with longer duration of PD. In contrast, anger scores did not worsen after Vim DBS in ET patients, despite longer disease duration in this group. These results have not yet been replicated, and their impact on the patients' daily life is unknown.

Finally, Burkard et al. observed a high rate of suicide (6/140 patients, 4.3%) in a large retrospective series of patients with movement disorders treated with DBS [156]. Apparent risk factors included a previous history of severe depression and multiple successive DBS surgeries, but there was no relationship with the underlying condition (PD, ET or dystonia), the DBS target (STN, GPi or Vim), stimulation parameters, or modifications of treatment. Paradoxically, all patients experienced an excellent motor outcome following the procedure. While the spread of the current to non-motor, associative or limbic, parts of the STN or GPi may play a role in acute mood changes occasionally observed in some cases, it appears less likely to be the cause of increased suicide in this series as suicide completion occurred years after DBS surgery, could not be related to recent parameter modifications, and was also observed with stimulation of the Vim. It seems than, rather than causing the suicidal ideation, DBS may have facilitated the decision to act –out in patients at risk. This underlines the need for a thorough screening of DBS candidates, with the exclusion of high suicide risk patients from the procedure. With similar conclusions, Houeto et al. reported worsening of pre-existing psychiatric disorders in patient undergoing BL STN for DBS, as well as improvement of personality traits in some patients without a previous psychiatric history, underlining, once again, the importance of appropriate patient screening [157]. In addition, Weintraub et al. reported no increase in suicidality 6 months post DBS compared to BMT, as well as no difference in suicidality between STN DBS and GPi DBS in a prospective randomized controlled trial of 255 PD patients [158].

B. Patients Screening and Selection

Not all PD patients are candidates for DBS, and a thorough multidisciplinary screening process is required to determine those who are good candidates [159, 160]. In a retrospective chart review of 233 PD patients who were candidates for DBS, Abboud et al. reported that 41.2% were not implanted after completing the screening process, advocating, like many other authors, the need for thorough screening to avoid implanting poor candidates that will either not benefit enough from DBS, or poorly tolerate it [161].

In the current context of reducing unnecessary expenses, this screening process can be staged to help reduce costs and improve its efficiency (Figure 1) [53]. Patients should first undergo a thorough clinical evaluation from the neurologist to ascertain the diagnosis and exclude other causes of parkinsonism, such as vascular parkinsonism or atypical parkinsonism that are refractory to DBS. The neurologist should optimize medical management before offering DBS. Patients should then discuss at length with the neurologist and neurosurgeon to assess their understanding of the risk/benefits ratio of the surgery. If the patients then clearly understand this commitment and wish to proceed, the ON levodopa/OFF levodopa motor testing can be performed. In the ON/OFF testing, the patient is asked to withhold all PD medications for 12 hours before undergoing examination with the United Parkinson's Disease Rating Scale (UPDRS). The patient is then given his regular dose of levodopa and the UPDRS is administered again after the patient reports feeling the full effect of this dose. ON and OFF UPDRS scores are compared and an improvement of at least 30% after medication intake is typically recommended to proceed to the next step. Indeed, only the symptoms that improve with levodopa are expected to improve with DBS, with the notable exception of medication refractory tremor that can still improve after surgery. DBS should thus be offered to patients with levodopa-responsive symptoms [162]. At that point, if the patient is still considered a good candidate for surgery, brain MRI, neuropsychological testing and psychiatry evaluation would be pursued.

In addition to insuring appropriate patient selection, following this algorithm will decrease the cost of medical expenses by delaying costly evaluation such as MRI and neuropsychological evaluation until after thorough neurological and neurosurgical clinical evaluations and open discussion with the patient. However, this can increase the patient's inconvenience and direct cost given that it might imply multiple trips to a health care facility. These draw back could be decreased by scheduling all the procedures and visits within a 48-hour window and in the order suggested in the algorithm, and, if at any step in the process the patient is found not to be a good DBS candidate, the process can be terminated and the remaining visits or procedures cancelled [161]. Finally, we recommend paying close attention to social factors (such as family support, travel and distance from the center, financial stability, and so on) when screening patients as these are instrumental for post-operative programming visits that will occur monthly early on and then at least 4 times a year.

Age

While most of the randomized controlled trials excluded patients older than 75 years of age, and surgeons are often resistant to perform surgery in an older patient for fear of increased post-operative complications, DeLong et al. conducted a retrospective non-controlled study on 1757 DBS patients, 7% of which were 75 years or older at the time of surgery, and showed no increase in the frequency of complications or in duration of hospital stay with increasing age at the time of surgery [163]. It thus seems that older age should not be an exclusion criterion by itself, but the same screening steps detailed above should apply to all DBS candidates, regardless of age.

Target Selection

Once a patient is determined to be a good candidate for DBS, a target for the procedure has to be selected. Ablative surgery or DBS of the ventral intermediate (Vim) nucleus of the thalamus is being used for essential and other secondary causes of tremor. However, because it does not address the other cardinal motor symptoms of PD, Vim DBS is rarely used for that disorder [164]. The two main targets considered for DBS in PD are the STN and the GPi (Table 4).

Anderson et al. conducted the first randomized controlled trial comparing STN DBS and GPi DBS. This trial included only 20 patients followed for 12 months and showed both targets to be equally effective for improving PD motor symptoms and dyskinesia. It also showed a greater decrease in dopaminergic medication use in the STN group (p=0.08) as well as cognitive and behavioral complications exclusively in that group [165].

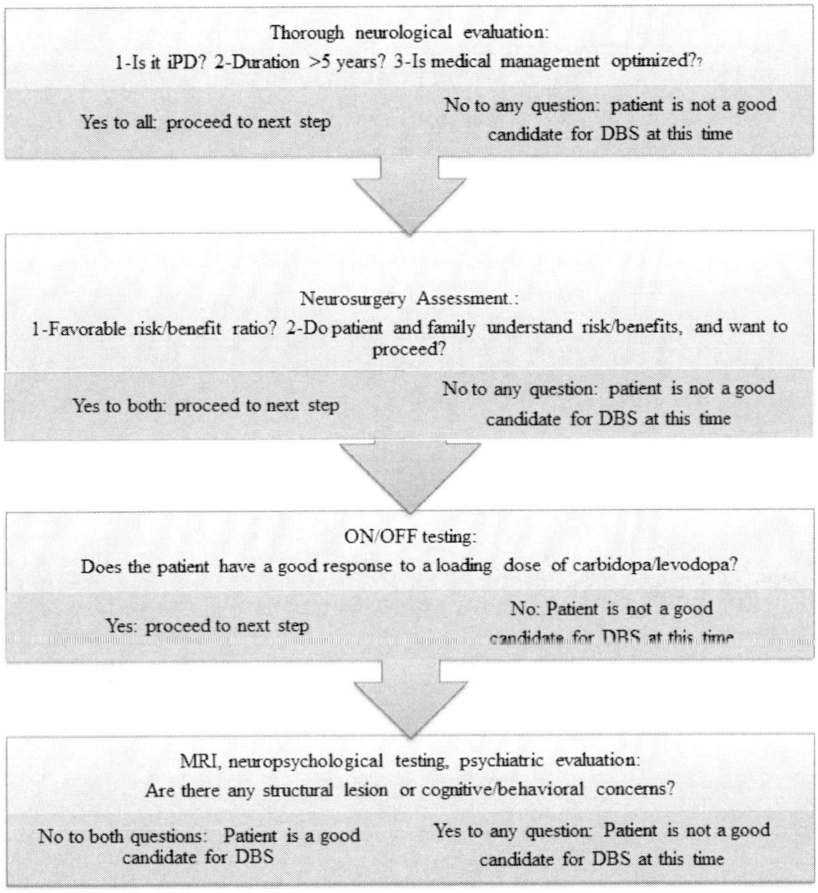

Figure 1. Suggested staging of the screening process for patients with Parkinson disease being evaluated for deep brain stimulation (DBS).

The COMPARE trial included 45 patients with unilateral GPI or STN DBS who were followed for 7 months [166]. The 2 targets were similar in motor control improvement and side effects profiles including mood and cognition, except for worsening of verbal fluency in the STN DBS group GPi DBS patients had a bigger improvement in their quality of life compared to STN patients (38 vs. 14%, respectively; P = 0.03) with decrease in verbal fluency potentially contributing to less improvement in the STN patients [167]. However, decrease in verbal fluency was not statistically significant between the 2 groups once correction for multiple analyses was made [112]. In a follow up to the COMPARE trial including 52 patients, unilateral STN DBS implant carried a 5.2 times increased risk to require a contralateral DBS implant at 3 years, when compared to unilateral GPi DBS implant [168].

In a large multicenter randomized control trial, Follett et al. [58] followed 299 patients for 2 years. GPi and STN DBS were similar in motor control improvement and side effects profiles, except for requiring lower doses of dopaminergic medications in STN DBS patients (p=0.03 and 0.02 respectively). The level of depression reportedly improved in the GPi DBS group while it worsened in STN DBS patients, but the difference between both groups was not significant after correction for multiple analyzes. Finally, the authors reported severe decline in visuomotor processing in the STN group, but this also was not statistically significant after correction for multiple analyzes [112]. At the 3-year follow-up of the same group, including 159 patients, Weaver et al. [169] showed that the 2 targets were similar in motor control improvement and side-effect profiles, except for worse cognitive performance in the STN group at 3 years (p=0.01). This study also confirmed the greater reduction in dopaminergic drugs in the STN group.

The most recent double blinded randomized controlled trial comparing STN and GPi DBS included 128 patients and reproduced the lack of significant difference in quality of life improvement between the 2 targets at 1 year [170]. However, there was greater improvement in the OFF phase motor score and disability in STN DBS patients (p=0.03). This study also confirmed a greater decrease in dopaminergic medication doses in the STN group (p=0.01). However, there was no difference in cognitive, psychiatric and behavioral side-effects between the 2 groups.

Table 4. Randomized controlled trials comparing STN and GPi DBS

Author, year	Number of patients	Follow up	Side	Similar results	Differences in results, after correction for multiple analysis when needed.
Anderson et al., 2005[165]	20	12 months	Bilateral	• Motor symptoms	• Greater decrease in dopaminergic drug dosage with STN. • Cognitive and behavioral complications exclusively with STN.
Okun et al., 2009[166]	45	7 months	Unilateral	• Motor symptoms. • Side effects including mood and cognition.	• Greater improvement in QOL with GPi [117]. • Higher risk to require controlateral DBS implant in STN group [112].
Follett et al., 2010[58]	299	24 months	Bilateral	• Motor symptoms. • Side effects profile.	• Greater decrease in dopaminergic drug dosage with STN.
Weaver et al., 2012[169]	159	36 months	Bilateral	• Motor symptoms. • Side effects profile.	• Greater decrease in dopaminergic drug with STN. • Worse cognitive performance with STN
Odekerken et al., 2013[170]	128	12 months	Bilateral	• Quality of life. • Cognitive, psychiatric and behavioral side effects	• Greater decrease in dopaminergic drug dosage with STN. • Greater improvement in the OFF phase motor score with STN • Greater improvement in disability with STN

Legend: STN: subthalamic nucleus; GPi: Globus pallidum pars interna; DBS: deep brain stimulation; QOL: quality of life.

Adapted from Mehanna et al. [53] with permission from the authors.

Table 5. Studies comparing cognitive outcome between GPi and STN DBS in PD patients

Author, year	N STN/GPi	Laterality	F/u (mo)	Status of stimulation/ medication at cognitive assessment	Cognitive measures assessed	Differences between GPI and STN
Rothlind et al., 2007 [172]	19/23	UL	6	ON/ON	A/C,E,L,V,M	None
Rothlind et al., 2007 [172]	14/15	BL	21	ON/ON	A/C,E,L,V,M	None
Okun et al., 2009 [166]	22/23	UL	7	ON/OFF	L	None
Follett et al., 2010 [58]	147/152	BL	24	ON/OFF	GC, L, V, E, M	None
Weaver et al., 2012 [169]	70/89	BL	36	ON/OFF	GC, L, V, E,M	M worse with STN
Odekerken et al., 2013 [170]	63/65	BL	12	ON/Integrated ON and OFF	Composite test	None
Rothlind et al., 2014 [141]	84/80	BL	6	ON/ON	A/C, E, GC, L, M	None

Legend: PD: Parkinson's disease; GPi: globus pallidus interna; STN: subthalamic nucleus; N: number of patients; mo: months; UL: unilateral; BL: bilateral; A/C: Attention/Concentration; E: Executive; GC: Global Cognition; L: language; M: Memory; V: Visual.

Adapted from Mehanna [112] with permission from the author.

While multiple studies did not show any difference in the rate of depression between GPi and STN DBS [58, 166, 167], a meta-analysis of 4 randomized controlled trials [58, 165, 167, 170] comparing GPI to STN DBS in PD patients reported similar improvement in UPDRS ON medications, less depression after GPi DBS (RR=0.53, 95% CI 0.31 to 0.90, p=0.02) and no difference in the frequency of confusion/delirium, intracranial haemorrhage, dysarthria/speech problems, balance disorder or stroke/TIA [171]. The higher frequency of depression after STN might be secondary to the greater decrease in dopaminergic drugs after surgery in that group.

A current tendency is to prefer GPi DBS for patients with mild cognitive impairment for fear that STN DBS is associated with more cognitive side effects. It is unclear why STN DBS might have a higher rate of cognitive decline in some studies, but both current spreading to limbic regions as well as the decreased dose of dopaminergic drugs have been presented as possibly contributory [111].

While there is more data reporting cognitive worsening after STN DBS, this data is markedly imbalanced as the published studies on this topic have evaluated 15 times more STN DBS than GPi DBS patients [112]. Therefore, a closer and more critical look at head to head comparison between the 2 targets is needed.

To our knowledge, 6 studies have compared head to head the cognitive impact of STN and GPi DBS (Table 5) [58, 112, 166, 169, 170, 172, 141]. Only one [166] reported correction for multiple analyses. After corrections were applied when needed, only Weaver et al. reported worsening on one memory test 3 years after STN DBS compared to GPi DBS, in 159 patients [169]. The other studies, totaling 678 subjects (335 STN and 343 GPi) followed up to 2 years, could not detect any statistically significant difference between the 2 targets. While this discrepancy might be explained by the longer follow up in the study of Weaver et al., it is interesting to note that it did not report any worse decline in language, fluency, attention or executive function in the STN group, as would have been expected form the open labeled and nonsurgical patient matched series discussed earlier in this chapter.

Regarding the specific issue of gait and balance problems in PD, there is no definitive data to suggest whether the GPi target or the STN target is preferable, but a meta-analysis revealed a slightly superior effect of STN-DBS compared with GPi-DBS on these symptoms within the first postoperative year [173] and a multicenter study demonstrated a trend toward a stronger anti-akinetic effect of STN DBS at 6 years [174]. However, in a double-blind study comparing 14 STN BDS patients to 14 GPi DBS patients, all with PD, St George et al. reported that, although gait and balance were better in the GPi group when patient were OFF stimulation and medication, both groups had similar improvement of gait and balance with stimulation only ON, as well as when both stimulation and medications were ON [175].

Taking all these data into consideration, the current tendency is to prefer targeting the STN because of a greater improvement in the OFF phase motor symptoms as well as a higher chance to decrease the medication dosage and a lower battery consumption linked to the use of lower voltage in the STN compared to the GPi DBS. Lower battery consumption correlates with longer battery life and thus less frequent surgery to replace it [170]. However, the cost of therapy in the first 36 months after surgery, which is usually before the first battery replacement, seems to be similar between the 2 targets [176]. On the other hand, GPi DBS has a direct anti-dyskinestic effect when stimulation is delivered to the ventral part of the nucleus, while decrease in LID after STN DBS can be achieved through the decrease in medication dose. For that reason, GPi can be the preferred target if LID is the main complaint. Indeed, 3 patients with severe dystonia and LID 8 years after STN DBS improved after GPi DBS [177].

Because of its role in locomotion, the pedunculopontine nucleus (PPN) has been suggested as a DBS target to address gait difficulty and freezing of gait, which are typically resistant to STN or GPi DBS. A few small observational or open labeled studies have been conducted, evaluating PPN DBS as an add-on to STN DBS [79, 178-183]. Precise anatomical lead locations as well as results were controversial, and speech deterioration was noted in one series [184]. One study reported some improvement in gait initiation in 10 PD patients after unilateral PPN DBS, without STN DBS [185]. In addition, 2 patients with PD and Pisa syndrome, a postural disorder clinically defined as the sustained lateral bending of the trunk, were reported to have improvement of their Pisa syndrome after PPN DBS. One patient was implanted ipsilateraly to his trunkal bending [186], and the other contralaterally [187]. Unfortunately, the improvement was only transient in both cases. In conclusion, PPN DBS cannot be recommended at this point.

Because of its dense reciprocal interconnections to the PPN, the Substancia Nigra pars reticulata (SNr) has also been investigated for treatment resistant gait difficulties. Exclusive SNr stimulation was not beneficial [188]. Combined SNr-DBS and STN DBS was proven to be safe and without clinically relevant neuropsychiatric side effects but overall not superior to STN-DBS alone in a randomized double-blinded, cross-over trial including 12 patients [189]. However, freezing of gait was improved in the combined group, and larger studies are needed. At this time, add on SNr DBS after STN DBS cannot be recommended for treatment resistant gait difficulties.

Timing of Surgery

Currently, patients are not considered for DBS unless they do not tolerate levodopa, become resistant to medications or have complications from medical therapy, while still being medically and psychologically fit for surgery. Some authors suggest that exhausting all pharmacological options before considering DBS can delay the surgery to a time when the patient is no longer fit because of disease progression [190, 191].

A small randomized trial of bilateral STN DBS in 10 patients with early PD (mean duration of 7 years) compared to 10 matched medically treated controls showed a significant benefit from DBS on quality of life, motor control and decrease in levodopa doses [192]. More recently, Schüpbach et al. conducted EARLYSTIM, a randomized controlled trial comparing bilateral STN DBS to optimal medical management in 251 PD patients aged less than 60 years, with PD for more than 4 years but with motor fluctuations and dyskinesia for 3 years or less and a Hoehn and Yahr below Stage III when ON medications [193]. Patients had levodopa therapy duration of 4.9 years and fluctuations and/or dyskinesia present for 1.5 or 1.7 years respectively. At 2 years follow up, quality of life and motor control, but also emotion, cognition and communication were superior in the DBS group. Prevalence of moderate to serious adverse events was comparable between the 2 groups, except for a higher frequency of depression in the surgical group, despite an overall improvement in mood at the end of the trial.

With a mean age of onset of 52 years as compared with 59 to 62 years in other trials [56, 57, 77, 170] and a mean duration of PD of 7.5 years, as compared with 10.8 to 13.8 years [54, 56, 57, 58, 170] this study demonstrated the added benefit of early DBS in PD symptoms control, when medical treatment is still effective. However, some authors raised concerns that offering DBS within 5 years of symptoms onset might include patients with atypical parkinsonism who are unlikely to benefit from it, and that complications of surgery such as stroke or intracerebral hemorrhage might have a bigger socio-economic impact on younger patients [194].

More recently, a small pilot randomized controlled trial assessed DBS at an even earlier stage of PD, involving 15 patients treated with STN DBS and optimal drug therapy to 15 patients treated with optimal drug therapy alone [195]. Patients were 50 to 75 years old, had a Hoehn and Yahr Stage II when off medications, were treated with antiparkinsonian medications for greater than six months but less than or equal to four years, and had no current or prior history of motor fluctuations. This study aimed at assessing safety and tolerability of STN DBS very early in PD, and reported no difference in various motor and quality of life scales in both OFF medication/stimulation and ON medication/stimulation at 2 years, but a greater decrease in medication dosage in the DBS group. There were also no differences in cognitive side effects, but one patient in the DBS group had a basal ganglia stroke with permanent cognitive deficit and transient motor deficit. While this small study shows the safety and tolerability of DBS even before motor fluctuations develop, it does not support the use of DBS that early and more studies are needed.

In addition, an analytic model of STN DBS, defined by off time and applied at an early versus delayed stage, concluded that early DBS increases quality-adjusted life years and reduces treatment costs [196]. However, further studies in this area are warranted before recommending early DBS placement in PD patients. In addition, it would be wise to wait 5 years after the onset of symptoms before performing the surgery, in order to rule out any atypical parkinsonism.

One should keep in mind, however, that the study assessing survival after DBS compared to BMT detailed previously in this chapter, Ngoga et al., reported a statistically significant improvement in survival when surgery was offered during the first 10 years of the disease progression compared to longer durations [70].

C. Programming in PD

Suggested Algorithm

There is no randomized clinical trial proving the superiority of one algorithm over another. However, it is very important to have a clear plan when starting to program a patient, keeping an open mind so it can always be modified based on the patient's feedback. Following an algorithm allows a programming specialist (physician or other) to know what steps have likely already been tried by looking at the patient's present settings, without having to go through huge amounts of prior programming summaries to see what has already been tried. We here provide the one we follow (Figure 2). On a side note, although many centers utilize specially trained nurses or physician assistant to program their patients, while physicians manage the medical treatment, it is our experience that optimal patient management requires that the same person, in this case the physician, manages both in order to better integrate these 2 complementary but not identical treatment modalities.

Programming starts on the first post-surgical visit, usually 4 weeks after DBS implant to allow any potential clinical benefit induced by the edema created during implant, known as microlesion effect, to subside. Patient should present OFF medication for at least 12 hours, to fully assess the benefit of stimulation without the confounding factor of motor fluctuations or LID induced by medications. This first visit lasts around one hour per side stimulated. It is also known as monopolar review as all 4 monopolar configurations (using the IPG as anode and each of the 4 contacts on the electrode as cathodes successively) should be tested. Electrode impedance is checked to rule out any open circuit (broken wire) or short circuit (unwanted and unexpected flow of current between two electrode contacts). If such a situation is identified, programming should avoid using the involved contact(s). A fixed pulse width (usually 60 or 90 microsecs) and frequency (usually 130 Hz or above) are selected and kept constant throughout the visit. Of note, it has been reported than frequency at or above 130Hz control tremor much better than frequency around 60Hz [197], but no studies could demonstrate an inter-individual reproducible optimal frequency for improvement of bradykinesia or rigidity.

Starting with a monopolar configuration at contact 0 (recorded as C+0-, where C stands for Case which is the implanted program stimulator, or battery), response to stimulation at an increasing voltage is noted on tremor, bradykinesia and rigidity. Rigidity is the most reliable sign to examine serially as bradykinesia can be effort dependent and tremor can spontaneously fluctuate. Typical increases in voltage would be of the order of 0.5 V. Two important thresholds have to be recorded: the therapeutic threshold at which clinically

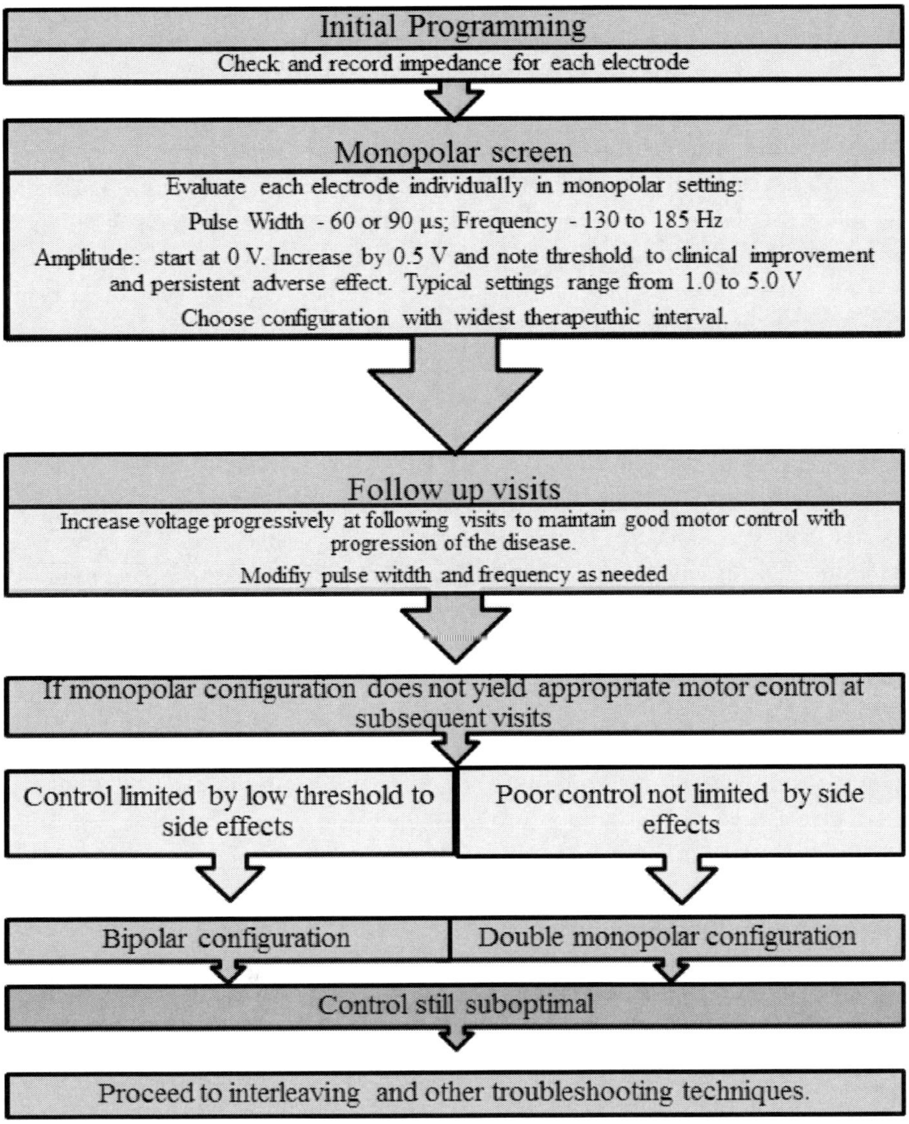

Figure 2. Suggested algorithm for DBS programming in PD patients.

significant improvement is seen, and the adverse effect threshold at which clinically significant side effects (muscle twitching/contraction, visual changes, persistent paresthesia or other subjective changes such as dizziness) are detected. It should be noted that patients frequently report transient paresthesia just after voltage increase that usually resolves within a few seconds. While important to note, these do not usually define the adverse event threshold as they are transient. The voltage difference between the therapeutic threshold and adverse event threshold constitute a therapeutic interval.

The wider this interval, the better, as it gives more room for increase in voltage with the progression of the disease. It is thus very important to continue testing at higher voltages until the adverse event threshold is found, and not to stop just after clinical benefit is noted. Once the review of one monopolar configuration is complete, the voltage is brought back to zero, which means stimulation is stopped. The following monopolar configuration is set (C+1-) but the steps detailed above should not be re-initiated until the PD symptoms come back to their baseline, to avoid any residual effect from the previous stimulation [198]. This usually requires around 5 minutes, but sometimes a little bit longer. These steps are repeated for all monopolar configurations. At the end of the monopolar review, the physician will have 4 therapeutic intervals, corresponding to the 4 monopolar configurations, and should choose the configuration with the largest interval. The type of side effect encountered may also affect the choice of the configuration, as patients tend to develop tolerance to subjective side effects (persistent paresthesia or other subjective changes such as dizziness) but not to muscle twitching/contraction or visual changes, making the latter less desirable. Initiating the stimulation will generally require a decrease in total dopamine equivalent dosage, especially in STN DBS, to avoid LID. However, one should be careful not to decrease it too low and too fast so as not to lose symptom control.

Over successive visits, voltage can be increased as needed to control motor symptoms, but usually not more than 0.4V per side of stimulation and per encounter, to avoid severe side effects from too much stimulation, effects than can sometimes take a few days to develop and not be visible in clinic. With newer IPG that allow to store more than one program created by the physician in clinic, and in between which the patient can switch using the patient's hand held device at home, it is useful to have the habit of always saving the previous settings (if they were well tolerated) as a "program B" and instruct the patient to switch back to that program if intolerable and persistent side effects were to develop at home. This would avoid many panicky urgent visits to the clinic or even to the emergency room. Similarly, new programmers give the physician the option to delegate some control of the parameters to the patient: if the patient is reliable, the physician can choose one variable (pulse width, amplitude or frequency) and set a lower and upper limit in between the patient can modify the variable in case of side effects or little benefits.

If benefits from the best monopolar configuration, as determined by the monopolar review, are not enough despite successive increase in voltage over multiple visits, one should consider increasing the pulse width and /or the frequency. The STN being a smaller target, we would not recommend going above 90 microsecs of pulse width as it will most likely cause side effects by current spreading to unwanted nearby structures. The GPi, being as larger structure, can tolerate higher pulse width, up to 240 microsecs as seen in some patient with dystonia. However, such high numbers are unlikely to be needed in PD patients. Once the amplitude of 5 volts, frequency of 180HZ and pulse width of 90 microsecs (for the STN) have been reached, and control of previously dopamine responsive symptoms by the combination of DBS and medications is not satisfactorily, then the second best monopolar configuration, as determined by the monopolar review, should be selected and the steps above repeated. If control is still unsatisfactory, but without limiting side effects at low threshold, then a double monopolar configuration should be used, to enlarge the stimulation field. In this configuration, the IPG is selected as the anode, and the 2 best contacts, as determined by the monopolar review and with the input of the first configuration tried, are selected as cathodes. One should use a lower voltage in this configuration to avoid too much current spread, and the increase at each visit should be limited to 0.2 V (that would be 0.2 V at each cathode, for a total of 0.4 V). Of note, dorsal stimulation of the GPi has a strong anti-bradykinesia effect and can in fact induce dyskinesia similar to STN stimulation. Inversely, ventral stimulation of the GPi can worsen akinesia while suppressing dyskinesia and improving rigidity. This anatomical difference should be taken into consideration and correlated to the clinical picture, with more ventral contacts selected when dyskinesia is the main complaint, and more dorsal contacts selected if akinesia is most bothersome.

On the other hand, if side effects are limiting the increase in voltage without good symptom control, then a bipolar stimulation should be considered. It this configuration, the contact with the best symptom control will be selected as cathode, and the 2nd best contact as anode. This creates a smaller field, concentrating it in the target and preventing current spread to adjacent structures. Voltage requirement are typically higher than in a monopolar configuration because of the more condensed field.

If monopolar, double monopolar or bipolar settings do not yield satisfactory results, intereleaving can be considered. Interleaving allows a clinician to define two stimulation programs that automatically alternate. It can sometimes be used to provide differential therapeutic benefits with the possibility of fewer side effects. It is most likely to be useful in two clinical scenarios: 1) when different contacts are beneficial for specific symptoms, but each at a different stimulation amplitude. For example, Wojtecki et al. reported a PD patient whose rigidity and bradykinesia responded to STN stimulation at contact 1 at 3.9 V, but whose tremor responded best to stimulation at contact 3 at 1.5 V [199]. Using double monopolar stimulation (in which both contact have to use the same amplitude) at 3 V or higher (to control rigidity and bradykinesia) lead to unacceptable dysarthria. However, interleaving between these 2 programs allowed good control of the 3 symptoms without side effects. 2) When symptoms are resolved incompletely and further voltage increase is limited by side effects. In this case, interleaving between 2 partially successful stimulation programs might allow better symptom control without side effects. The exact mechanism of action of interleaving is unknown, but it is speculated that the 2 programs can potentially create an effective field that is the results of the 2 individual fields, although the pulses from these 2 programs are offset from each other [200]. However, interleaving may drain the neurostimulator battery faster than the conventional settings, and its maximal frequency is limited to 125Hz, which may be suboptimal for tremor control [201].

If all the above fail, then poor positioning of the DBS lead must be suspected and surgical revision might need to be considered. DBS troubleshooting will be detailed in chapter 10.

Gait Issues

Gait, traditionally resistant or occasionally worsened by DBS, deserves special mention.

Although STN DBS has been reported to improve postural instability and gait disorders in many small studies [202-206], usually to the extent of the improvement observed with levodopa [174], other small studies did not replicate these results [197] and gait was not specifically and individually assessed it large trials. Postoperative worsening of gait has been reported in up to 40% of patients in some series despite overall improvement of outcome scores [207].

Moreau et al. reported on 13 bilateral STN DBS patients that the combination of low frequency (Mean 60 Hz) and high voltage (Mean 3.7V) might help decrease the frequency of freezing of gait in advanced PD, while a high frequency (Mean 130 Hz) and low voltage (mean 3V) might actually worsen freezing in those patients [208]. Later on, Xie et al. reported

2 PD patients who developed freezing of gait immediately upon activation of the newly placed STN DBS, that was alleviated by switching frequency from 130 Hz to 60 Hz and without changing any other stimulation parameters [209]. More recently, Phibbs et al. reported on 20 bilateral STN DBS that low frequency stimulation (60Hz) was not superior to high frequency stimulation (130Hz) if the decrease in frequency was not compensated by an increase in voltage to try to maintain the same amount of energy delivered [210]. Then, in a study on 7 PD patients with bilateral STN DBS and freezing on gait, Xie et al. reported a 57% decrease in aspiration frequency on modified barium swallow as well as a significant improvement in freezing of gait with a stimulation frequency of 60hz compared to 130 Hz without change in voltage but with patients ON medications [211]. The apparent contradiction between the last 2 studies might be explained by the ON medication status that alleviated the need for a higher voltage in the study from Xie et al., while patients in the study of Phibbs et al. required higher voltages to compensate for being OFF medications. However, in a study on 19 patients, Vallabhajosula et al. reported that total UPDRS-III score, step length and velocity during gait initiation, as well as gait speed significantly improved during low frequency (60 Hz) and high frequency (>100 Hz) stimulation conditions when compared to no stimulation [206]. But there were no statistically significant differences between low frequency and high frequency stimulation with the same voltage, or between high frequency stimulation at a lower voltage and low frequency stimulation at a higher voltage. Finally, in a study on 10 PD patients with STN or GPI DBS, Dhall et al. reported that stimulation frequency of 80 Hz led to improvement of gait variables in more patients than a frequency of 30 HZ or 130 hz, but the number was very small and the difference was not statistically significant. In addition, STN and GPi patient were lumped together, and no information regarding target specific frequency was available [212].

In conclusion, is seems that switching from high (130Hz) to low (60Hz) frequency, with an increase in voltage to maintain a similar amount of energy delivered, could improve gait in PD patients who experience severe gait deterioration after high frequency STN-DBS. However, not all such patients might improve [213] and this switch should also not be expected to improve gait in those who do not experience this gait worsening. One should also remember that low frequency has a lesser beneficial impact on tremor than high frequency stimulation [197, 210]. No studies assessing programming strategies to improve gait after GPi have been reported.

Another approach is that post DBS worsening of gait can be caused by an unfavorable stimulation setting that accentuates lower limbs asymmetry and thus interferes with inter-limb coordination [214]. Reducing asymmetry by decreasing stimulation of the better controlled side can be attempted when facing a patient with stimulation-resistant gait freezing [174]. One study also reported that stimulation of more dorsal contacts might improve step velocity, step length, and balance more so than ventral stimulation [215], but another study concluded the opposite, advocating the use of more ventral contacts in the STN to improve gait [216]. No conclusion can be drawn on this point specifically for gait, but one should remember that dorsal contacts are usually optimal for high-frequency STN DBS [217, 218].

On a side note, hypophonia and dysarthria, typically resistant to DBS, might improve on low frequency (60Hz) compared to high freq (130Hz) or OFF stimulation in PD patients with STN DBS [219], but this has not yet been replicated

CONCLUSION

For the last 50 years, levodopa has been the cornerstone of PD management. However, a majority of patients develop motor fluctuations and/or LID about 5years after the initiation of therapy. DBS of the STN or the GPi grants to PD patient improved quality of life and decreased motor complications, and has been approved as such by the Food and Drug Administration in the US in 2002. The success of DBS surgery depends on the accurate placement of the leads and meticulous programming of the stimulation. Therefore, it is best accomplished by an experienced team of neurosurgeon, neurologist, and support staff dedicated to the treatment.

REFERENCES

[1] Tanner, CM; Aston, DA. Epidemiology of Parkinson's disease and akinetic syndromes. *Curr Opin Neurol*, 2000, 13, 427-430.

[2] Mehanna, R; Jankovic, J. Respiratory problems in neurologic movement disorders. *Parkinsonism Relat Disord.*, 2010, 16, 628-638.

[3] Jankovic, J; Mehanna, R. Pathophysiology and clinical assessment. In Handbook of Parkinson's Disease. 5th edition. Edited by PahwaR & Lyons K. Florida, CRC press, 2013, 61-91.

[4] Fahn, S. The spectrum of levodopa-induced dyskinesias. *Ann Neurol*, 2000, 47, (Suppl 1), S2-S9.

[5] Fahn, S. Description of Parkinson's disease as a clinical syndrome. *Ann N Y Acad Sci*, 2003, 991, 1-14.

[6] Okun, M. Deep brain stimulation for Parkinson's disease. *N Engl J Med*, 2012, 367, 1529-1538.

[7] Findley, LJ. The economic impact of Parkinson's disease. *Parkinsonism Relat Disord*, 2007, 13(Suppl), S8-S12.

[8] Vossius, C; Nilsen, OB; Larsen, JP. Parkinson's disease and nursing home placement, the economic impact of the need for care. *Eur J Neurol*, 2009, 16, 194-200.

[9] Winter, Y; Balzer-Geldsetzer, M; Spottke, A; Reese, JP; Baum, E; Klotsche, J; Rieke, J; Simonow, A; Eggert, K; Oertel, WH; Dodel, R. Longitudinal study of the socioeconomic burden of Parkinson's disease in Germany. *Eur J Neurol*, 2010, 17, 1156-1163.

[10] Weintraub, D; Comella, CL; Horn, S. Parkinson's disease. Part 1, Pathophysiology, symptoms, burden, diagnosis and assessment. *Am J Manag Care*, 20081, 14, S40-S48.

[11] Chen, JJ. Parkinson's disease; health-related quality of life; economic cost, and implications of early treatment. *Am J Manag Care*, 2010, 16 (Suppl Implications), S87-S93.

[12] Mehanna, R; Jankovic, J. Movement disorders in cerebrovascular disease. *Lancet Neurology*, 2013, 12, 597-608.

[13] Diederich, NJ; Parent, A. Parkinson's disease, acquired frailty of archaic neural networks? *J Neurol Sci*, 2012, 314, 143–151.

[14] Brunenberg, EJ; Moeskops, P; Backes, WH; Pollo, C; Cammoun, L; Vilanova, A; Janssen, ML; Visser-Vandewalle, VE; ter Haar Romeny; BM; Thiran, JP; Platel, B. Structural and resting state functional connectivity of the subthalamic nucleus; identification of motor STN parts and the hyperdirect pathway. *PLoS One*, 2012, 7, e39061.

[15] Bergman, H; Wichmann, T; DeLong, MR. Reversal of experimental parkinsonism by lesions of the subthalamic nucleus. *Science*, 1990, 249, 1436–1438.

[16] Lintas, A; Silkis, IG; Albéri, L; Villa, AE. Dopamine deficiency increases synchronized activity in the rat subthalamic nucleus. *Brain Res*, 2012, 1434, 142–151.

[17] Dostrovsky, JO; Hutchinson, WD; Lozano, AM. The globus pallidus; deep brain stimulation and Parkinson's disease. *Neuroscientist*, 2002, 8, 284–290.

[18] Brown, P. Abnormal oscillatory synchronisation in the motor system leads to impaired movement. *Curr Opin Neurobiol*, 2007, 17, 656–664.

[19] Hammond, C; Bergman, H; Brown, P. Pathological synchronization in Parkinson's disease; networks, models and treatments. *Trends Neurosci*, 2007, 30, 357–364.

[20] Boecker, H; Brooks, DJ. Resting tremor in Parkinson disease: is the pallidum to blame? *Ann Neurol*, 2011, 69, 229–231.

[21] Bartolic´, A; Pirtosek, Z; Rozman, J; Ribaric, S. Tremor amplitude and tremor frequency variability in Parkinson's disease is dependent on activity and synchronisation of central oscillators in basal ganglia. *Med Hypotheses*, 2010, 74, 362–365.

[22] Kühn, AA; Kupsch, A; Schneider, GH; Brown, P. Reduction in subthalamic 8-35 Hz oscillatory activity correlates with clinical improvement in Parkinson's disease. *Eur J Neurosci*, 2006, 23, 1956–1960.

[23] Ray, NJ; Jenkinson, N; Wang, S; Holland, P; Brittain, JS; Joint, C. Stein, JF; Aziz, T. Local field potential beta activity in the subthalamic nucleus of patients with Parkinson's disease is associated with improvements in bradykinesia after dopamine and deep brain stimulation. *Exp Neurol*, 2008, 213, 108–113.

[24] McIntyre, CC; Hahn, PJ. Network perspectives on the mechanisms of deep brain stimulation. *Neurobiol Dis*, 2010, 38, 329-337.

[25] Vitek, JL. Mechanisms of deep brain stimulation, excitation or inhibition. *Mov Disord*, 2002, 17(Suppl 3), S69-S72.

[26] Goldberg, J; Boraud, T; Bergman, H. Microrecording in the primate MPTP model. In Microelectrode recording in movement disorder surgery. Edited by Israel, Z; Burchiel, K. *New York*, *Thieme*, 2004, 46-62.

[27] Farmer, S. Neural rhythms in Parkinson's disease. *Brain*, 2002, 125, 1175–1176.

[28] Levy, R; Ashby, P; Hutchison, WD; Lang, AE; Lozano, AM; Dostrovsky, JO. Dependence of subthalamic nucleus oscillations on movement and dopamine in Parkinson's disease. *Brain*, 2002, 125, 1196–1209.

[29] Priori, A; Foffani, G; Pesenti, A; Tamma, F; Bianchi, AM; Pellegrini, M; Locatelli, M; Moxon, KA; Villani, RM. Rhythm-specific pharmacological modulation of subthalamic activity in Parkinson's disease. *Exp Neurol*, 2004, 189, 369–379.

[30] Silberstein, P; Pogosyan, A; Kühn, AA; Hotton, G; Tisch, S; Kupsch, A; Dowsey-Limousin, P; Hariz, MI; Brown, P. Cortico-cortical coupling in Parkinson's disease and its modulation by therapy. *Brain*, 2005, 128, 1277–1291.

[31] McIntyre, CC; Savasta, M; Kerkerian-Le Goff, L; Vitek, JL. Uncovering the mechanism(s) of action of deep brain stimulation, activation, inhibition, or both. *Clin Neurophysiol.*, 2004, 115, 1239–1248.

[32] Wichmann, T; DeLong, MR; Guridi, J; Obeso, JA. Milestones in research on the pathophysiology of Parkinson's disease. *Mov Disord*, 2011, 26, 1032-1041.

[33] Tawfik, VL; Chang, SY; Hitti, FL; Roberts, DW; Leiter, JC; Jovanovic, S; Lee, KH. Deep brain stimulation results in local glutamate and adenosine release, investigation into the role of astrocytes. *Neurosurgery*, 2010, 67, 367-375.

[34] Lee, KH; Chang, SY; Roberts, DW; Kim, U. Neurotransmitter release from high-frequency stimulation of the subthalamic nucleus. *J Neurosurg*, 2004, 101, 511-517.

[35] Lee, KH; Hitti, FL; Chang, SY, Lee, DC; Roberts, DW; McIntyre, CC; Leiter, JC. High frequency stimulation abolishes thalamic network oscillations; an electrophysiological and computational analysis. *J Neural Eng*, 2011, 8, 046001.

[36] Vedam-Mai, V; van Battum, EY; Kamphuis, W; Feenstra, MG; Denys, D; Reynolds, BA; Okun, MS; Hol, EM. Deep brain stimulation and the role of astrocytes. *Mol Psychiatry*, 2012, 17, 124-131.

[37] Bandettini, PA; Wong, EC; Hinks, RS; Tikofsky, RS; Hyde, JS. Time course EPI of human brain function during task activation. *Magnetic resonance in medicine*, 1991, 25, 390-397.

[38] Kwong, KK; Belliveau, JW; Chesler, DA; Goldberg, IE; Weisskoff, RM; Poncelet, BP; Kennedy, DN; Hoppel, BE; Cohen, MS; Turner, R; et al. Dynamic magnetic resonance imaging of human brain activity during primary sensory stimulation. *Proceedings of the National Academy of Sciences*, 1992, 89, 5675-5679.

[39] Ogawa, S; Lee, T; Kay, A; Tank, D. Brain magnetic resonance imaging with contrast dependent on blood oxygenation. *Proc Natl Acad Sci U S A*, 1990, 87, 9868-9872.

[40] Phelps, ME. PET: the merging of biology and imaging into molecular imaging. *J Nucl Med*, 2000, 41, 661-681.

[41] Heiss, W-D; Herholz, K. Brain receptor imaging. *J Nucl Med*, 2006, 47, 302-312.

[42] Asanuma, K; Tang, C; Ma, Y; Dhawan, V; Mattis, P; Edwards, C; Kaplitt, MG; Feigin, A; Eidelberg, D. Network modulation in the treatment of Parkinson's disease. *Brain*, 2006, 129, 2667-2678.

[43] Boertien, T; Zrinzo, L; Kahan, J; Jahanshahi, M; Hariz, M; Mancini, L; Limousin, P; Foltynie, T. Functional imaging of subthalamic nucleus deep brain stimulation in Parkinson's disease. *Mov Disord*, 2011, 26, 1835-1843.

[44] Geday, J; Ostergaard, K; Johnsen, E; Gjedde, A. STN-stimulation in Parkinson's disease restores striatal inhibition of thalamocortical projection. *Hum Brain Mapp*, 2009, 30, 112-121.

[45] Haslinger, B; Kalteis, K; Boecker, H; Alesch, F; Ceballos-Baumann, AO. Frequency-correlated decreases of motor cortex activity associated with subthalamic nucleus stimulation in Parkinson's disease. *Neuroimage*, 2005, 28, 598-606.

[46] Hilker, R; Voges, J; Weisenbach, S; Kalbe, E; Burghaus, L; Ghaemi, M; Lehrke, R; Koulousakis, A; Herholz, K; Sturm, V; Heiss, WD. Subthalamic nucleus stimulation restores glucose metabolism in associative and limbic cortices and in cerebellum:evidence from a FDG-PET study in advanced Parkinson's disease. *J Cereb Blood Flow Metab*, 2004, 24, 7-16.

[47] Hilker, R; Voges, J; Weber, T; Kracht, LW; Roggendorf, J; Baudrexel, S; Hoevels, M; Sturm, V; Heiss, WD. STN-DBS activates the target area in Parkinson disease An FDG-PET study. *Neurology*, 2008, 71,708-713.

[48] Jech, R; Urgosík, D; Tintera, J; Nebuzelský, A; Krásenský, J; Liscák, R; Roth, J; Růzicka, E. Functional magnetic resonance imaging during deep brain stimulation: a pilot study in four patients with Parkinson's disease. *Mov Disord*, 2001, 16, 1126-1132.

[49] Jech, R. Functional imaging of deep brain stimulation: fMRI: SPECT: and PET. In: Deep Brain Stimulation in Neurological and Psychiatric Disorders. *Springer*, 2008, 179-201.

[50] Albaugh, DL; Shih, YY. Neural Circuit Modulation during Deep Brain Stimulation at the Subthalamic Nucleus for Parkinson's Disease: What Have We Learned from Neuroimaging Studies? *Brain Connect.*, 2013 Oct 22., [Epub ahead of print]

[51] Ceballos-Baumann, AO; Boecker, H; Bartenstein, P; von Falkenhayn, I; Riescher, H; Conrad, B; Moringlane, JR; Alesch, F. A positron emission tomographic study of subthalamic nucleus stimulation in Parkinson disease: enhanced movement-related activity of motor-association cortex and decreased motor cortex resting activity. *Arch Neurol*, 1999, 56, 997.

[52] Scherfler, C; Seppi, K; Mair, KJ; Donnemiller, E; Virgolini, I; Wenning, GK; Poewe, W. Left hemispheric predominance of nigrostriatal dysfunction in Parkinson's disease. *Brain*, 2012, 135, 3348-3354.

[53] Mehanna, R; Lai, EC. Deep brain stimulation in Parkinson's disease. *Transl Neurodegener.*, 2013 Nov 18, 2(1), 22.

[54] Deuschl, G; Schade-Brittinger, C; Krack, P; Volkmann, J; Schäfer, H; Bötzel, K; Daniels, C; Deutschländer, A; Dillmann, U; Eisner, W; Gruber, D; Hamel, W; Herzog, J; Hilker, R; Klebe, S; Kloss, M; Koy, J; Krause, M; Kupsch, A; Lorenz, D; Lorenzl, S; Mehdorn, HM; Moringlane, JR; Oertel, W; Pinsker, MO; Reichmann, H; Reuss, A; Schneider, GH; Schnitzler, A; Steude, U; Sturm, V; Timmermann, L; Tronnier, V; Trottenberg, T; Wojtecki, L; Wolf, E; Poewe, W; Voges, J. German Parkinson Study Group: Neurostimulation Section: A randomized trial of deep-brain stimulation for Parkinson's disease. *N Engl J Med*, 2006, 355, 896-908.

[55] Weaver, FM; Follett, K; Stern, M; Hur, K; Harris, C; Marks, WJ; Jr. Rothlind, J; Sagher, O; Reda, D; Moy, CS; Pahwa, R; Burchiel, K; Hogarth, P; Lai, EC; Duda, JE; Holloway, K; Samii, A; Horn, S; Bronstein, J; Stoner, G; Heemskerk, J; Huang, GD. CSP 468 Study Group: Bilateral deep brain stimulation vs best medical therapy for patients with advanced Parkinson disease: a randomized controlled trial. *JAMA*, 2009, 301, 63-73.

[56] Williams, A; Gill, S; Varma, T; Jenkinson, C; Quinn, N; Mitchell, R; Scott, R; Ives, N; Rick, C; Daniels, J; Patel, S; Wheatley, K. PD SURG Collaborative Group: Deep brain stimulation plus best medical therapy versus best medical therapy alone for advanced Parkinson's disease (PD SURG trial): a randomized: open-label trial. *Lancet Neurol*, 2010, 9, 581-591.

[57] Okun, MS; Gallo, BV; Mandybur, G; Jagid, J; Foote, KD; Revilla, FJ; Alterman, R; Jankovic, J; Simpson, R; Junn, F; Verhagen, L; Arle, JE; Ford, B; Goodman, RR; Stewart, RM; Horn, S; Baltuch, GH; Kopell, BH; Marshall, F; Peichel, D; Pahwa, R; Lyons, KE; Tröster, AI; Vitek, JL; Tagliati, M. SJM DBS Study Group: Subthalamic

deep brain stimulation with a constant-current device in Parkinson's disease: an open-label randomized controlled trial. *Lancet Neurol*, 2012, 11, 140-149.

[58] Follett, KA; Weaver, FM; Stern, M; Hur, K; Harris, CL; Luo, P; Marks, WJ; Jr. Rothlind, J; Sagher, O; Moy, C; Pahwa, R; Burchiel, K; Hogarth, P; Lai, EC; Duda, JE; Holloway, K; Samii, A; Horn, S; Bronstein, JM; Stoner, G; Starr, PA; Simpson, R; Baltuch, G; De Salles, A; Huang, GD; Reda, DJ. CSP 468 Study Group; Pallidal versus subthalamic deep-brain stimulation for Parkinson's disease. *N Engl J Med*, 2010, 362, 2077-2091.

[59] Desouza, R; Moro, E; Lang, A; Schapira, A. Timing of deep brain stimulation in Parkinson's disease: A need for reappraisal? *Ann Neurol.*, 2013, 73, 565-575.

[60] Amara, AW; Standaert, DG; Guthrie, S; Cutter, G; Watts, RL; Walker, HC. Unilateral subthalamic nucleus deep brain stimulation improves sleep quality in Parkinson's disease. *Parkinsonism Relat Disord.*, 2012, 18, 63-68.

[61] Okun, MS; Foote, KD. Enough is enough: moving on to deep brain stimulation in patients with fluctuating Parkinson disease. *Arch Neurol*, 2009, 66, 778-780.

[62] Spieles-Engemann, AL; Behbehani, MM; Collier, TJ; Wohlgenant, SL; Steece-Collier, K; Paumier, K; Daley, BF; Gombash, S; Madhavan, L; Mandybur, GT; Lipton, JW; Terpstra, BT; Sortwell, CE. Stimulation of the rat subthalamic nucleus is neuroprotective following significant nigral dopamine neuron loss. *Neurobiol Dis*, 2010, 39, 105-115.

[63] Maesawa, S; Kaneoke, Y; Kajita, Y; Usui, N; Misawa, N; Nakayama, A; Yoshida, J. Long-term stimulation of the subthalamic nucleus in hemiparkinsonian rats. neuroprotection of dopaminergic neurons. *J Neurosurg*, 2004, 100, 679-687.

[64] Harnack, D; Meissner, W; Jira, JA; Winter, C; Morgenstern, R; Kupsch, A. Placebo-controlled chronic high-frequency stimulation of the subthalamic nucleus preserves dopaminergic nigral neurons in a rat model of progressive Parkinsonism. *Exp Neurol*, 2008, 210, 257-260.

[65] Zhao, XD; Cao, YQ; Liu, HH; Li, FQ; You, BM; Zhou, XP. Long term high frequency stimulation of STN increases dopamine in the corpus striatum of hemiparkinsonian rhesus monkey. *Brain Res*, 2009, 1286, 230-238.

[66] Wallace, BA; Ashkan, K; Heise, CE; Foote, KD; Torres, N; Mitrofanis, J; Benabid, AL . Survival of midbrain dopaminergic cells after lesion or deep brain stimulation of the subthalamic nucleus in MPTP-treated monkeys. *Brain*, 2007, 130, 2129- 2145.

[67] Shaw, VE; Keay, KA; Ashkan, K; Benabid, AL; Mitrofanis, J. Dopaminergic cells in the periaqueductal grey matter of MPTP-treated monkeys and mice: patterns of survival and effect of deep brain stimulation and lesion of the subthalamic nucleus. *Parkinsonism Relat Disord*, 2010, 16, 338-344.

[68] Warnke, PC. STN stimulation and neuroprotection in Parkinson's disease-when beautiful theories meet ugly facts. *J Neurol Neurosurg Psychiatry*, 2005, 76, 1186-1187.

[69] Hilker, R; Portman, AT; Voges, J; Staal, MJ; Burghaus, L; van Laar, T; Koulousakis, A; Maguire, RP; Pruim, J; de Jong, BM; Herholz, K; Sturm, V; Heiss, WD; Leenders, KL. Disease progression continues in patients with advanced Parkinson's disease and effective subthalamic nucleus stimulation. *J Neurol Neurosurg Psychiatry*, 2005, 76, 1217-1221.

[70] Ngoga, D; Mitchell, R; Kausar, J; Hodson, J; Harries, A; Pall, H. Deep brain stimulation improves survival in severe Parkinson's disease. *J Neurol Neurosurg Psychiatry.*, 2014 Jan, 85(1), 17-22.

[71] Mehanna, R; Jankovic J. Respiratory problems in neurologic movement disorders. *Parkinsonism Relat Disord*, 2010, 16, 628–38.

[72] Lengerer, S; Kipping, J; Rommel, N; et al. Deep-brain-stimulation does not impair deglutition in Parkinson's disease. *Parkinsonism Relat Disord*, 2012, 18, 847–53.

[73] Ciucci, MR; Barkmeier-Kraemer, JM; Sherman, SJ. Subthalamic nucleus deep brain stimulation improves deglutition in Parkinson's disease. *Mov Disord*, 2008, 23, 676–83.

[74] Silbergleit, AK; LeWitt, P; Junn, F; et al. Comparison of dysphagia before and after deep brain stimulation in Parkinson's disease. *Mov Disord*, 2012, 27, 1763–8.

[75] Kitashima, A; Umemoto, G; Tsuboi, Y; et al. Effects of subthalamic nucleus deep brain stimulation on the swallowing function of patients with Parkinson's disease. *Parkinsonism Relat Disord*, 2013, 19, 480–2.

[76] Asahi, T; Inoue, Y; Hayashi, N; et al. Alleviation of dysphagia after deep brain stimulation; results from a Parkinson's disease patient. *Mov Disord*, 2012, 27, 325–6.

[77] Krack, P; Batir, A; Van Blercom, N; Chabardes, S; Fraix, V; Ardouin, C; Koudsie, A; Limousin, PD; Benazzouz, A; LeBas, JF; Benabid, AL; Pollak, P. Five-year follow-up of bilateral stimulation of the subthalamic nucleus in advanced Parkinson's disease. *N Engl J Med*, 2003, 349, 1925-1934.

[78] Fasano, A; Romito, LM; Daniele, A; Piano, C; Zinno, M; Bentivoglio, AR; Albanese, A. Motor and cognitive outcome in patients with Parkinson's disease 8 years after subthalamic implants. *Brain*, 2010, 133, 2664-2676.

[79] Moro, E; Lozano, AM; Pollak, P; Agid, Y; Rehncrona, S; Volkmann, J; Kulisevsky, J; Obeso, JA; Albanese, A; Hariz, MI; Quinn, NP; Speelman, JD; Benabid, AL; Fraix, V; Mendes, A; Welter, ML; Houeto, JL; Cornu, P; Dormont, D; Tornqvist, AL; Ekberg, R; Schnitzler, A; Timmermann, L; Wojtecki, L; Gironell, A; Rodriguez-Oroz, MC; Guridi, J; Bentivoglio, AR; Contarino, MF; Romito, L; Scerrati, M; Janssens, M; Lang, AE. Long-term results of a multicenter study on subthalamic and pallidal stimulation in Parkinson's disease. *Mov Disord*, 2010, 25, 578- 586.

[80] Zibetti, M; Merola, A; Rizzi, L; Ricchi, V; Angrisano, S; Azzaro, C; Artusi, CA; Arduino, N; Marchisio, A; Lanotte, M; Rizzone, M; Lopiano, L. Beyond nine years of continuous subthalamic nucleus deep brain stimulation in Parkinson's disease. *Mov Disord*, 2011, 2, 2327-2334.

[81] Castrioto, A; Lozano, AM; Poon, YY; Lang, AE; Fallis, M; Moro, E. Ten-year outcome of subthalamic stimulation in Parkinson disease: a blinded evaluation. *Arch Neurol*, 2011, 68, 1550-1556.

[82] Bang Henriksen, M; Johnsen, EL; Sunde, N; Vase, A; Gjelstrup, MC; Ostergaard, K. Surviving 10 years with deep brain stimulation for Parkinson's disease - a follow-up of 79 patients. *Eur J Neurol.*, 2014 Dec 9. doi; 10.1111/ene.12614. [Epub ahead of print]

[83] Rizzone, MG; Fasano, A; Daniele, A; Zibetti, M; Merola, A; Rizzi, L; Piano, C; Piccininni, C; Romito, LM; Lopiano, L; Albanese, A. Long-term outcome of subthalamic nucleus DBS in Parkinson's disease: from the advanced phase towards the late stage of the disease? *Parkinsonism Relat Disord.*, 2014 Apr, 20(4), 376-81.

[84] Hely, MA; Reid, WG; Adena, MA; Halliday, GM; Morris, JG. The Sydney multicenter study of Parkinson's disease: the inevitability of dementia at 20 years. *Mov Disord*, 2008, 23, 837-844.

[85] Vercruysse, S; Vandenberghe, W; Münks, L; Nuttin, B; Devos, H; Nieuwboer, A. Effects of deep brain stimulation of the subthalamic nucleus on freezing of gait in Parkinson's disease: a prospective controlled study. *J Neurol Neurosurg Psychiatry.*, 2014 Aug, 85(8), 871-7. Doi: 10.1136/jnnp-2013-306336. Epub 2014 Jan 6.

[86] Lilleeng, B; Gjerstad, M; Baardsen, R; Dalen, I; Larsen, JP. Motor symptoms after deep brain stimulation of the subthalamic nucleus. *Acta Neurol Scand.*, 2014 Oct 23.

[87] Nazzaro, JM; Pahwa, R; Lyons, KE. The impact of bilateral subthalamic stimulation on nonmotor symptoms of Parkinson's disease. *Parkinsonism Relat Disord*, 2011, 17, 606-609.

[88] Strutt, AM; Simpson, R; Jankovic, J; York, MK. Changes in cognitive-emotional and physiological symptoms of depression following STN-DBS for the treatment of Parkinson's disease. *Eur J Neurol*, 2012, 19, 121-127.

[89] Halim, A; Baumgartner, L; Binder, DK. Effect of deep brain stimulation on autonomic dysfunction in patients with Parkinson's disease. *J Clin Neurosci*, 2011, 18, 804-806.

[90] Witjas, T; Kaphan, E; Régis, J; Jouve, E; Chérif, AA; Péragut, JC; Azulay, JP. Effects of chronic subthalamic stimulation on nonmotor fluctuations in Parkinson's disease. *Mov Disord*, 2007, 22, 1727-1734.

[91] Cury, RG; Galhardoni, R; Fonoff, ET; Dos Santos Ghilardi, MG; Fonoff, F; Arnaut, D; Myczkowski, ML; Marcolin, MA; Bor-Seng-Shu, E; Barbosa, ER; Teixeira, MJ; Ciampi de Andrade, D. Effects of deep brain stimulation on pain and other nonmotor symptoms in Parkinson disease. *Neurology.*, 2014 Oct 14, 83(16), 1403-9.

[92] Pellaprat, J; Ory-Magne, F; Canivet, C; Simonetta-Moreau, M; Lotterie, JA; Radji, F; Arbus, C; Gerdelat, A; Chaynes, P; Brefel-Courbon, C. Deep brain stimulation of the subthalamic nucleus improves pain in Parkinson's disease. *Parkinsonism Relat Disord.*, 2014 Jun, 20(6), 662-4.

[93] Buhmann, C; Maintz, L; Hierling, J; Vettorazzi, E; Moll, CK; Engel, AK; Gerloff, C; Hamel, W; Zangemeister, WH. Effect of subthalamic nucleus deep brain stimulation on driving in Parkinson disease. *Neurology.*, 2014 Jan 7, 82(1), 32-40.

[94] Halpern, CH; Rick, JH; Danish, SF; Grossman, M; Baltuch, GH. Cognition following bilateral deep brain stimulation surgery of the subthalamic nucleus for Parkinson's disease. *Int J Geriatr Psychiatry*, 2009, 24, 443-451.

[95] Mehanna, R; Ondo, W. Sleep problems in Parkinson's disease patients. *Neurodegenerative disease management.*, 2011, 1, 307-321.

[96] Amara, AW; Watts, RL; Walker, HC. The effects of deep brain stimulation on sleep in Parkinson's disease. *Ther Adv Neurol Disord*, 2011, 4, 15-24.

[97] Okun, MS; Tagliati, M; Pourfar, M; Fernandez, HH; Rodriguez, RL; Alterman, RL; Foote, KD. Management of referred deep brain stimulation failures: a retrospective analysis from 2 movement disorders centers. *Arch Neurol*, 2005, 62, 1250-1255.

[98] Ellis, TM; Foote, KD; Fernandez, HH; Sudhyadhom, A; Rodriguez, RL; Zeilman, P; Jacobson, CE; 4th, Okun, MS. Reoperation for suboptimal outcomes after deep brain stimulation surgery. *Neurosurgery*, 2008, 63, 754-760.

[99] McIntosh, E. Perspective on the Economic Evaluation of Deep Brain Stimulation. *Front Integr Neurosci.*, 2011, 5, 19.

[100] Valldeoriola, F; Morsi, O; Tolosa, E; Rumia, J; Marti, MJ; Martinez-Martin, P; Prospective comparative study on cost-effectiveness of subthalamic stimulation and best medical treatment in advanced Parkinson's disease. *Mov Disord*, 2007, 22, 2183-2191.

[101] Spottke, EA; Volkmann, J; Lorenz, D; Krack, P; Smala, AM; Sturm, V; Gerstner, A; Berger, K; Hellwig, D; Deuschl, G; Freund, HJ; Oertel, WH; Dodel, RC. Evaluation of healthcare utilization and health status of patients with Parkinson's disease treated with deep brain stimulation of the subthalamic nucleus. *J Neurol*, 2002, 249, 759-766.

[102] Fraix, V; Houeto, JL; Lagrange, C; Le Pen, C; Krystkowiak, P; Guehl, D; Ardouin, C; Welter, ML; Maurel, F; Defebvre, L; Rougier, A; Benabid, AL; Mesnage, V; Ligier, M; Blond, S; Burbaud, P; Bioulac, B; Destée, A; Cornu, P; Pollak, P. SPARK Study Group: Clinical and economic results of bilateral subthalamic nucleus stimulation in Parkinson's disease. *Neurol Neurosurg Psychiatry*., 2006, 77, 443-449.

[103] Voges, J; Waerzeggers, Y; Maarouf, M; Lehrke, R; Koulousakis, A; Lenartz, D; Sturm, V. Deep-brain stimulation: long-term analysis of complications caused by hardware and surgery — experiences from a single centre. *J Neurol Neurosurg Psychiatry*, 2006, 77, 868-872.

[104] Sillay, KA; Larson, PS; Starr, PA. Deep brain stimulator hardware-related infections incidence and management in a large series. *Neurosurgery*, 2008, 62, 360-366.

[105] Fenoy, AJ; Simpson, RK. Management of device-related wound complications in deep-brain stimulation surgery. *J Neurosurg*, 2012, 116, 1324-1332.

[106] Zrinzo, L; Foltynie, T; Limousin, P; Hariz, MI. Reducing hemorrhagic complications in functional neurosurgery: a large case series and systematic literature review. *J Neurosurg*, 2012, 116, 84-94.

[107] Coley, E; Farhadi, R; Lewis, S; Whittle, IR. The incidence of seizures following deep brain stimulating electrode implantation for movement disorders; pain and psychiatric conditions. *Br J Neurosurg*, 2009, 23, 179-183.

[108] Voon, V; Krack, P; Lang, AE; Lozano, AM; Dujardin, K; Schüpbach, M; D'Ambrosia, J; Thobois, S; Tamma, F; Herzog, J; Speelman, JD; Samanta, J; Kubu, C; Rossignol, H; Poon, YY; Saint-Cyr, JA; Ardouin, C; Moro, E. A multicentre study on suicide outcomes following subthalamic stimulation for Parkinson's disease. *Brain*, 2008, 131, 2720-2728.

[109] Temel, Y. Limbic effects of high-frequency stimulation of the subthalamic nucleus. *Vitam Horm*, 2010, 82, 47-63.

[110] Parsons, TD; Rogers, SA; Braaten, AJ; Woods, SP; Troster, AI. Cognitive sequelae of subthalamic nucleus deep brain stimulation in Parkinson's disease: a metaanalysis. *Lancet Neurol*, 2006, 5, 578-588.

[111] Tagliati, M. Turning tables: should GPi become the preferred DBS target for Parkinson disease? *Neurology*., 2012, 79, 19-20.

[112] Mehanna, R. Cognitive changes after deep brain stimulation in Parkinson's disease: a critical review. *Brain Disord Ther*, 2014, 3, 2.

[113] Cilia, R; Siri, C; Marotta, G; De Gaspari, D; Landi, A; et al. Brain networks underlining verbal fluency decline during STN-DBS in Parkinson's disease: an ECD-SPECT study. *Parkinsonism Relat Disord*, 2007, 13, 290-294.

[114] York, MK; Dulay, M; Macias, A; Levin, HS; Grossman, R; et al. Cognitive declines following bilateral subthalamic nucleus deep brain stimulation for the treatment of Parkinson's disease. *J Neurol Neurosurg Psychiatry*, 2009, 79, 789-795.

[115] Alberts, JL; Voelcker-Rehage, C; Hallahan, K; Vitek, M; Bamzai, R; et al. Bilateral subthalamic stimulation impairs cognitive-motor performance in Parkinson's disease patients. *Brain*, 2008, 131, 3348-3360.

[116] Aybek, S; Gronchi-Perrin, A; Berney, A; Chiuvé, SC; Villemure, JG; et al. Long-term cognitive profile and incidence of dementia after STN-DBS in Parkinson's disease. *Mov Disord*, 2007, 22, 974-981.

[117] Krack, P; Batir, A; Van Blercom, N; et al. Five-year follow-up of bilateral stimulation of the subthalamic nucleus in advanced Parkinson's disease. *N. Engl J Med*, 2003, 349, 1925–1934.

[118] De Gaspari, D; Siri, C; Landi, A; Cilia, R; Bonetti, A; et al. Clinical and neuropsychological follow up at 12 months in patients with complicated Parkinson's disease treated with subcutaneous apomorphine infusion or deep brain stimulation of the subthalamic nucleus. *J Neurol Neurosurg Psychiatry*, 2006, 77, 450-453.

[119] Funkiewiez, A; Ardouin, C; Caputo, E; Krack, P; Fraix, V; et al. Long term effects of bilateral subthalamic nucleus stimulation on cognitive function; mood; and behaviour in Parkinson's disease. *J Neurol Neurosurg Psychiatry*, 2004, 75, 834-839.

[120] Schüpbach, WM; Chastan, N; Welter, ML; Houeto, JL; Mesnage, V; et al. Stimulation of the subthalamic nucleus in Parkinson's disease: a 5 year follow up. *J Neurol Neurosurg Psychiatry*, 2005, 76, 1640-1644.

[121] Whelan, BM; Murdoch, BE; Theodoros, DG; Hall, B; Silburn, P. Defining a role for the subthalamic nucleus within operative theoretical models of subcortical participation in language. *J Neurol Neurosurg Psychiatry*, 2003, 74, 1543-1550.

[122] Ardouin, C; Pillon, B; Peiffer, E; Bejjani, P; Limousin, P; et al. Bilateral subthalamic or pallidal stimulation for Parkinson's disease affects neither memory nor executive functions: a consecutive series of 62 patients. *Ann Neurol*, 1999, 46, 217-223.

[123] Gironell, A; Kulisevsky, J; Rami, L; Fortuny, N; García-Sánchez, C; et al. Effects of pallidotomy and bilateral subthalamic stimulation on cognitive function in Parkinson disease. A controlled comparative study. *J Neurol.*, 2003, 250, 917-923.

[124] Hilker, R; Voges, J; Weisenbach, S; Kalbe, E; Burghaus, L; et al. Subthalamic nucleus stimulation restores glucose metabolism in associative and limbic cortices and in cerebellum:evidence from a FDG-PET study in advanced Parkinson's disease. *J Cereb Blood Flow Metab*, 2004, 24, 7-16.

[125] Morrison, CE; Borod, JC; Perrine, K; Beric, A; Brin, MF; et al. Neuropsychological functioning following bilateral subthalamic nucleus stimulation in Parkinson's disease. *Arch Clin Neuropsychol*, 2004, 19, 165-181.

[126] Castelli, L; Rizzi, L; Zibetti, M; Angrisano, S; Lanotte, M; et al. Neuropsychological changes 1-year after subthalamic DBS in PD patients; A prospective controlled study. *Parkinsonism Relat Disord*, 2010, 16, 115-118.

[127] Williams, AE; Arzola, GM; Strutt, AM; Simpson, R; Jankovic, J; et al. Cognitive outcome and reliable change indices two years following bilateral subthalamic nucleus deep brain stimulation. *Parkinsonism Relat Disord*, 2011, 17, 321-327.

[128] Witt, K; Granert, O; Daniels, C; Volkmann, J; Falk, D; et al. Relation of lead trajectory and electrode position to neuropsychological outcomes of subthalamic

neurostimulation in Parkinson's disease: results from a randomized trial. *Brain* 2013, 136, 2109-2119.

[129] Witt, K; Daniels, C; Reiff, J; Krack, P; Volkmann, J; et al. Neuropsychological and psychiatric changes after deep brain stimulation for Parkinson's disease: a randomized: multicentre study. *Lancet Neurol*, 2008, 7, 605-614

[130] Smeding, HM; Speelman, JD; Koning-Haanstra, M; Schuurman, PR; Nijssen, P; et al. Neuropsychological effects of bilateral STN stimulation in Parkinson disease: a controlled study. *Neurology*, 2006, 66, 1830-1836.

[131] Sáez-Zea, C; Escamilla-Sevilla, F; Katati, MJ; Mínguez-Castellanos, A. *Cognitive Effects of Subthalamic Nucleus Stimulation in Parkinson's Disease: A Controlled Study Eur Neurol*, 2012, 68, 361-366.

[132] Zangaglia, R; Pacchetti, C; Pasotti, C; Mancini, F; Servello, D. Deep brain stimulation and cognitive functions in Parkinson's disease: A three-year controlled study. *Mov Disord*, 2009, 24, 1621-1628.

[133] Moretti, R; Torre, P; Antonello, RM; Capus, L; Marsala, SZ; et al. Neuropsychological changes after subthalamic nucleus stimulation: a 12 month follow- up in nine patients with Parkinson's disease. *Parkinsonism Relat Disord*, 2003, 10, 73-79.

[134] Daniele, A; Albanese, A; Contarino, MF; Zinzi, P; Barbier, A; et al. Cognitive and behavioural effects of chronic stimulation of the subthalamic nucleus in patients with Parkinson's disease. *J Neurol Neurosurg: Psychiatry*, 2003, 74, 175-182.

[135] Kumar, R; Lang, AE; Rodriguez-Oroz, MC; Lozano, AM; Limousin, P; et al. Deep brain stimulation of the globus pallidus pars interna in advanced Parkinson's disease. *Neurology*, 2000, 55, S34-39.

[136] Tsai, ST; Lin, SH; Lin, SZ; Chen, JY; Lee, CW; et al. Neuropsychological effects after chronic subthalamic stimulation and the topography of the nucleus in Parkinson's disease. *Neurosurgery*, 2007, 61, E1024-1029.

[137] Smith, KM; O'Connor, M; Papavassiliou, E; Tarsy, D; Shih, LC. Phonemic verbal fluency decline after subthalamic nucleus deep brain stimulation does not depend on number of microelectrode recordings or lead tip placement. *Parkinsonism Relat Disord.*, 2014 Apr, 20(4), 400-4.

[138] Wojtecki, L; Timmermann, L; Jörgens, S; Südmeyer, M; Maarouf, M; et al. Frequency-dependent reciprocal modulation of verbal fluency and motor functions in subthalamic deep brain stimulation. *Arch Neurol*, 2006, 63, 1273-1276.

[139] Schoenberg, MR; Mash, KM; Bharucha, KJ; Francel, PC; Scott, JG. Deep brain stimulation parameters associated with neuropsychological changes in subthalamic nucleus stimulation for refractory Parkinson's disease. *Stereotact Funct Neurosurg*, 2008, 86, 337-344.

[140] Trepanier, LL; Kumar, R; Lozano, AM; Trépanier, LL; Kumar, R; et al. Neuropsychological outcome of GPi pallidotomy and GPi or STN deep brain stimulation in Parkinson's disease. *Brain Cogn*, 2000, 42, 324-347.

[141] Hershey, T; Revilla, FJ; Wernle, A; Gibson, PS; Dowling, JL; et al. Stimulation of STN impairs aspects of cognitive control in PD. *Neurology*, 2004, 62, 1110-1114.

[142] Saint-Cyr, JA; Albanese, A. STN DBS in PD: selection criteria for surgery should include cognitive and psychiatric factors. *Neurology*, 2006, 66, 1799-1800.

[143] Castelli, L; Perozzo, P; Zibetti, M; Crivelli, B; Morabito, U ; et al. Chronic deep brain stimulation of the subthalamic nucleus for Parkinson's disease: effects on cognition: mood: anxiety and personality traits. *Eur Neurol*, 2006, 55, 136-144.

[144] Jahanshahi, M; Ardouin, CM; Brown, RG; Rothwell, JC; Obeso, J; et al. The impact of deep brain stimulation on executive function in Parkinson's disease. *Brain*, 2000, 123, 1142-1154.

[145] Rothlind, JC; York, MK; Carlson, K; Luo, P; Marks, WJ; Jr. Weaver, FM; Stern, M; Follett, K; Reda, D. for the CSP-468 Study Group. Neuropsychological changes following deep brain stimulation surgery for Parkinson's disease: comparisons of treatment at pallidal and subthalamic targets versus best medical therapy. J Neurol Neurosurg Psychiatry. 2014 Sep 2. Pii: jnnp-2014-308119. doi: 10.1136/jnnp-2014-308119. [Epub ahead of print]

[146] Broen, M; Duits, A; Visser-Vandewalle, V; Temel, Y; Winogrodzka, A. Impulse control and related disorders in Parkinson's disease patients treated with bilateral subthalamic nucleus stimulation: a review. *Parkinsonism & Related Disorders*, 2011, 17, 413–7.

[147] Demetriades, P; Rickards, H; Cavanna, AE. Impulse control disorders following deep brain stimulation of the subthalamic nucleus in Parkinson's disease: clinical aspects. *Parkinsons Dis*, 2011, 2011, 658415.

[148] Hariz, MI; Rehncrona, S; Quinn, NP; Speelman, JD; Wensing, C. Multicenter study on deep brain stimulation in Parkinson's disease: an independent assessment of reported adverse events at 4 years. *Mov Disord*, 2008, 23, 416–21

[149] Lhommée, E; Klinger, H; Thobois, S; Schmitt, E; Ardouin, C; Bichon, A; Kistner, A; Fraix, V; Xie, J; Aya Kombo, M; Chabardès, S; Seigneuret, E; Benabid, AL; Mertens, P; Polo, G; Carnicella, S; Quesada, JL; Bosson, JL; Broussolle, E; Pollak, P; Krack, P. Subthalamic stimulation in Parkinson's disease: restoring the balance of motivated behaviours. *Brain.*, 2012 May, 135(Pt 5), 1463-77.

[150] Krack, P; Pollak, P; Limousin, P; Hoffmann, D; Xie, J; Benazzouz, A; et al. Subthalamic nucleus or internal pallidal stimulation in young onset. Parkinson's disease. *Brain*, 1998, 121, 451–7.

[151] Lim, SY; O'Sullivan, SS; Kotschet, K; Gallagher, DA; Lacey, C; Lawrence, AD; et al. Dopamine dysregulation syndrome: impulse control disorders and punding after deep brain stimulation surgery for Parkinson's disease. *J Clin Neurosci*, 2009, 16, 1148–52.

[152] Castrioto, A; Funkiewiez, A; Debû, B; Cools, R; Lhommée, E; Ardouin, C; Fraix, V; Chabardès, S; Robbins, TW; Pollak, P; Krack, P. Iowa gambling task impairment in Parkinson's disease can be normalised by reduction of dopaminergic medication after subthalamic stimulation. *J Neurol Neurosurg Psychiatry.*, 2014 May 23. pii: jnnp-2013-307146. doi; 10.1136/jnnp-2013-307146. [Epub ahead of print]

[153] Bejjani, P; Damier, P; Arnulf, I; et al. Transient acute depression induced by high-frequency deep-brain stimulation. *N Engl J Med*, 1999, 340, 1476–1480.

[154] Berney, A; Vingerhoets, F; Perrin, A; et al. Effect on mood of subthalamic DBS for Parkinson's disease. *Neurol*, 2002, 59, 1427–1429.

[155] Kulisevsky, J; Berthier, ML; Gironell, A; et al. Mania following deep brain stimulation for Parkinson's disease. *Neurology*, 2002, 59(9),1421–1424.1424.

[156] Romito, LM; Raja, M; Daniele, A; et al. Transient mania with hypersexuality following surgery for high frequency stimulation of the subthalamic nucleus in Parkinson's disease. *Move Disord*, 2002, 19 ,1371–4
[157] Welter, ML; Schüpbach, M; Czernecki, V; Karachi, C; Fernandez-Vidal, S; Golmard, JL; Serra, G; Navarro, S; Welaratne, A; Hartmann, A; Mesnage, V; Pineau, F; Cornu, P; Pidoux, B; Worbe, Y; Zikos, P; Grabli, D; Galanaud, D; Bonnet, AM; Belaid, H; Dormont, D; Vidailhet, M; Mallet, L; Houeto, JL; Bardinet, E; Yelnik, J; Agid, Y. Optimal target localization for subthalamic stimulation in patients with Parkinson disease. *Neurology.*, 2014 Apr 15, 82(15), 1352-61
[158] Okun, MS; Green, J; Saben, R; Gross, R; Foote, KD; Vitek, JL. Mood changes with deep brain stimulation of STN and GPi: results of a pilot study. *J Neurol Neurosurg Psychiatry*, 2003, 74, 1584–1586.
[159] Burdick, AP; Foote, KD; Wu, S; Bowers, D; Zeilman, P; Jacobson, CE; Ward, HE; Okun, MS. Do patient's get angrier following STN; GPi; and thalamic deep brain stimulation. *Neuroimage.*, 2011 Jan, 54 Suppl 1, S227-32.
[160] Burkard, PR; Vingerhoets, FJ; Berney, A; et al. Suicide after successful deep brain stimulation for movement disorders. *Neurology*, 2004. 63, 2170–2172.
[161] Houeto, JL; Mesnage, V; Mallet, L; et al. Behavioural disorders; Parkinson's disease and subthalamic stimulation. *J Neurol Neurosurg Psychiatry*, 2002, 72(6), 701–707.
[162] Weintraub, D; Duda, JE; Carlson, K; Luo, P; Sagher, O; Stern, M; et al. Suicide ideation and behaviours after STN and GPi DBS surgery for Parkinson's disease: results from a randomized: controlled trial. *J Neurol Neurosurg Psychiatry*, 2013 May 10.
[163] Okun, MS; Fernandez, HH; Pedraza, O; Misra, M; Lyons, KE; Pahwa, R; Tarsy, D; Scollins, L; Corapi, K; Friehs, GM; Grace, J; Romrell, J; Foote, KD; Development and initial validation of a screening tool for Parkinson disease surgical candidates. *Neurology*, 2004, 63, 161-163.
[164] Okun, MS; Foote, KD. Parkinson's disease DBS: what: when: who and why? The time has come to tailor DBS targets. *Expert Rev Neurother*, 2010, 10, 1847-1857.
[165] Abboud, H; Mehanna, R; Machado, A; Ahmed, A; Gostkowski, M; Cooper, S; Itin, I; Sweeney, P; Pandya, M; Kubu, C; Floden, D; Ford, PJ; Fernandez, HH. Comprehensive; Multidisciplinary Deep Brain Stimulation Screening for Parkinson Patients; No Room for "Short Cuts." *Movement disdorders clinical practice. E Pub*, 10 Oct 2014.
[166] Okun, MS; Fernandez, HH; Rodriguez, RL; Foote, KD. Identifying candidates for deep brain stimulation in Parkinson's disease: the role of the primary care physician. *Geriatrics*, 2007, 62, 18-24.
[167] DeLong, MR; Huang, KT; Gallis, J; Lokhnygina, Y; Parente, B; Hickey, P; Turner, DA; Lad, SP. Effect of advancing age on outcomes of deep brain stimulation for Parkinson disease. *JAMA Neurol.*, 2014 Oct, 71(10), 1290-5
[168] Pedrosa, DJ; Timmermann, L. Review: management of Parkinson's disease. *Neuropsychiatr Dis Treat.*, 2013, 9, 321-340.
[169] Anderson, VC; Burchiel, KJ; Hogarth, P; Favre, J; Hammerstad, JP. Pallidal vs subthalamic nucleus deep brain stimulation in Parkinson disease. *Arch Neurol*, 2005, 62, 554–560.

[170] Okun, MS; Fernandez, HH; Wu, SS; Kirsch-Darrow, L; Bowers, D; Bova, F; Suelter, M; Jacobson, CE; 4th. Wang, X; Gordon, CW; Jr. Zeilman, P; Romrell, J; Martin, P; Ward, H; Rodriguez, RL; Foote, KD. Cognition and mood in Parkinson's disease in subthalamic nucleus versus globus pallidus interna deep brain stimulation: the COMPARE trial. *Ann Neurol*, 2009, 65, 586-595.

[171] Zahodne, LB; Okun, MS; Foote, KD; Fernandez, HH; Rodriguez, RL; Wu, SS; Kirsch-Darrow, L; Jacobson, CE; 4th, Rosado, C; Bowers, D. Greater improvement in quality of life following unilateral deep brain stimulation surgery in the globus pallidus as compared to the subthalamic nucleus. *J Neurol*, 2009, 256, 1321–1329.

[172] Taba, HA; Wu, SS; Foote, KD; Hass, CJ; Fernandez, HH; Malaty, IA; Rodriguez, RL; Dai, Y; Zeilman, PR; Jacobson, CE; Okun, MS. A closer look at unilateral versus bilateral deep brain stimulation: results of the National Institutes of Health COMPARE cohort. *J Neurosurg*, 2010, 113, 1224-1229.

[173] Weaver, FM; Follett, KA; Stern, M; Luo, P; Harris, CL; Hur, K; Marks, WJ; Jr. Rothlind, J; Sagher, O; Moy, C; Pahwa, R; Burchiel, K; Hogarth, P; Lai, EC; Duda, JE; Holloway, K; Samii, A; Horn, S; Bronstein, JM; Stoner, G; Starr, PA; Simpson, R; Baltuch, G; De Salles, A; Huang, GD; Reda, DJ. CSP 468 Study Group: Randomized trial of deep brain stimulation for Parkinson disease: thirty-six month outcomes. *Neurology*, 2012, 79, 55- 65.

[174] Odekerken, VJ; van Laar, T; Staal, MJ; Mosch, A; Hoffmann, CF; Nijssen, PC; Beute, GN; van Vugt, JP; Lenders, MW; Contarino, MF; Mink, MS; Bour, LJ; van den Munckhof, P; Schmand, BA; de Haan, RJ; Schuurman, PR; de Bie, RM. Subthalamic nucleus versus globus pallidus bilateral deep brain stimulation for advanced Parkinson's disease (NSTAPS study): a randomised controlled trial. *Lancet Neurol.*, 2013, 12, 37-44.

[175] Sako, W; Miyazaki, Y; Izumi, Y; Kaji, R. Which target is best for patients with Parkinson's disease? A meta-analysis of pallidal and subthalamic stimulation. *J Neurol Neurosurg Psychiatry.*, 2014 Sep, 85(9), 982-6.

[176] Rothlind, JC; Cockshott, RW; Starr, PA; Marks, WJ; Jr. (2007) Neuropsychological performance following staged bilateral pallidal or subthalamic nucleus deep brain stimulation for Parkinson's disease. *J Int Neuropsychol Soc*, 13, 68-79.

[177] Bakker, M; Esselink, RA; Munneke, M; Limousin-Dowsey, P; Speelman, HD; Bloem, BR. Effects of stereotactic neurosurgery on postural instability and gait in Parkinson's disease. *Mov Disord*, 2004, 19, 1092–1099.

[178] Pötter-Nerger, M; Volkmann, J. Deep brain stimulation for gait and postural symptoms in Parkinson's disease. *Mov Disord.*, 2013 Sep 15, 28(11), 1609-15.

[179] St George, RJ; Carlson-Kuhta, P; Nutt, JG; Hogarth, P; Burchiel, KJ; Horak, FB. The effect of deep brain stimulation randomized by site on balance in Parkinson's disease. *Mov Disord.*, 2014 Jun, 29(7), 949-53.

[180] Stroupe, KT; Weaver, FM; Cao, L; Ippolito, D; Barton, BR; Burnett-Zeigler, IE; Holloway, RG; Vickrey, BG; Simuni, T; Follett, KA. Cost of deep brain stimulation for the treatment of Parkinson's disease by surgical stimulation sites. *Mov Disord.*, 2014 Nov, 29(13), 1666-74. doi; 10.1002/mds.26029. Epub 2014 Sep 15.

[181] Minafra, B; Fasano, A; Pozzi, NG; Zangaglia, R; Servello, D; Pacchetti, C. Eight-years failure of subthalamic stimulation rescued by globus pallidus implant. *Brain Stimul.*, 2014 Mar-Apr, 7(2), 179-81.

[182] Hamani, C; Moro, E; Lozano, AM. The pedunculopontine nucleus as a target for deep brain stimulation. *J Neural Transm.*, 2011, 118, 1461–1468.

[183] Stefani, A; Lozano, AM; Peppe, A; Stanzione, P; Galati, S; Tropepi, D; Pierantozzi, M; Brusa, L; Scarnati, E; Mazzone, P. Bilateral deep brain stimulation of the pedunculopontine and subthalamic nuclei in severe Parkinson's disease. *Brain.*, 2007, 130, 1596–1607.

[184] Stefani, A; Pierantozzi, M; Ceravolo, R; Brusa, L; Galati, S; Stanzione, P. Deep brain stimulation of pedunculopontine tegmental nucleus (PPTg) promotes cognitive and metabolic changes: a target-specific effect or response to a low-frequency pattern of stimulation? *Clin EEG Neurosci.*, 2010, 41, 82–86.

[185] Costa, A; Carlesimo, GA; Caltagirone, C; Mazzone, P; Pierantozzi, M; Stefani, A; Peppe, A. Effects of deep brain stimulation of the peduncolopontine area on working memory tasks in patients with Parkinson's disease. *Parkinsonism Relat Disord.*, 2010, 16, 64–67.

[186] Ferraye, MU; Debu, B; Fraix, V; Goetz, L; Ardouin, C; Yelnik, J; Henry- Lagrange, C; Seigneuret, E; Piallat, B; Krack, P; Le Bas, JF; Benabid, AL; Chabardes, S; Pollak, P. Effects of pedunculopontine nucleus area stimulation on gait disorders in Parkinson's disease. *Brain*, 2010, 133, 205–214.

[187] Moro, E; Hamani, C; Poon, YY; Al-Khairallah, T; Dostrovsky, JO; Hutchison, WD; Lozano, AM. Unilateral pedunculopontine stimulation improves falls in Parkinson's disease. *Brain*, 2010, 133, 215–224.

[188] Pinto, S; Ferraye, M; Espesser, R; Fraix, V; Maillet, A; Guirchoum, J; Layani-Zemour, D; Ghio, A; Chabardès, S; Pollak, 7; Debû, B. Stimulation of the pedunculopontine nucleus area in Parkinson's disease: effects on speech and intelligibility. *Brain.*, 2014 Oct, 137(Pt 10), 2759-72.

[189] Mazzone, P; Paoloni, M; Mangone, M; Santilli, V; Insola, A; Fini, M; Scarnati, E. Unilateral deep brain stimulation of the pedunculopontine tegmental nucleus in idiopathic Parkinson's disease: effects on gait initiation and performance. *Gait Posture.*, 2014 Jul, 40(3), 357-62.

[190] Ricciardi, L; Piano, C; Bentivoglio, AR; Fasano, A. Long-term effects of pedunculopontine nucleus stimulation for pisa syndrome. *Parkinsonism Relat Disord.*, 2014 Oct 14, 20(12), 1445-1446. doi:10.1016/j.parkreldis.2014.10.006. [Epub ahead of print]

[191] Shih, LC; Vanderhorst, VG; Lozano, AM; Hamani, C; Moro, E. Improvement of Pisa syndrome with contralateral pedunculopontine stimulation. *Mov Disord*, 2013, 28, 555e6.

[192] Chastan, N; Westby, GW; Yelnik, J; et al. Effects of nigral stimulation on locomotion and postural stability in patients with Parkinson's disease. *Brain*, 2009, 132(pt 1), 172–184.

[193] Weiss, D; Walach, M; Meisner, C; et al. Nigral stimulation for resistant axial motor impairment in Parkinson's disease? A randomized controlled trial. *Brain*, 2013, 136, 2098–2108

[194] Moro, E; Allert, N; Eleopra, R; Houeto, JL; Phan, TM; Stoevelaar, H. A decision tool to support appropriate referral for deep brain stimulation in Parkinson's disease. *J Neurol*, 2009, 256, 83-88.

[195] Wachter, T; Minguez-Castellanos, A; Valldeoriola, F; Herzog, J; Stoevelaar, H. A tool to improve pre-selection for deep brain stimulation in patients with Parkinson's disease. *J Neurol*, 2011, 258, 641-646.

[196] Schüpbach, WM; Maltête, D; Houeto, JL; du Montcel, ST; Mallet, L; Welter, ML; Gargiulo, M; Béhar, C; Bonnet, AM; Czernecki, V; Pidoux, B; Navarro, S; Dormont, D; Cornu, P; Agid, Y. Neurosurgery at an earlier stage of Parkinson disease: a randomized: controlled trial. *Neurology*, 2007, 68, 267-271.

[197] Schüpbach, WM; Rau, J; Knudsen, K; Volkmann, J; Krack, P; Timmermann, L; Hälbig, TD; Hesekamp, H; Navarro, SM; Meier, N; Falk, D; Mehdorn, M; Paschen, S; Maarouf, M; Barbe, MT; Fink, GR;

[198] Kupsch, A; Gruber, D; Schneider, GH; Seigneuret, E; Kistner, A; Chaynes, P; Ory-Magne, F; Brefel Courbon, C; Vesper, J; Schnitzler, A; Wojtecki, L; Houeto, JL; Bataille, B; et al.; Neurostimulation for Parkinson's disease with early motor complications. *N Engl J Med.*, 2013, 368, 610-622.

[199] Mestre, TA; Espay, AJ; Marras, C; Eckman, MH; Pollak, P; Lang, AE. Subthalamic nucleus-deep brain stimulation for early motor complications in Parkinson's disease-the EARLYSTIM trial: Early is not always better. *Mov Disord.*, 2014 Dec, 29(14), 1751-6.

[200] Charles, D; Konrad, PE; Neimat, JS; Molinari, AL; Tramontana, MG; Finder SG; Gill, CE; Bliton, MJ; Kao, C; Phibbs, FT; Hedera, P; Salomon, RM; Cannard, KR; Wang, L; Song, Y; Davis, TL. Subthalamic nucleus deep brain stimulation in early stage Parkinson's disease. *Parkinsonism Relat Disord.*, 2014 Jul, 20(7), 731-7.

[201] Espay, AJ; Vaughan, JE; Marras, C; Fowler, R; Eckman, MH. Early versus delayed bilateral subthalamic deep brain stimulation for parkinson's disease: a decision analysis. *Mov Disord*, 2010, 25, 1456-1463.

[202] Stegemöller, EL; Vallabhajosula, S; Haq, I; Hwynn, N; Hass, CJ; Okun, MS. Selective use of low frequency stimulation in Parkinson's disease based on absence of tremor. *NeuroRehabilitation*, 2013, 33(2), 305e12.

[203] Mehanna, R; Machado, AG; Oravivattanakul, S; Genc, G; Cooper, SE. Comparing two deep brain stimulation leads to one in refractory tremor. *Cerebellum.*, 2014 Aug, 13(4), 425-32.

[204] Wojtecki, L; Vesper, J; Schnitzler, A. Interleaving programming of subthalamic deep brain stimulation to reduce side effects with good motor outcome in a patient with Parkinson's disease. *Park Relat Disord*, 2011, 17(4), 293e4.

[205] Montgomery, EB. Deep brain stimulation programming: principles and practice. Oxford University Press: 2010.

[206] Miocinovic, S; Khemani, P; Whiddon, R; Zeilman, P; Martinez-Ramirez, D; Okun, MS; Chitnis, S. Outcomes, management, and potential mechanisms of interleaving deep brain stimulation settings. *Parkinsonism Relat Disord.*, 2014 Oct 22, 20(12), 1434-1437. doi; 10.1016/j.parkreldis.2014.10.011. [Epub ahead of print]

[207] Limousin, P; Pollak, P; Benazzouz, A; et al. Bilateral subthalamic nucleus stimulation for severe Parkinson's disease. *Mov Disord*, 1995, 10, 672–674.

[208] Limousin, P; Krack, P; Pollak, P; et al. Electrical stimulation of the subthalamic nucleus in advanced Parkinson's disease. *N Engl J Med*, 1998, 339, 1105–1111.

[209] Liu, W; McIntire, K; Kim, S; et al. Bilateral subthalamic stimulation improves gait initiation in patients with Parkinson's disease. *Gait Posture*, 2006, 23(4), 492e8.

[210] Crenna, P; Carpinella, I; Rabuffetti, M; et al. Impact of subthalamic nucleus stimulation on the initiation of gait in Parkinson's disease. *Exp Brain Res*, 2006, 172(4), 519e32.

[211] Vallabhajosula, S; Haq, IU; Hwynn, N; Oyama, G; Okun, M; Tillman, MD; Hass, CJ. Low-frequency Versus High-frequency Subthalamic Nucleus Deep Brain Stimulation on Postural Control and Gait in Parkinson's Disease: A Quantitative Study. *Brain Stimul.*, 2015 Jan-Feb, 8(1), 64-75.

[212] van Nuenen, BF; Esselink, RA; Munneke, M; Speelman, JD; van Laar, T; Bloem, BR. Postoperative gait deterioration after bilateral subthalamic nucleus stimulation in Parkinson's disease. *Mov Disord*, 2008, 23, 2404–2406.

[213] Moreau, C; Defebvre, L; Destée, A; et al. STN-DBS frequency effects on freezing of gait in advanced Parkinson disease. *Neurology*, 2008, 71(2), 80e4.

[214] Xie, T; Kang, UJ; Warnke, P. Effect of stimulation frequency on immediate freezing of gait in newly activated STN DBS in Parkinson's disease. *J Neurol Neurosurg Psychiatry.*, 2012 Oct, 83(10), 1015-7

[215] Phibbs, FT; Arbogast, PG; Davis, TL. 60-Hz frequency effect on gait in Parkinson's disease with subthalamic nucleus deep brain stimulation. *Neuromodulation*, 2014 Dec, 17(8), 717-20.

[216] Xie, T; Vigil, J; MacCracken, E; Gasparaitis, A; Young, J; Kang, W; Bernard, J; Warnke, P; Kang, UJ. Low-frequency stimulation of STN-DBS reduces aspiration and freezing of gait in patients with PD. Neurology. 2014 Dec 24. pii:10.1212/WNL.0000000000001184. [Epub ahead of print]

[217] Dhall, R; Krishnamurthi, N; Deep, A; Lieberman, A; Wilhem, K; Akhtar, S. Gait abnormalities in Parkinson's Disease: does subthalamic nucleus or globus pallidus internus variable frequency deep brain stimulation help? *Abstract at the 28th annual symposium of Parkinson's study group, St Louis, USA*, September 19th, 2104.

[218] Brozova, H; Barnaure, I; Alterman, RL; Tagliati, M. STN-DBS frequency effects on freezing of gait in advanced Parkinson disease. *Neurology.*, 2009 Feb 24, 72(8), 770.

[219] Fasano, A; Herzog, J; Seifert, E; et al. Modulation of gait coordination by subthalamic stimulation improves freezing of gait. *Mov Disord*, 2009, 26, 844–851.

[220] Johnsen, EL; Sunde, N; Mogensen, PH; Ostergaard, K. MRI verified STN stimulation site—gait improvement and clinical outcome. *Eur J Neurol*, 2010, 17, 746–753.

[221] Khoo, HM; Kishima, H; Hosomi, K; Maruo, T; Tani, N; Oshino, S; Shimokawa, T; Yokoe, M; Mochizuki, H; Saitoh, Y; Yoshimine, T. Low-frequency subthalamic nucleus stimulation in Parkinson's disease: a randomized clinical trial. *Mov Disord.*, 2014 Feb, 29(2), 270-4.

[222] Benarroch, EE. Subthalamic nucleus and its connections: anatomic substrate for the network effects of deep brain stimulation. *Neurology*, 2008, 70, 1991-1995.

[223] Aravamuthan, BR; Muthusamy, KA; Stein, JF; Aziz, TZ; Johansen- Berg, H. Topography of cortical and subcortical connections of the human pedunculopontine and subthalamic nuclei. *Neuroimage*, 2007, 37, 694-705.

[224] Moreau, C; Pennel-Ployart, O; Pinto, S; Plachez, A; Annic, A; Viallet, F; Destée, A; Defebvre, L. Modulation of dysarthropneumophonia by low-frequency STN DBS in advanced Parkinson's disease. *Mov Disord.*, 2011 Mar, 26(4), 659-63. doi; 10.1002/mds.23538 Nov 18, 2(1), 22.

In: Deep Brain Stimulation
Editor: Raja Mehanna

ISBN: 978-1-63483-282-3

Chapter 7

DEEP BRAIN STIMULATION FOR ESSENTIAL TREMOR

Jessika Suescun, MD, Allison Boyle, MD and Mya Schiess, MD
University of Texas Health Science Center at Houston, Houston, Texas

ABSTRACT

Essential tremor is one of the most common movement disorders in adults. Tremor is also among the most difficult movement disorders to treat, control or suppress pharmacologically. Deep Brain Stimulation (DBS) is the most effective therapy for the control of medication resistant distal hand tremor. In this chapter, we define essential tremor clinically and describe the known pathophysiology, epidemiology, genetics and medical treatment options. We then discuss the choices and selection of targets for placing DBS electrodes and review the available literature on efficacy and side effects using ON/OFF DBS improvement as an outcome or pre and post DBS tremor improvement as an outcome. The process of patient selection is described and the basic steps for initial DBS programming and optimization of effect are outlined as an algorithm.

INTRODUCTION

The term *tremore semplice essenziale* (simple essential tremor) was first used by Burresi in Italy in 1874 and it was used to describe an 18-year-old man with a severe isolated action tremor; by the early 20th century the term began to appear frequently in medical literature. For many years Essential Tremor (ET) was referred to as "benign essential tremor"; however, the adjective "benign" has been abandoned due to the clear disabling nature of the disorder.

Essential tremor is the second most common movement disorder among adults after restless legs syndrome. There is a worldwide prevalence of 0.4-0.9% among the general population and a significant increase in prevalence to 4.6% in people 65 years of age and older [1]. The prevalence is slightly higher among men, and the incidence is around 23.7 per 100,000 people per year [2, 3]. Although ET can present at any age, including childhood, it has been shown to have one late life peak around 65 years of age. ET is associated with significant physical and psychosocial disability [4].

Essential tremor is most commonly characterized by several defining features: [1,4,5]

(a) Postural and kinetic tremor with a variable amplitude and a frequency of 4-12 Hz (inversely related to age) typically seen on finger-nose-finger maneuvers in approximately 50% of the cases.
(b) Tremor involving specific joints in specific directions (e.g. wrist tremor is greater than metacarpal tremor; wrist flexion-extension tremor is greater than wrist rotation tremor).
(c) Tremor affecting either proximal or distal musculature including upper extremities in 95% of the patients, head in 34%, lower extremities in 20%, voice in 12%, face/jaw in 7% and trunk in 5%. Arm tremor usually precedes cranial tremor, of which there is a female preponderance.
(d) Tremor is present during voluntary movement and may rarely be present at rest (late feature that can occur in 20% of patients).
(e) Tremor may increase in severity and in the distribution of affected body parts over time with an annual increase in tremor severity estimated between 3.1-5.3%.
(f) Co-occurrence of cerebellar features in addition to the tremor (e.g. gait ataxia in almost 50% of the cases, as well as oculomotor deficits).

Tremor in ET typically increases with anxiety or stress and is commonly relieved for approximately 3 hours with small amounts of alcohol (by its action on GABA receptors) in 50-70% of patients. ET is a progressive and heterogeneous disorder, that severely affects activities of daily living and quality of life (QoL). Activities that can be affected include: eating, drinking, writing, dressing, personal hygiene, social activities and employment [1, 3, 6]. Approximately 90% of ET patients who seek medical attention for tremor report disability [3]. A variety of different features such as: neurological deficits (bradykinesia, cerebellar dysfunction, dysfunction in ocular movements, dysarthria, sensory abnormalities and gait abnormalities like tandem walking), cognitive deficits (deficit in attention, executive functions and memory) and neuropsychiatric symptoms (depression, anxiety and personality disturbances) can be associated with ET or an essential –like tremor [3]. Diagnostic criteria are based on the consensus statement of the movement disorder society on tremor (MDS) [7].

ET has been found to be an inherited disorder with an autosomal dominant pattern with a high genetic penetrance before age 65. There are two well defined risk factors for ET: age and a family history of ET. To date, three genes associated with increased risk for ET have been identified: SLC1A, LINGO1 and LINGO2. The mechanism by which these genetic variant alleles confer risk is unknown [4, 8]. Although many patients with family histories consistent with an autosomal dominant inheritance have been described, no other genes have been identified as yet [3]. It is thought that the onset of essential tremor may be influenced by both genetic and environmental factors based on the considerable clinical, genetic and pharmacological heterogeneity among ET patients. An estimated 30-50% of ET patients report a first or second degree relative that is affected by the disease [3].

The pathophysiology of ET is thought to be the result of the pacemaking neurons in the inferior olivary nucleus of the cerebellum. These neurons typically begin firing in a rhythmic manner at 4-12Hz via gamma amino butyric acid (GABA) mediated gap junctions. The signal is then transmitted to the cerebellar cortex and subsequently distributed along the ascending cerebello-thalamic pathway and the descending brainstem medial reticular formation to manifest as tremor, and is further modulated by peripheral (muscle) adrenoreceptors [9, 10]. Although the pathophysiology of essential tremor can be understood in terms of cerebellar systems dysfunction, the neuropathology of ET is quite controversial and there is an unresolved debate as to whether an underlying cerebellar neurodegenerative process exists in ET. In several studies comparing postmortem examination of ET patients to age-matched controls, a variety of changes in the cerebellum, most commonly in the Purkinje cells, has been described including decreased density of Purkinje cells and a torpedo shaped swelling of proximal portion of the Pukinje cell axons, thusly referred to as torpedoes. Neuropathological changes have been reported in the surrounding neuronal populations, including the presence of lower brainstem Lewy bodies and intranuclear inclusions in the cerebellum [5, 11].

Currently, no curative treatment exists for ET and management is typically aimed at symptomatic control. There are several treatments aimed at symptomatic improvement, and the first line therapy typically is pharmacological and involves enhancing of the GABA-ergic system. Based on the concept of the widespread neuronal oscillation, anticonvulsants are thought to act through ion channels and benzodiazepines through GABA receptor modulation. Calcium channel blockers can be used by targeting low-threshold calcium currents active in membrane oscillation. β- adrenergic blockers (beta blockers) are thought to reduce the stretch-reflex sensitivity [8]. The American Academy of Neurology (AAN) practice parameters established a level A recommendation for efficacy of the β- adrenergic blocker propranolol and the anticonvulsant, primidone; level B recommendations include: alprazolam, atenolol, gabapentin (monotherapy), sotalol and topiramate. However, recent evidence suggests topiramate will likely be raised to a level A recommendation . Propranolol is the only medication that is approved by the FDA to treat ET. However, 30-60% of patients with ET will not respond to treatment and the remaining percentage has a variable or only partial response [5]. Once patients fail level A medical treatments, they should be considered for surgical treatment with Deep Brain Stimulation therapy (DBS).

DBS therapy has been an FDA approved treatment for tremor since 1997 and is a level C recommendation by the AAN for the management of ET if the following criteria are met.

- Medically refractory ET patients who have tried at least a β- adrenergic blocker and primidone without satisfactory resolution
- Disabling tremor: interfering with daily life activities and/or independence
- Patients do not suffer from dementia or significant comorbidities such as severe cardiac or pulmonary conditions that make them a surgical risk.

DBS therapy has become a mainstay treatment for severe and medically intractable ET. Even though DBS therapy has shown stable efficacy over the last two decades, the manner in which DBS accomplishes tremor control remains unclear. One hypothesis suggests axonal or synaptic failure by disruption of the oscillatory activity in a pathway from the cerebellum to the ventrolateral thalamus, and consequent excitation of the thalamo-cortical loop [12]. The electrodes used for DBS implantation are usually well tolerated in patients long term. Autopsy studies have shown minimal gliosis and lymphocytic infiltration of tissue immediately adjacent to the DBS leads [1].

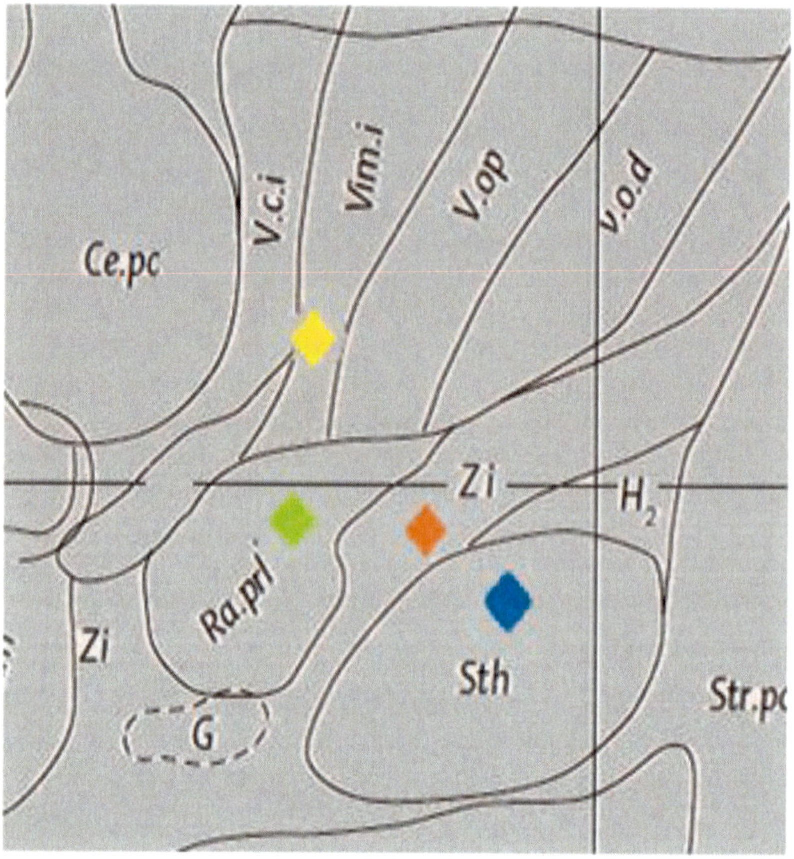

Figure 1. Surgical targets for Essential tremor. A sagittal cut from the Schaltenbrand-Wahren atlas is used to roughly show possible locations of stimulation. The targets include: nucleus ventrointermedius of the thalamus (Vim, yellow diamond), the posterior subthalamic area (PSA) including both, caudal zona incerta (cZi, orange diamond) and prelemniscal radiation (Ra.prl, green diamond) and the subthalamic nucleus (Sth, blue diamond).

A. Review of Evidence

There are currently 3 main targets for DBS surgery in ET patients: the ventrointermedius nucleus of the thalamus (Vim), the posterior subthalamic area (PSA) including both zona incerta and prelemniscal radiation, and the subthalamic nucleus (STN) (Figure 1). Among these, only the Vim is approved by US and European regulatory agencies as a target for DBS surgery in ET patients.

Ventrointermedius Nucleus of the Thalamus (Vim)

The Vim is currently the surgical target of choice. This nucleus receives primarily cerebellar afferents with projections to the motor cortex and adjoining cortical areas involved in movement initiation and fine motor control. Within the Vim, there is a clear homunculus representation with kinesthetic leg cells situated laterally, arm cells located medially, and facial cells situated adjacent to the central thalamic nucleus [13].

The efficacy and safety of Vim DBS for ET treatment has been demonstrated widely in short and long term studies (> 5 years) including data on long term satisfaction and mortality rates [14-38]. In this chapter, the authors report change in tremor using the Fahn-Tolosa-Marin (FTM) tremor scale as the primary outcome in the majority of studies, the remainder of the studies using the essential tremor-rating scale (ETRS).

These studies report two different methods of assessing DBS therapy outcomes: comparing tremor score ON and OFF DBS, or tremor score before and after DBS. The first group includes 16 studies that compared patients post operatively with DBS switched on and then off. In this group, hand tremor improved significantly with DBS ON, with an improvement range between 33 and 87%, while TADLS (tremor activities of daily living scale) improved by 31-70%, head tremor improved by 38-80%, and voice tremor improved by 28-83%. Both head and voice tremor control had an intermediate response with unilateral Vim but gained full clinical response from bilateral implantation. For hand tremor, Vim was implanted either unilaterally and contralateral to the tremor dominant side, or bilaterally. One of the studies yielded a total survival above 80% and continued satisfaction of tremor control 10 years after implantation [37]. (Table 1A).

The second group includes 8 studies that compared tremor before DBS surgery and after the surgical procedure with DBS turned on. Arm tremor improvement ranged from 31-75% while head and voice tremor improved by 50-60%. However, one of the studies reported a decline in semantic verbal fluency as a result of DBS surgery [24]. (Table 1B).

The most common side effects of unilateral thalamic stimulation include: dysarthria (3-18% of the patients), paraesthesias (6-36%), dystonia (2-9%), balance disturbance (3-8%), ataxia (6%) and limb weakness (4-8%). Most side effects were mild in all studies and could be potentially improved by changes in the stimulation settings and parameters. Hardware complications (skin erosions, infections, lead fractures and connection-cable malfunctions) occurred in nearly 20% of the patients. Perioperative complications included intracerebral bleeding, ischemic stroke, and infection; and the 30-day mortality rate of DBS surgery for all the patients was estimated to be 0.4%.

The key limiting factor in effective suppression of tremor with the Vim target is the high incidence (50-75%) of dysarthria and imbalance with bilateral implantation. Bilateral implantation is required in most cases that involve head and voice tremor. Other side effects or limiting factors include: no significant change on balance and gait disorders with unilateral or bilateral implants, development of tolerance with progressively higher stimulation settings over time and diminished effect over time. Data show an average overall improvement of 50% 5 years post implantation. However, despite tremor progression, patients still perceive substantial benefit based on Activity of Daily Living (ADL) and Quality of Life (QoL) scales in long term studies [25, 34, 35-38].

Tremor emanating predominantly in the proximal part of the upper extremity or in the axial part of the body (neck or lower limbs) and cerebellar outflow tremor do not respond well to Vim DBS, with only one third of patients showing significant improvement. In some cases, even if the distal tremor resolves with Vim DBS, residual proximal tremor of the kinetic or postural type can impair activities of daily life. In these specific cases, literature has demonstrated that stimulation of the posterior subthalamic area (PSA) involving the zona incerta (Zi) and prelemniscal radiation (Raprl) remarkably improved proximal tremor.

Posterior Subthalamic Area

The posterior subthalamic area (PSA) involves the zona incerta (Zi) and prelemniscal radiation (Raprl) and is surrounded by the subthalamic nucleus anteriorly, the ventral thalamic nucleus superiorly, the dorsal border of the subtantia nigra inferiorly, the medial lemniscus posteriorly and the posterior limb of the internal capsule laterally (Figure 1). This target has been described as a 'bottle neck' of axons projecting to the thalamus. The Zi consists of a caudal (cZi) and a rostral part, in which the caudal component is the motor component and is considered to be an extension of the reticular/thalamic nucleus. Raprl is a bundle of fibers containing neurons from the mesencephalic reticular formation that project to the thalamus, as well as ascending cerebello-thalamic fibers [39, 40]. cZi is an effective target for tremor control based on its GABA-ergic connections with both the basal ganglia and the cerebellar thalamo-cortical loops, in addition to brainstem motor effectors through which tremor oscillation may be transmitted [39].

Placement of DBS in the PSA has been found to be both safe and efficacious. In review of current data, placement in the PSA can yield a reduction in tremor ranging from 60-95% and improvement of ADL's by 60-88% [41-51]. The side effects reported are similar to that with Vim placement, but with a few differences. Placement in the PSA has been found to have a long lasting effect that can be achieved at lower stimulation strengths and without any apparent development of tolerance in patients followed 4 years post implantation. Patients with bilateral PSA placement have not been found to have side effects of persistent dysphagia, dysarthria or disequilibrium as reported in patients with bilateral Vim placement (Table 2).

A total of 4 case studies have compared targets for the treatment of ET: 3 of the studies compared PSA vs Vim and 1 study compared PSA vs STN [43, 47-48]. The data from the studies report the same conclusion: PSA stimulation is more efficient in treating ET, but Vim targeting can be as equally effective with higher stimulation. These findings may be explained by the difference in cell types being stimulated in each target. Assuming that fiber stimulation (in PSA) needs less current than soma/dendrite stimulation (in Vim) and that the same amplitude is used in both targets, the stimulation in the Vim would not affect as many afferent neurons as stimulation in the PSA, thus leading to less efficient tremor suppression when stimulating Vim compared to PSA. Interestingly, in one study, patients were implanted with both Vim and PSA leads in an effort to choose the target with the best effect on an individualized basis. The results were based on patient response to stimulation and found no measurable difference between stimulation of either Vim or PSA [51].

Currently, there are a few limiting factors for choosing the PSA as a target for patients with ET. These factors include: lack of long term safety and efficacy studies beyond 4 years, variable locations of stimulation electrodes labeled as PSA in the published studies, and the limited number of patients and lack of controlled clinical trials that compare this target with the others available.

At this time, PSA cannot be formally recommended as a target for DBS in ET, and has not been approved as such by US and European regulatory agencies.

Table 1A. Studies of Vim DBS in ET with comparison of tremor score ON and OFF DBS as outcome

Author(year)	N	Assessment	Outcome/improvement (DBS ON/OFF)	Mean follow up (in months)	Complications subsequent to DBS programming*
Carpenter et al. (1998) [14].	7	Voice tremor	• 4/7 show reduction in voice tremor (1-3 points change in 5 scale) • 24 -60% difference in relative amplitude	18	Tingling, numbness and dysarthria
Lyons et al. (1998) [15].	22	Activities of Daily Living Scale	• 58% improvement in self-rated TADLS score • 54% in clinician rated TADLS scores	11	None reported
Ondo et al. (1998) [16].	14	Arm tremor	• 83% reduction in contralateral arm tremor	3	Disequilibrium, paresthesia, dysarthria, headache, nausea, diplopia and transient altered mental status.
Koller et al. (1999) [17].	38	Head tremor	• 3 months: improved in 71% of patients, unchanged in 26%, and worsened in 3%. • 6 months: improved in 68% of patients, unchanged in 23%, and worsened in 9%. • One year: improved in 75% of patients, unchanged in 20% and worsened in 5%.	12	Paresthesia, headache, dysarthria, paresis, attention/cognitive deficits, gait disorders, facial weakness, dystonia, hypophonia, nausea, depression, and dizziness.
Obwegeser et al. (2000) [19].	27	Arm, head, voice, tongue, and face tremor.	• 82% total contralateral arm tremor reduction. • Unilateral: 38%-head, 28%-voice, 93% tongue and 65% face improvement • Bilateral: 95%-head, 83%-voice and 100% tongue improvement	12	Disequilibrium, dysarthria, and paresthesias
Koller et al. (2001) [20].	25	Arm tremor	• 97% contralateral arm tremor reduction	40	Paresthesia, headache, paresis, dysarthria, nausea, disequilibrium, facial weakness, gait disorder, dystonia, mild attention/cognitive deficit, dizziness, hypophonia, anxiety, syncope, drooling and vomiting.

Table 1A. (Continued)

Author(year)	N	Assessment	Outcome/improvement (DBS ON/OFF)	Mean follow up (in months)	Complications subsequent to DBS programming*
Ondo et al. (2001) [21].	11	Unilateral vs Bilateral Vim DBS	• Midline tremors (face and head) improved only after the second side implantation in 80%.	3	Dysarthria, gait or disequilibrium problems, paresthesias and neck pain.
Vaillancourt et al. (2003) [23].	6	Hand tremor	• DBS reduced the amplitude and the regularity of tremor	3	None reported
Sydow et al. (2003) [25].	19	Long-Term Efficacy in arm, head and voice tremor	• 41% improvement on tremor's impact on activities of daily living • Non-significant trend in head and voice tremor reduction after 6 years.	72	Paraesthesia, dysarthria, gait disorders, dystonia, headaches, chest pain, local pain at pocket site and connector site.
Rehncrona et al. (2003) [26]	19	Long-Term Efficacy	• Tremor in upper extremity was significantly reduced (P=0.025) 7 years after the procedure.	72	Paraesthesias
Bryant et al. (2003) [27].	16	Activities of Daily Living	• 44% improvement in the patient-rated TADLS • 45.2% improvement in the clinician-rated TADLS. • 33.9% improvement in the TRS.	13	Paresthesia, dysarthria, diplopia and disequilibrium.
Putzke et al. (2004) [28].	22	Long-term Efficacy	• 87% improvement on hand tremor • 70% improvement on ADL	36	Dysarthria, disequilibrium, motor disturbances, paresthesias
Pahwa et al. (2006) [30].	23	Long-Term Efficacy in arm, head and voice tremor	• Unilateral: 75% improvement hand tremor • Bilateral: 65-85% improvement.	60	Paresthesia, pain, dysarthria and balance difficulties.
De Oliveira et al. (2012) [35].	26	Long- Term benefits	• 79% tremor improvement • 55% QOL improvement.	41	None reported

Author(year)	N	Assessment	Outcome/improvement (DBS ON/OFF)	Mean follow up (in months)	Complications subsequent to DBS programming*
Peng-cheng et al. (2013) [36].	22	Long-Term Efficacy	• 40% tremor improvement • 67% ADL improvement.	40.8	Mental decline, motor symptoms, aphasia, gait impairment and mania.
Borretzen et al. (2014) [37].	26	Long- Term satisfaction and mortality	• No significant increase in mortality. • Long term satisfaction. • 10 years survival above 80%	72	Dysarthria, headache, paresthesia, abnormal taste, dizziness, tongue discomfort , reduced balance.
Baizabal-Carvallo et al. (2014) [38].	13	Long-Term Efficacy	• 37.2% tremor improvement • 31.7% ADL improvement	96	Dysarthria, disequilibrium and gait ataxia.

* In clinical practice, most of these complications can be alleviated with changes in the stimulation parameters.

Table 1B. Studies of Vim DBS in ET with comparison of tremor score before and after DBS as outcome

Author(year)	N	Assessments	Outcome/improvement (Before/after DBS)	Follow up in months (mean)	Complications subsequent to DBS programming*
Taha et al. (1999) [18].	15	Head and voice tremor	• 90% of patients with head tremor improved between 50-75%. • 86% of patients with voice tremor improved 50%.	10	Dysarthria, disequilibrium, memory loss
Hariz et al. (2002) [22].	27	Health-related quality of life	• 47% improvement of TRS scores • For 70% patients DBS met their expectations.	12	Disequilibrium, dysarthria, headache and depression
Fields et al. (2003) [24].	40	Quality of life	• Improvements on: cognitive measures, fine visuomotor, visuoperceptual functions, verbal memory, mood state, and QoL. • Semantic verbal fluency declined significantly in 10% of the patients.	12	None reported
Lee and Kondziolka (2005) [29].	18	Arm tremor and handwriting	• 75.8% tremor improvement • 64% improvement in handwriting.	27	Tingling

Table 1B. (Continued)

Author(year)	N	Assessments	Outcome/improvement (Before/after DBS)	Follow up in months (mean)	Complications subsequent to DBS programming*
Blomstedt et al. (2007) [31].	19	Long-Term Efficacy in arm, head and voice	• 60.3% hand tremor improvement • 35.4% hand function improvement • 60% improvement on head tremor	86	None reported
Pilitsis et al. (2008) [32].	26	Long-Term Efficacy	• 75.3% tremor improvement • 73.8% handwriting improvement	40	None reported
Zhang et al. (2010) [33].	34	Long-Term Efficacy	• 80.4% tremor improvement • 69.7% handwriting improvement	56.9	Tingling, numbness, eye movement disorders, weakness, gait instability, slurring of speech, and drooling.
Nazarro et el (2012) [34].	91	Long- Term benefits in quality of life	• 31% tremor improvement • 36.9% ADL improvement.	108	None reported

* In clinical practice, most of these complications can be alleviated with changes in the stimulation parameters.

Table 2. PSA (zona incerta and prelemniscal radiation) in ET

Author(year)	N	Assessments	Outcome/improvement	Mean follow up(in months)	Complications subsequent to DBS programming*
Murata et al.* (2003) [41].	8	Arm tremor	DBS before/after: • Contralateral tremor improved by 81%	22	Paresthesia, limb ataxia
Plaha et al. (2004) [42].	4	Arm and head tremor	DBS before/after: • 80% tremor improvement (ETRS) • ADL improve by 88.8%	12	No related complications.
Herzog et al. (2007) [43].	10	PSA vs VIM	DBS before/after • PSA led to a mean reduction of the lateralized tremor rating scale by 15.8 points which was significantly superior to thalamus (P<0 05).	14	Paresthesia, sensory dysfunction, nystagmus, dysarthria, urinary incontinence, slight visual disturbance, oculomotor paresis, dysarthria.
Hamel et al. (2007) [44].	8	Efficacy of different subthalamic areas	DBS before/after: • Tremor on the left and right side of the body was improved by 68% and 73% respectively.	12	Paresthesia, dysarthria, gait ataxia.
Blomstedt et al. (2010) [45].	21	Efficacy of PSA stimulation	DBS before/after: • 60% reduction in total ETRS • 66% ADL improvement	12	Expressive dysphasia, clumsiness, blurred vision, dizziness
Plaha et al. (2011) [46].	15	Quality of life	DBS before/after: • The total tremor score improved by 73.8% (p<0.0001). • The SF-36 physical component score improved by 23.7% and the mental component score by 22.4% (p<0.0001).	32	Dysarthria and hypophonia.
Barbe et al. (2011) [47].	21	PSA vs VIM	DBS on/off: • PSA stimulation may be more efficient compared to thalamic but equally effective when patients individual stimulation parameters are used.	3	Paresthesia and dysarthria.

Table 2. (Continued)

Author(year)	N	Assessments	Outcome/improvement	Mean follow up(in months)	Complications subsequent to DBS programming*
Blomstedt et al. (2011) [48].	4	PSA vs STN	DBS on/off: • PSA is more efficient than STN for ET treatment.	12	Dysarthria, dystonia, dizziness and blurred vision
Sandvik et al. (2011) [49].	36	PSA vs VIM	DBS before/after: • ETRS was reduced by 48.4% in VIM and by 58.2% in the PSA group.	12	None reported
Sandvik et al. (2012) [50].	16	Quality of life	DBS before/after: • 95% hand tremor improvement • 71% improvement on ADL	12	Vertigo and speech quality impacted
Fytagoridis et al. (2012) [40].	18	Long term efficacy	DBS on/off: • 52.4% decrease on the ETRS score • ADL improved by 65.8%	48	Expressive dysphasia, clumsiness, blurred vision, dizziness
Chang et al. (2013) [51].	5	PSA vs VIM	DBS before/after: • TETRAS scores improved 94% for postural tremor and 76% for kinetic tremor. • There was no statistically significant difference between PSA and VIM in terms of benefits.	12	None reported

* In clinical practice, most of these complications can be alleviated with changes in the stimulation parameters.

Subthalamic Nucleus

STN seems to improve tremor in ET patients through tonic activation of adjacent cerebello-thalamic fibers, thus leading to a tonic activation of Vim neurons which causes a disruption of tremor synchronous activity. Studies looking at STN as a target for ET are limited. The majority of case reports are actually patients with PD that have comorbid ET [52-53]. To date, there is one case series that includes 12 ET patients treated with STN stimulation [54]. In this study, 3 of the patients were followed for 9 years, and the remainder were followed for 3 years. In the long term group (9 years) the authors report excellent tremor control with unchanged, or only slightly increased, stimulation intensity over time. The study did report several side effects that were more commonly seen in patients older than 70 years of age and that included dystonic posture of the neck, dysarthria, balance disturbances and a reported long latency for tremor control. Currently, there is not enough literature to support the use of STN placement for the treatment of ET (Table 3), and this target is not approved by US and European regulatory agencies.

B. Patient Selection

The severity of tremor in patients with ET varies widely from a minimal low amplitude tremor in the hands to a severely disabling tremor of the hands, head, voice and trunk. DBS surgery should be considered for patients that experience moderate to severe tremor that is either refractory to medical management, limited by medication side effects or impairs activities of daily living. When determining which patients are candidates for surgical intervention, it is important to address several factors including proper diagnosis and pharmacologic management.

The first step when evaluating a patient for potential surgical intervention is determining if they meet the clinical criteria for the diagnosis of ET. It has been estimated that between 30-50% of patients with ET are misdiagnosed with other tremor disorders [55-56]. There are several established sets of criteria for the diagnosis of ET. The most commonly used set of criteria in the past was the TRIG criteria. However, in 1998, the Movement Disorders Society (MDS) proposed consensus criteria for the diagnosis of ET that are more widely used today. The MDS consensus criteria for the diagnsosis of ET include: 1. Bilateral, largely symmetric postural or kinetic tremor involving hands and forearms that is visible and persistent and 2. Additional or isolated tremor of the head may occur, but in the absence of abnormal posture. There are secondary clinical criteria to help further facilitate diagnosis, that include: 1. Long duration (>3yrs) 2. Positive family history and 3. Beneficial response to alcohol. Exclusion criteria include other abnormal neurolgic signs especially dystonia, presence of known causes of enhanced physiologic tremor, sudden onset and progression of tremor, and isolated/focal tremor [55, 57].

After proper diagnosis is established, the next step in the selection process is to review the past and present medications prescribed to the patient for the treatment of tremor. There are two main medications that have been proven to be the most effective treatments of ET: propranolol and primidone. Both medications have similar efficacy, but may be limited by side effects. Propranolol can be associated with hypotension, bradycardia, exercise intolerance and drowsiness. Primidone may be limited by nausea, drowsiness and balance difficulty. There are several other medications that have shown benefit for ET, though are less studied, including benzodiazepines, topiramate and gabapentin.

Patients that have had adequate medication trials, i.e. maximal titrations and preferably combinations of a beta blocker, primidone, and possibly a benzodiazepine or topiramate and do not achieve adequate tremor control or are limited by medication side effects should be considered for DBS therapy [15, 55].

Patients should undergo neuropsychological evaluation to identify cognitive deficits and mood changes, that include verbal fluency tests, memory, attention and executive function, depression and anxiety screening [2].

Patients should then be evaluated by a neurosurgeon for assessment of their surgical risk, and determining the type of DBS pulse generator that will be implanted. Overall, patients undergo a multidisciplinary evaluation, with an emphasis on setting realistic expectations from the surgery [55].

After a patient is determined to be a good candidate for DBS therapy, the next step is to determine if he/she would benefit from unilateral or bilateral placement in an effort to achieve good tremor control. The decision for unilateral versus bilateral placement of DBS should be based on the outcome goal, severity of tremor and location of tremor. Patients with severe tremor of the dominant hand that are not limited by tremor elsewhere may only need unilateral placement, whereas patients with severe bilateral hand tremor and tremor of head, trunk or legs may require bilateral placement [55].

After a patient undergoes surgical implantation of DBS, the next step in care is effective and efficient post-operative programming.

Table 3. STN in ET

Author(year)	N	Assessments	Outcome/improvement (Before/after DBS)	Mean follow up (in months)	Complications subsequent to DBS programming
Requejo et al. (2004)[52]	1	Arm tremor	• 82.4% improvement of arm tremor	18	None reported
Stover et al. (2005)[53]	1	Arm tremor	• Complete suppression of the action and postural tremor	36	None reported
Lind et al. (2008)[54]	12	Short and long term results	• STN is a good target for long-term treatment	45	None reported

C. PROGRAMMING IN ET

Effective DBS programming corresponds to creating a sufficient neuronal response in the intended target without spread of electrical stimulation to unintended nearby structures. This is achieved by a judicious choice of active electrode configuration and by determining an effective combination of electrical parameters in order to obtain tremor control without causing side effects. Each DBS lead has a variety of variables that can be modified in an effort to achieve the most effective treatment. The variables that can be adjusted are the electrode configuration (monopolar or bipolar), voltage, pulse width and rate. The electrical charge generated during the DBS pulse dissipates with distance from the electrode and the electrical charge is highest near the active electrode contact. The active electrodes can be configured as monopolar, bipolar and multi-polar. The monopolar configuration has a single negative electrode (cathode) and the metal case of the implanted neurostimulator acts as the positive electrode (anode). In the bipolar configuration a single electrode is negative and another electrode is positive. In the multi-polar configuration there are one or more negative electrodes and one or more positive electrodes. The distance between the positive and negative electrodes affects the intensity of the electric field, the closer they are together the more intense the signal. The monopolar configuration is broad resulting in a less intense, but larger electrical field; whereas the bipolar or multipolar configurations lead to a smaller, more intense electrical field. The electrical field can be further modified by adjusting the stimulation parameters (voltage, pulse width and rate). The number and location of axons that are stimulated can be adjusted by changes in the voltage. Higher voltages can stimulate more axons by increasing the spatial extent of the electrical field intensities. Within the electrical field, increasing the voltage can increase the number of axons stimulated. The type of axon that is stimulated can be manipulated by changes in the pulse width. Axons with larger diameters are stimulated by shorter pulse widths, whereas small diameter axons are stimulated by longer pulse widths. The effects of different rates (frequency) of DBS on neuronal activities are less straightforward. In the past, it was thought that high frequency inhibits the stimulated target and low frequency excites the target; however, there are many cases in which low frequency is therapeutic [55, 58].

The effects of stimulation are dependent on the location of the active electrode, stimulation parameters and type of neuronal tissue that is being stimulated. The first step for initial programming is to assess the efficacy and adverse effects of stimulation by screening each individual electrode (Figure 2). Typical initial stimulation parameters begin with amplitude of 0 volts, pulse width of 60 or 90 microseconds and frequency of 130-160 Hz. During the initial screening, the electrodes are screened typically in the monopolar configuration and the amplitude is slowly increased to maximally tolerated voltages (typically 4-5V) while the patient is observed for both benefits and adverse effects. The electrode with the best tremor control and fewest side effects is then chosen for continued programming and fine tuning and may stay monopolar or may need to be adjusted to a bipolar configuration. Typical final settings for VIM DBS are: amplitude 1-4 V, pulse width of 60-120 us and rate of 130-185 Hz.

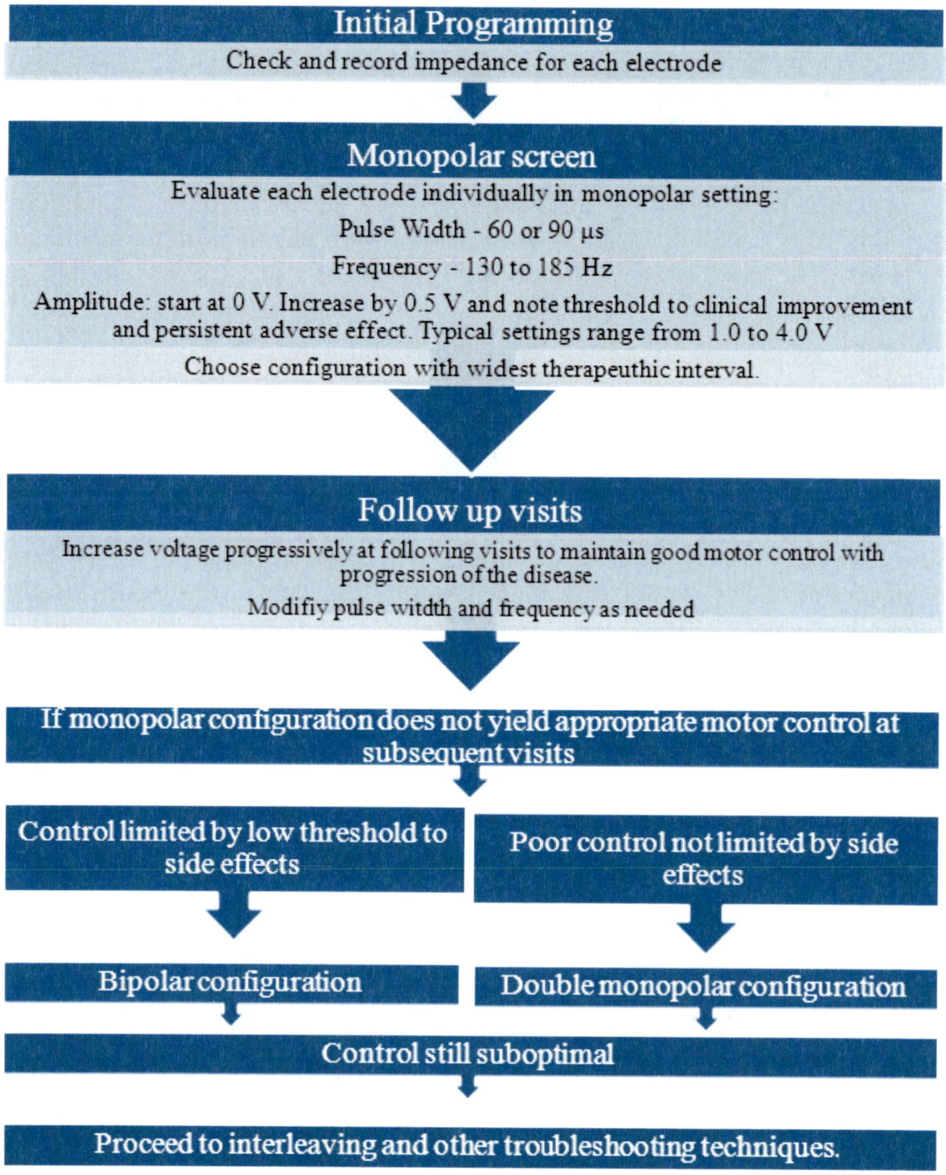

Figure 2. Suggested algorithm for DBS programming in ET patients.

Troubleshooting Techniques

For patients that have not had an optimal response to DBS programming there are a few techniques that can be used in an effort to obtain optimal tremor control. For most patients, the efficacy of DBS is based on high frequency stimulation and the majority of patients with ET have rate of stimulation between 130 – 185 Hz. Low stimulation (below 50 Hz) has been found to cause stimulation induced worsening of tremor. In ET patients that have a tremor that is refractory to programming, trial of using a higher than average rate may be effective [55]. Another technique used for refractory tremor patients is that of Interleaved stimulation

(ILS). ILS as a relatively new technique used to optimize the stimulation field to provide the best possible symptomatic control while minimizing side effects. With ILS, two programs are interleaved in an alternating fashion on the same lead. The two programs are able to drive their own combination of active electrodes, pulse width, and amplitude in an effort to provide symptom control. There are limited data comparing outcomes of patients with ILS versus traditional programming but the information available indicates that ILS theoretically may have advantages for patients with tremor, especially patients with suboptimal response [59]. Troubleshooting techniques will be discussed in further details in chapter 10.

Conclusion

ET is a common movement disorder that is frequently refractory to medical management. DBS therapy appears to be a safe and effective therapy option for these cases (achieving improvement of greater than 70%). Unilateral Vim is the most widely used target and its short term and long term benefit in upper extremity tremor has been demonstrated. Bilateral Vim is associated with a higher prevalence of side effects including dysarthria, dysphagia and balance difficulties and is commonly used to achieve better results in head and voice tremor. Targeting PSA for DBS appears to be safe and effective in short term studies and is an available option for axial and cerebellar outflow tremors that are poorly responsive to Vim targeting. However, long term studies are needed and this target has not been approved by US and European regulatory agencies for the treatment of ET. Case reports have shown PSA to be a more effective target than Vim with the advantage of fewer side effects when implanted bilaterally. However, further comparative studies and randomized control trials are needed to assess the true advantage of using this target instead of Vim. There is no substantial evidence for the use of STN in ET (kinetic tremor) management. The algorithm for programming DBS targeting Vim is fairly straightforward with emphasis placed on avoiding the stimulation of adjacent structures that could cause adverse effects while emphasizing optimal tremor control. DBS efficacy in the treatment of ET has been shown to be maintained over time.

References

[1] Nazarro, J; Lyons, K; Rajesh, P. Deep brain stimulation for essential tremor. Lozano and Hallet. *Handbook of clinical neurology.*, 2013, 116, 155-166. Elsevier B.V.

[2] Bermejo-Pareja, F. Essential tremor- a neurodegenerative disorder associated with cognitive defects? *Rev. Neurol.* 2011, 7, 273-282.

[3] Benito-Leon, J; Louis, E. Update on essential tremor. *Minerva med*, 2011, 102, 417-440.

[4] Elbe, Rodger. What is essential tremor?. *Curr Neurol Neurosci Rep.*, 2013, 13, 353.

[5] Louis Elan.'Essential tremor' or the esssential tremors: is this one disease or a family of diseases?. *Neuroepidemiology*, 2014, 42, 81-89.

[6] Sandvik, U; Hariz, G; Blomstedt. Quality of life following DBS in the caudal zona incerta in patients with essential tremor. *Acta Neurochir.*, 2012, 154, 495-499.

[7] Deuschl, G; Bain, P; Brin, M; et al. Consensus statement of the movement disorder society on tremor. *Movement disorders*., 1998, 13(3), 2-23.

[8] Deuschl, G; Raethjen, J; Hellriegel, H; Elbe, R. Treatment of patients with essential tremor. *Lancet Neurol*., 2013, 10, 148-161.

[9] Louis, Elan. Rethinking the biology of essential tremor: from models to morphology. *Parkinsonism and Related disorders*., 2014, S88-S93.

[10] Plaha, P; Javed, S; Agombar, D; O'Farrell, G; et al. Bilateral caudal zona incerta nucleus stimulation for essential tremor: outcome and quality of life. *J Neurol neurosurg psychiatry*., 2011, 82, 899-904

[11] Louis, Elan. Understanding essential tremor: progress on the biological front. *Curr Neurol neurosci Rep*., 2014, 14, 450.

[12] Elble, R. Mechanism of deep brain stimulation for essential tremor. *Brain*, 2014, 137, 4-5.

[13] Hamani, C; Dostrovsky, JO; Lozano, AM. The motor thalamus in neurosurgery. *Neurosurgery*., 2006, 58, 146-158.

[14] Carpenter, MA; Pahwa, R; Miyawaki, KL; Wilkinson, SB; Searl, JP; et al. Reduction in voice tremor under thalamic stimulation. *Neurology*., 1998, 50 (3), 796-798.

[15] Lyons, KE; Pahwa, R; Busenbark, KL; Tröster, AI; Wilkinson, S; et al. Improvements in daily functioning after deep brain stimulation of the thalamus for intractable tremor. *Mov Disord*., 1998, 13(4), 690-692.

[16] Ondo, W; Jankovic, J; Schwartz, K; Almaguer, M; Simpson, RK. Unilateral thalamic deep brain stimulation for refractory essential tremor and Parkinson's disease tremor. *Neurology*., 1998, 51(4), 1063-1069.

[17] Koller, WC; Lyons, KE; Wilkinson, SB; Pahwa, R. Efficacy of unilateral deep brain stimulation of the VIM nucleus of the thalamus for essential head tremor. *Mov Disord*., 1999, 14(5), 847-850.

[18] Taha, JM; Janszen, MA; Favre, J. Thalamic deep brain stimulation for the treatment of head, voice, and bilateral limb tremor. *J Neurosurg*., 1999, 91(1), 68-72.

[19] Obwegeser, AA; Uitti, RJ; Turk, MF; Strongosky, AJ; Wharen, RE. Thalamic stimulation for the treatment of midline tremors in essential tremor patients. *Neurology*., 2000, 54(12), 2342-2344.

[20] Koller, WC; Lyons, KE; Wilkinson, SB; Troster, AI; Pahwa, R. Long-term safety and efficacy of unilateral deep brain stimulation of the thalamus in essential tremor. *Mov Disord*., 2001, 16(3), 464-468.

[21] Ondo, W; Almaguer, M; Jankovic, J; Simpson, RK. Thalamic deep brain stimulation: comparison between unilateral and bilateral placement. *Arch Neurol*. 2001, 58(2), 218-222.

[22] Hariz, GM; Lindberg, M; Bergenheim, AT. Impact of thalamic deep brain stimulation on disability and health-related quality of life in patients with essentialtremor. *J Neurol Neurosurg Psychiatry*., 2002, 72(1), 47-52.

[23] Vaillancourt, DE; Sturman, MM; Verhagen, Metman, L; Bakay, RA; Corcos, DM. Deep brain stimulation of the VIM thalamic nucleus modifies several features of essential tremor. *Neurology*., 2003, 61(7), 919-925.

[24] Fields, JA; Tröster, AI; Woods, SP; Higginson, CI; Wilkinson, SB; et al. Neuropsychological and quality of life outcomes 12 months after unilateral thalamic stimulation for essentialtremor. *J Neurol Neurosurg Psychiatry*., 2003, 74(3), 305-311.

[25] Sydow, O; Thobois, S; Alesch, F; Speelman, JD. Multicentre European study of thalamic stimulation in essential tremor: a six year follow up. *J Neurol Neurosurg Psychiatry.*, 2003, 74(10), 1387-1391.

[26] Rehncrona, S; Johnels, B; Widner, H; Törnqvist, AL; Hariz, M; Sydow, O. Long-term efficacy of thalamic deep brain stimulation for tremor: double-blind assessments. *Mov Disord.*, 2003, 18(2), 163-70.

[27] Bryant, JA; De Salles, A; Cabatan, C; Frysinger, R; Behnke, E; et al. The impact of thalamic stimulation on activities of daily living for essential tremor. *Surg Neurol.*, 2003, 59(6), 479-484.

[28] Putzke, JD; Wharen, RE; Jr. Obwegeser, AA; Wszolek, ZK; Lucas, JA; Turk, MF; Uitti, RJ. Thalamic deep brain stimulation for essential tremor: recommendations for long-term outcome analysis. *Can J Neurol Sci.*, 2004, 31(3), 333-342.

[29] Lee, JY; Kondziolka, D. Thalamic deep brain stimulation for management of essential tremor. *J Neurosurg.*, 2005, 103(3), 400-403.

[30] Pahwa, R; Lyons, KE; Wilkinson, SB; Simpson, RK; Jr. et al. Long-term evaluation of deep brain stimulation of the thalamus. *J Neurosurg.*, 2006, 104(4), 506-512.

[31] Blomstedt, P; Hariz, GM; Hariz, MI; Koskinen, LO. Thalamic deep brain stimulation in the treatment of essential tremor: a long-term follow-up. *Br J Neurosurg.*, 2007, 21(5), 504-509.

[32] Pilitsis, JG; Metman, LV; Toleikis, JR; Hughes, LE; Sani, SB; Bakay, RA. Factors involved in long-term efficacy of deep brain stimulation of the thalamus for essential tremor. *J Neurosurg.*, 2008, 109(4), 640-646.

[33] Zhang, K; Bhatia, S; Oh, MY; Cohen, D; Angle, C; Whiting, D. Long-term results of thalamic deep brain stimulation for essential tremor. *J Neurosurg.*, 2010, 112(6), 1271-1276.

[34] Nazzaro, JM; Pahwa, R; Lyons, KE. Long-term benefits in quality of life after unilateral thalamic deep brain stimulation for essential tremor. *J Neurosurg.*, 2012, 117(1), 156-161.

[35] De Oliveira, TH; Ginsberg, MR; Cooper, S; Nowacki, A; Rezai, A; et al. Long-term effects of deep brain stimulation for essential tremor with subjective and objective quantification via mailed-in questionnaires. *Stereotact Funct Neurosurg.*, 2012, 90(6), 394-400.

[36] Peng-Chen, Z; Morishita, T; Vaillancourt, D; Favilla, C; et al. Unilateral thalamic deep brain stimulation in essential tremor demonstrates long-term ipsilateral effects. *Parkinsonism Relat Disord.*, 2013, 19(12), 1113-1117.

[37] Børretzen, MN; Bjerknes, S; Sæhle, T; Skjelland, M; et al. Long-term follow-up of thalamic deep brain stimulation for essential tremor - patient satisfaction and mortality. *BMC Neurol.*, 2014, (5)14, 120.

[38] Baizabal-Carvallo, JF; Kagnoff, MN; Jimenez-Shahed, J; et al. The safety and efficacy of thalamic deep brain stimulation in essential tremor: 10 years and beyond. *J Neurol Neurosurg Psychiatry.*, 2014, 85(5), 567-572.

[39] Xie, T; Bernard, J; Warnke, P. Post subthalamic area deep brain stimulation for tremors: a mini-review. *Transl Neurodegener.*, 2012, 1(1), 20

[40] Fytagoridis, A; Sandvik, U; Aström, M; Bergenheim, T; et al. Long term follow-up of deep brain stimulation of the caudal zona incerta for essential tremor. *J Neurol Neurosurg Psychiatry.*, 2012, 83(3), 258-262.

[41] Murata, J; Kitagawa, M; Uesugi, H; Saito, H; et al. Electrical stimulation of the posterior subthalamic area for the treatment of intractable proximal tremor. *J Neurosurg.*, 2003, 99(4), 708-715.
[42] Plaha, P; Patel, NK; Gill, SS. Stimulation of the subthalamic region for essential tremor. *J Neurosurg.*, 2004, 101(1), 48-54.
[43] Herzog, J; Hamel, W; Wenzelburger, R; Pötter, M; et al. Kinematic analysis of thalamic versus subthalamic neurostimulation in postural and intention tremor. *Brain.*, 2007,130(6), 1608-1625.
[44] Hamel, W; Herzog, J; Kopper, F ; Pinsker, M; et al. Deep brain stimulation in the subthalamic area is more effective than nucleus ventralis intermedius stimulation for bilateral intention tremor *Acta Neurochir* (Wien) (2007) 149, 749–758.
[45] Blomstedt, P; Sandvik, U; Tisch, S. Deep brain stimulation in the posterior subthalamic area in the treatment of essential tremor. *Mov Disord.*, 2010, 25(10), 1350-1356.
[46] Plaha, P; Javed, S; Agombar, D; O' Farrell, G; et al. Bilateral caudal zona incerta nucleus stimulation for essential tremor: outcome and quality of life. *J Neurol Neurosurg Psychiatry.*, 2011, 82(8), 899-904.
[47] Barbe, MT; Liebhart, L; Runge, M; Deyng, J; Florin, E; et al. Deep brain stimulation of the ventral intermediate nucleus in patients with essential tremor: stimulation below intercommissural line is more efficient but equally effective as stimulation above. *Exp Neurol.*, 2011, 230(1), 131-137
[48] Blomstedt, P; Sandvik, U; Linder, J; Fredricks, A; et al. Deep brain stimulation of the subthalamic nucleus versus the zona incerta in the treatment of essential tremor. *Acta Neurochir* (Wien). 2011, 153(12), 2329-2335.
[49] Sandvik, U; Lars-Owe, K; Anders, L; Patric, B. Thalamic and Subthalamic DBS for Essential Tremor: Where Is the Optimal Target? *Neurosurgery.*, 2011.
[50] Sandvik, U ; Blomstedt, P. Quality of life following DBS in the caudal zona incerta in patients with essential tremor. *Acta Neurochir* (Wien). 2012, 154(3), 495-499.
[51] Chang, W; Chung, J; Kim, J; Chang, J. Simultaneous thalamic and posterior subthalamic electrode insertion with single deep btrain stimulation for essential tremor. *Nueromodulation.*, 2013, 16, 236-243.
[52] Requejo, H; Pastor, J; Sánchez, P; et al. Treatment of a case of essential tremor with subthalamic stimulation. *Rev Neurol.*, 2004, 38(7), 637-639
[53] Stover, NP; Okun, MS; Evatt, ML; Raju, DV; Bakay, RA; Vitek, JL. Stimulation of the subthalamic nucleus in a patient with Parkinson disease and essential tremor. *Arch Neurol.*, 2005, 62(1), 141-143.
[54] Lind, G; Schechtmann, G; Lind, C; Winter, J; Meyerson, BA; Linderoth, B. Subthalamic stimulation for essential tremor. Short- and long-term results and critical target area. *Stereotact Funct Neurosurg.*, 2008, 86(4), 253-8
[55] William, J. Marks, ed. Deep Brain Stimulation Management. Cambridge University Press. 2010.
[56] Jain, S; Lo, SE; Louis, ED. Common misdiagnosis of a common neurological disorder: how are we misdiagnosing essential tremor? *Arch Neurol.*, 2006, 63(8), 1100-4.
[57] Deuschl, G; Zimmermann, R; Gender, H; et al. Physiological classification of essential tremor. *Handbook of tremor disorders.*, 1995, 195-208
[58] Montgomery, EB; Jr. Gale, JT. Mechanisms of action of deep brain stimulation(DBS). *Neurosci Biobehav Rev.*, 2008, 32(3), 388-407

[59] Ramirez-Zamora, A; Kahn, M; Campbell, J; DeLaCruz, P; Pilitsis, JG. Interleaved programming of subthalamic deep brain stimulation to avoid adverse effects and preserve motor benefit in Parkinson's disease. *J Neurol.*, 2014 Dec 14.

In: Deep Brain Stimulation
Editor: Raja Mehanna

ISBN: 978-1-63483-282-3

Chapter 8

DEEP BRAIN STIMULATION FOR DYSTONIA

Jessika Suescun, MD[1], Erin Furr-Stimming, MD[1] and Neepa Patel, MD[2]
[1]University of Texas Health Science Center at Houston, Houston, Texas, US
[2]University of Texas-Southwestern, US

ABSTRACT

Dystonia is a heterogeneous movement disorder characterized by sustained or intermittent contraction of agonist and antagonist muscles producing abnormal postures. Dystonia can be focal, multifocal, segmental or generalized. Botulinum toxin injections are generally effective in treating focal dystonia. Oral medications can be effective in attenuating generalized and segmental dystonia, but have limitations. Generalized dystonia, however, is more often refractory to available medical therapies. Deep brain stimulation (DBS) has been established as an effective intervention to treat patients with dystonia refractory to medical therapy. This chapter describes the current accepted classification scheme for diagnosing dystonia, specific considerations for the phenomenology, etiology and treatment, and reviews the current literature evidence supporting the use of DBS in a variety of dystonia syndromes; it also provides general consideration for patient selection and recommendations for approach to programming DBS for the treatment of dystonia.

INTRODUCTION

The earliest descriptions of dystonia first appeared in the early 17th century when members of the British Civil Service reported task specific muscle spasms occurring in the hand, which is now recognized as writer's cramp. In the late 1800s additional descriptions of unusual facial and limb spasms began to appear in the literature and by 1901, Destarac introduced the term *torticollis spasmodique* to describe abnormal neck and pelvic dystonic posturing. Most physicians at this time considered these abnormal movements to be a form of hysteria and it was not until 1911 that Hermann Oppenheim suggested that this syndrome may be related to neurological dysfunction, coining the term *dystonia musculorum demformans* based on his description of 4 unrelated Jewish children from Galicia and Russia.

The term d*ystonia* is derived from the Latin *dys-* and Greek *–tonos and is now recognized as a neurological disorder resulting from abnormalities in the structural and/or functional connectivity of basal ganglia thalamic circuit (BGTC)* [1]. Dystonia is a heterogeneous movement disorder characterized by sustained or intermittent muscle contraction resulting in repetitive movements and abnormal postures; the movements are typically patterned, twisting and may be tremulous. Dystonic postures are often initiated or worsened by voluntary action, associated with overflow muscle activation and symptoms can often be transiently relieved by the use of alleviating maneuvers [2, 3]. Virtually any region of the body may be affected, from few isolated muscle groups to the entire body. Onset can be at any age and once symptoms rarely remit spontaneously.

Dystonia affects essentially all racial and ethnic groups. The prevalence of early-onset primary dystonia varies depending on the population with estimates as low as 0.7 per million or as high as 50 per million. Prevalence can even be higher in some subpopulations like Ashkenazi Jews with 111 cases per million due to presence of the DYT1 mutation [4, 5]. The America Academy of Neurology reported 250,000 people with a diagnosis of dystonia in the United States in 2013, but this could be an underestimation because of underdiagnosis and misdiagnosis.

The pathophysiology of dystonia remains elusive, as no distinct pathological correlates have been identified to date. Theories on the pathophysiology of dystonia include disruption of the functional or structural connectivity of the BGTC and the cerbellothalamocortical circuit (CBTC). Disruption of the BGTC results in: *(a)* impaired surrounding, spinal, brainstem and cortical inhibition, *(b)* alterations of synaptic plasticity within the basal ganglia and cortex, (c) impaired somatosensory processing and integration including altered globus pallidus internus (GPi) firing patterns and low frequency synchronized oscillations. CBTC involvement includes diminished integrity of the fiber tracts and decreased cerebellar inhibition [6-8].

An international consensus committee of movement disorders experts has recently updated its recommendations for classification of dystonia utilizing a two axes approach for evaluation: 1) clinical characteristics and 2) etiology. Clinical characteristics include age at onset, body distribution, temporal pattern and associated features whereas etiology takes into consideration inherited or acquired neuroanatomical pathology (Figure 1) [2].

Childhood or young adult onset dystonia typically begins with focal limb involvement and gradually progresses to a generalized form [9]. Patients with onset of dystonia after the age of 40 (late adult onset dystonia) nearly always remains focal or may progress to segmentally involve a single region of the body, but rarely progress to a generalized dystonia [10]. Dystonic movements can vary from stereotyped tonic posturing at rest to dynamic or phasic patterned movements that occur only during specific activities. Some patients may have a superimposed dystonic tremor (DT) that is characterized by coexisting postural/intention tremor in the same segment. This tremor is often focal with irregular and variable amplitude and frequency (typically below 7Hz). DT commonly presents as a head tremor in the context of cervical dystonia and can be more prominent than the dystonic posture itself. DT may also appear as an isolated task specific limb tremor [11, 12].

The phenomenology of dystonia is often described by the body areas affected and includes:

- Generalized: The trunk and at least 2 other sites are involved.
- Focal: Only one body region is affected and includes but is not limited to: blepharospasm, oromandibular dystonia, torticollis or cervical dystonia, spasmodic dysphonia, and writer's cramp.
- Segmental: Two or more contiguous body regions are affected; such as craniocervical dystonia (Meige syndrome) or bi-brachial dystonia.
- Multifocal: Two or more noncontiguous body regions are involved.
- Hemidystonia: More than one body regions restricted to one body side are involved. Most often associated with a structural lesion [13].

The presence of other movement disorders (i.e. myoclonus, parkinsonism, etc.) and presence of non-motor features (cognitive changes, psychiatric symptoms and metabolic derangements) may suggest a specific genetic or neurodegenerative syndrome [2]. Dopa responsive dystonia, for example, is a rare inherited disorder resulting from a defect in dopamine synthesis pathway. Patients generally have an excellent response to levodopa therapy at low doses. Therefore, clinicians should have a high index of suspicion when evaluating young individuals with focal or generalized dystonia [14].

In most cases of dystonia, treatment is symptomatic and directed towards improving abnormal postures and disabling movements thereby improving functionality and attenuating pain. Patients with dystonia often require a combination of several medications and treatments. Four classes of medications are typically used: anticholinergic, dopaminergic, muscle relaxants and intramuscular injection of botulinum neurotoxins.

Because of the potential limitations with available medications, surgical treatments or more specifically, deep brain stimulation (DBS) has evolved as an effective treatment option for patients with primarily generalized dystonia or medication refractory focal dystonia.

Deep brain stimulation was first introduced for the treatment of dystonia in 1977 [15]. Since then, several case reports and case series have described substantial improvement of dystonic symptoms with this therapy, expediting its approval in 2003 under humanitarian device exemption by the FDA for the aid in management of chronic, drug refractory primary dystonia, including generalized and segmental dystonia, hemidystonia, and cervical dystonia, for individuals 7 years of age and older. The posteroventro-lateral part of the internal globus pallidus (GPi) is the most studied target, although other targets within the basal ganglia thalalmic circuit (BGTC) are currently under investigation.

The therapeutic effects of GPi DBS are likely to be mediated through normalizing firing patterns and silencing pathological electrical activity. Electrical stimulation of brain structures with short duration pulses activates axons rather than somas based on their threshold charge density. This induces axonal spikes at the target nucleus that collide with intrinsic lower frequency orthodromic axons thus suppressing the spontaneous activity of the somas at the surrounding area. As a result, DBS activates axons and depresses somas, inhibiting the pathological oscillatory activity and propagating axonal spikes toward the corresponding cell bodies of distant structures, retrogradely affecting cortical and subcortical circuits in complex ways that reorganize a new neural circuitry [16, 17].

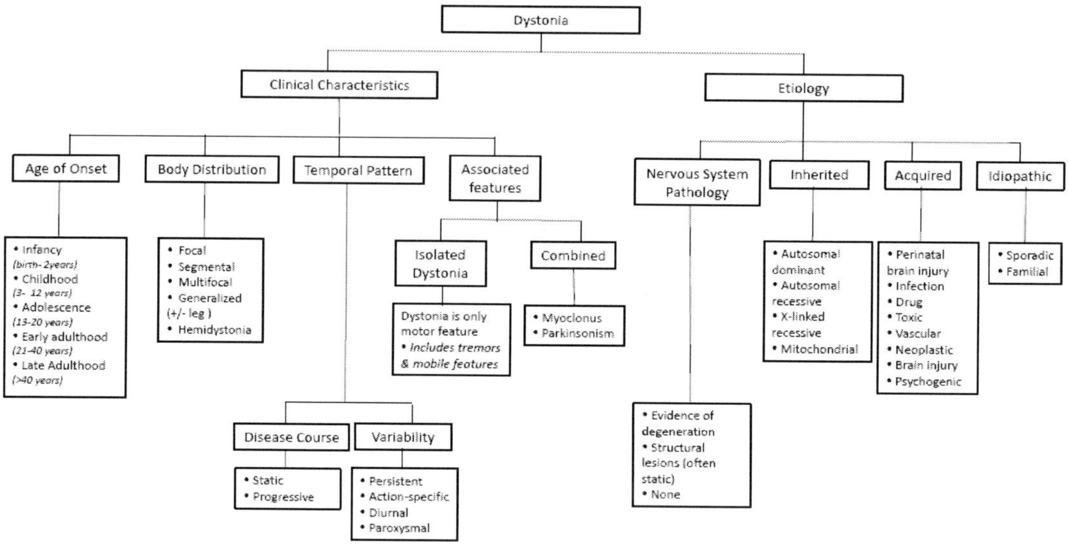

Adapted from Albanese et al. (2013) Phenomenology and Classification of Dystonia: A Consensus Update.

Figure 1. Classification of Dystonia.

A. Review of Evidence for DBS in the Treatment of Dystonia

Generalized Dystonia

Primary generalized dystonia is a progressive, disabling disorder that usually begins in child-hood, initially involving at least one leg, the trunk and another body region. DYT1 is the most commonly implicated gene and its mutation is responsible for a deletion of glutamate in Torsin A, a protein of unknown function that is highly concentrated in the substantia nigra. DYT1 accounts for 60% of patients with generalized dystonia in the general population and up to 90% in the Ashkenazi Jewish population [18-20]. There are three available clinical scales that may be employed to objectively assess patients with generalized dystonia: the Burke-Fahn-Marsden scale (BFM), the Unified Dystonia rating scale (UDRS) and the global dystonia rating scale (GDS).

To date, the safety and efficacy of high frequency stimulation has been reported in more than 400 patients with primary generalized dystonia (Table 1) [21-39]. Several retrospective case series, large scale randomized clinical trials and sham-stimulation-controlled studies have been done [23, 25, 27, 29, 40]. Early studies demonstrated the superiority of stimulation of the posteroventrolateral portion of the globus pallidus pars intera (GPi) compared to the ventrolateral portion of the thalamus (VLp) in generalized dystonia [41]. Thus, the GPi is the most studied target for the treatment of dystonia at this time, though there is emerging evidence suggesting the use of alternate targets in the treatment of specific dystonia syndromes.

Table 1. GPi in Generalized Dystonia

Author and year	N	Diagnosis	Outcome/improvement (before/after DBS)	Mean follow up (in months)	Complications	
					Subsequent to DBS programming*	Surgical complications
Krauss et al. 2003 [21].	2	Non-DYT1 generalized dystonia	• BFM motor score improved by 74% at 2 years.	24	Perioral tightness, dysarthria, dizziness.	Lead fracture
Yianni et al. 2003 [22].	25	Generalized dystonia and spasmodic torticollis	• BFM motor score improved by 47.6% • BFM disability score improved by 37.6%	12	None reported	Lead migration and infection
Coubes et al. 2004 [23].	31	Generalized dystonia	• BFM motor score improved by 79% at 2 years.	24	None reported	Local infection
Bittar et al. 2005 [24].	12	Generalized dystonia and spasmodic torticollis	• 46% improvement in the BFMDRS in the generalized dystonia group • 59% improvement in the total TWSTRS in the torticollis group.	24	None reported	Lead migration/damage, battery failure, neurological deterioration, infection
Vidailhet et al. 2005 [25].	22	Generalized dystonia	• The BFM motor score improved in 55% of patients at 12 months ($P<0.001$). • The BFM disability score improved in 43% of patients • General health and physical functioning were significantly improved at month 12	12	None reported	Edema of the frontal lobe, lead fracture, skin infection
Hälbig et al. 2005 [26].	15	Generalized dystonia and tardive dystonia	• No deterioration was observed in cognitive and neuropsychiatric measures. • 24.7 points average improvement on PDQ39	12	None reported	None reported

Table 1. (Continued)

Author and year	N	Diagnosis	Outcome/improvement (before/after DBS)	Mean follow up (in months)	Complications	
					Subsequent to DBS programming*	Surgical complications
Kupsch et al. 2006 [27].	40	Generalized or segmental dystonia	• 39.3% reduction in symptoms in the neurostimulation group as compared to a 4.9% reduction in the sham stimulation group. • 37.5% improvement in disability scores improvement in the neurostimulation group, compared to 8.3% in the sham-stimulation group. • 29.8% improvement in quality of life (SF-36) in the neurostimulation group, compared to 11.4% in the placebo group.	6	Dysarthria, Stuttering, worsening of dystonia, sleep disorder, facial weakness, gait disorder, dysesthesias	Infections at the stimulator site, lead dislodgment, lead breakage, seizures and seroma.
Egidi et al. 2007 [28].	69	Generalized Dystonia	• Mean BFM improved by 42% in both severity and disability score.	24	None reported	Lead fracture or displacement, infection, symptomatic hemorrhage and white matter edema.
Vidailhet et al. 2007 [29].	22	Generalized Dystonia	• BFM score improved by 51% and 58% at one and 3 years.	36	None reported	Unilateral lead fracture and local infection
Mueller et al. 2008 [30].	40	Generalized or segmental dyst-onia	• All SF-36 domain scores were significantly reduced compared to a normal population but did not differ significantly between the active and sham-stimulation group.	3	None reported	None reported
Mehrkens et al. 2009 [31].	9	Generalized dystonia	• BFM motor score improved by 39.4%, 42.5% and 46.8% at 3	60	Phosphenes, motor symptoms, psychological/	Local infection, subcutaneous hematoma, electrode dislocation and

Author and year	N	Diagnosis	Outcome/improvement (before/after DBS)	Mean follow up (in months)	Complications	
					Subsequent to DBS programming*	Surgical complications
			months, 12 months and long term follow up.		behavioral abnormalities and speech disturbance	breakage of the extension cable.
Isaias et al. 2009 [32].	23	Primary generalized dystonia	• BFM motor score improved by 79.6% and 82.5% at 1 and 2 years. • BFM disability score improved by 69.2% and 75.2% at 1 and 2 years.	24	Speech difficulties and transit blepharospasm.	Localized infection, fractured extension cable, scalp erosion
Cif et al. 2010 [33].	26	DYT1 positive generalized dystonia	• BFM motor score improved by 59% • BFM disability score improved by 50%	72	None reported	Cable breakages and local infection
Valldeoriola et al. 2010 [34].	22	Generalized dystonia	• BFM motor score improve by 59% • BFM disability score improve by 38% • 40% improvement in QoL	12	Dysphagia and dysarthria	Transient hemiparesia and scalp infection
Volkmann et al. 2012 [35].	40	Generalized dystonia	• Significant improvement on BFM motor scores of 64% at 3 and 5 years.	60	Dysarthria, dysesthesias and gait disorder	Subcutaneous infection, lead dislodgement, lead breakage and extension cable fracture.
Schjerling et al. 2013 [36].	12	Focal, multifocal and generalized dystonia (GPi vs STN)	• BFM score improved by 46% after 6 months of either STN or GPi stimulation. • TWSTRS improved by 4.8% and 50.9% with GPi and STN DBS	6	Depression, Hyperkinesia, hypomania, dysphagia and nausea.	Infection, reduce neck mobility

Table 1. (Continued)

Author and year	N	Diagnosis	Outcome/improvement (before/after DBS)	Mean follow up (in months)	Complications	
					Subsequent to DBS programming*	Surgical complications
			respectively (no statistical significance) • QoL improved by 41% and 68% with GPi and STNDBS respectively.			
Jahanshahi et al. 2014 [37].	14	Generalized dystonia	• BFM score improved by 69% • Deterioration in sustained attention • No significance change in QoL, depression and anxiety scales	12	None reported	None reported
Miri et al. 2014 [38].	9	DYT1 positive generalized dystonia	• BFM motor score improved by 73%	8	None reported	None reported
Sobstyl et al. 2014 [39].	12	Generalized dystonia: DYT1 positive vs DYT1 negative	• DYT1 positive patients improved functional and motor scores by 58% and 65% respectively. • DYT1 negative patients improved functional and motor scores by 59% and 51% respectively.	60	None reported	Lead breakage, skin erosion, sterile seromas bilaterally

* In clinical practice, most of these complications can be alleviated with changes in the stimulation parameters.

GPi stimulation (Table 1) has demonstrated a mean BFM motor improvement ranging from 39.3% to 74% in both short and long-term (> 5 years) follow up, in addition to a disability improvement within the same scale between 37.6-75%. Quality of life (QoL) assessed by SF-36 showed enhancement in both mental and physical categories.

Potential peri or post-operative complications include intracerebral hemorrhage, edema, infection, seizures, anxiety and depression. Hardware malfunction such as lead fracture, migration and connection-cable malfunction may also occur.

Recent studies have reported benefit from stimulation of the subthalamic nucleus (STN), but follow-up data was limited [42]. The only cross-over design study comparing stimulation of the STN and GPi for generalized, focal and multifocal dystonia demonstrated comparable improvement of dystonia and proposed that STN may provide earlier symptomatic relief [36]. Sun et al. proposes that STN stimulation in generalized dystonia is superior due to immediate symptomatic improvement after programming and use of lower stimulation parameters that allows longer battery life [43]. However, the results have not been superior to those achieved with GPi stimulation and further studies need to be performed to compare the efficacy of GPi DBS versus STN DBS for generalized dystonia.

Because conservative therapies are rarely sufficient in effectively treating generalized dystonia, GPi DBS is now a considered a standard therapy.

Focal/Segmental Dystonia

Focal dystonia is 10 times more common than generalized dystonia and may involve the neck, face, arm or leg. With the exception of writer's cramp, focal dystonia is more common in women. Focal dystonia typically progresses over one to two years and then follows a relatively static course, although it occasionally can spread to adjacent muscle groups and become segmental.

Cervical dystonia, the most common form of focal dystonia, can be a highly disabling condition and includes rotated and laterally or anteroposteriorly shifted head positions. The most frequently used rating scales include: the Toronto Western Spasmodic torticollis rating scales (TWSTRS), Tsui scale and the cervical dystonia severity scale. The beneficial effects of GPi DBS for cervical dystonia have been reported in several large scale blinded studies [51, 58-60]. To date, more than 150 patients with cervical dystonia treated with GPi DBS have been reported to have a significant improvement in the total TWSTRS ranging from 42% to 76%, as well as a 43-72% improvement in the BFMDRS. QoL measures using the SF-36 improved between 24-36%, with a follow up average of over 31 months (Table 2) [44, 46, 47, 50, 51, 56, 58-60]. The efficacy of STN stimulation has also been reported in a case series in which 20 patients were followed for a mean of one year (Table 3) [61-64]. Preliminary results of a cross-over design study comparing stimulation of STN and GPi demonstrated comparable improvement and propose that STN may provide earlier symptomatic relief [36]. Nonetheless, this topic requires further investigation.

Severe writer's cramp or task specific dystonia is a rare upper limb dystonia produced by excessive co-contraction of agonist and antagonistic muscles of the hand and forearm [65]. The ventral oris nucleus of the thalamus (Vo) has been reported to be an effective treatment based on preliminary observations with a single patient that improved with Vo thalamotomy [66-67]. In a case series of 5 patients with writer's cramp, DBS of the Vo was noted to have immediate and complete resolution of symptoms [68]. STN as an alternate target has also demonstrated efficacy in a small case series [69].

Segmental dystonia affects two or more adjacent parts of the body. Meige syndrome or cranial cervical dystonia is an example of segmental dystonia that includes blepharospasm, cervical dystonia and oromandibular dystonia. Onset occurs between the fifth and the sixth decade of life and is more common in females with a ratio of 3:1 [70]. Small case series and case reports of GPi stimulation have demonstrated sustained reduction of dystonic posturing with a range of improvement between 45-72% [45, 52-55, 57]. However, as is true for most forms of dystonia, improvement is not achieved immediately after the initial programming. The response is delayed and optimal results may not be apparent for up to 12 months. In some cases, delayed benefit beyond the first year has been reported [54, 55]. Best results were obtained using low stimulation intensity or a cyclical stimulation mode. (Table 2)

The efficacy of DBS has not been demonstrated for the remainder of the cranial dystonias, especially those affecting speech and swallowing [54].

Other Dystonias – Dystonia Plus Syndromes

Myoclonus dystonia (DYT 11) is an autosomal dominant relatively rare hyperkinetic disorder with prominent action myoclonus and dystonia that is most often cervical, although the trunk and limbs can also be affected. Onset is typically in childhood with a mean age of 6 years. Although genetically heterogeneous, up to 40% are caused by point mutations or large deletions in the epsilon sarcoglycan gene (SGCE) [74]. There are case series reporting sustained beneficial effects of DBS in various targets [75-77]. The benefits of ventral intermediate nucleus of the thalamus (Vim) and GPi DBS have both been promising [78-80]. In a meta-analysis of 17 reports describing 40 patients, Rughani et al. found that though both Vim and GPi DBS had up to 70% reduction in myoclonus, but that GPi was superior to Vim for the treatment of dystonic symptoms (60% improvement with GPi DBS vs 33% with Vim DBS) [81], suggesting that GPi may be the preferred target for the treatment of both myoclonus and dystonia in this rare syndrome. A dual stimulation of both the of GPi and Vim was safe and effective and may be considered for refractory cases [76].

Dystonic tremor (DT) is characterized by coexisting postural/intention tremor and abnormal dystonic posturing in the same segment. The most common form is head tremor in the context of cervical dystonia and is present in 68% of these patients. Vim DBS was noted to be effective in the treatment of dystonic tremors with up to 50% reduction in symptoms in one study [82]. In a retrospective analysis of 10 patients implanted at a single institution, Vim DBS provided an average of 80% reduction in tremor compared to 40% in the GPi DBS group; however Vim provided minimal relief of dystonic symptoms [83]. This implies that those patients with dystonic tremor with mild underlying dystonia may benefit from thalamic stimulation.

The benefit of DBS in status dystonicus and secondary dystonias such as dystonic-choreoathetotic cerebral palsy or other disorders is still under investigation and data are not conclusive [84-87]. A case of bilateral necrosis of the basal ganglia secondary to anoxic injury had marked improvement of dystonia with bilateral Vo stimulation suggesting that this

Table 2. GPi in Focal/segmental dystonia

Author, year	N	Diagnosis	Outcome/improvement (Before/after DBS)	Mean follow up (in months)	Complications	
					Subsequent to DBS programming*	Surgical complications
Bereznai et al. 2002 [44].	6	Segmental dystonia with cervical involvement	• BFM score improved by 72.5% • Tsui scale score improved by 63% • SF-36 improved by 36%	12	None reported	Skin infection, meningitis
Ostrem et al. 2007 [45].	6	Meige syndrome	• The total BFMDRS improved by 72% • The TWSTRS improved 54%	6	Worsening of handwriting, typing, balance and walking.	None reported
Kiss et al. 2007 [46].	10	Cervical dystonia	• The TWSTRS severity score improved in 42.8% at 12 months post-operatively ($P= 0.003$) • The disability and pain scores improved in 63.7% and 65.4% at 12 months, respectively (both $P<0.001$). • 24% improvement on SF-36	12	Swallowing difficulties, dysphagia, transient facial weakness, shingles.	Chronic subdural fluid collection, hemiparesis
Hung et al. 2007 [47].	10	Cervical dystonia	• TWSTRS severity score improved by 54.8% • TWSTRS disability score improved by 59.1% • TWSTRS pain score improved by 50.4%.	32	Dysarthria	Infection
Sensi et al. 2009 [48].	11	Segmental dystonia	• BFMDRS improved by 60% at 3 years.	36	Dysarthria and stiffness	Lead migration
Mehrkens et al. 2009 [49].	9	Focal and segmental dystonia	• Tsui score improved by 36.8%, 65.1% and 59.8% at 3 months, 12 months and long term follow up.	60	Phosphenes, motor symptom, psychological behavioral abnormalities and speech disturbance	Local infection, subcutaneous hematoma, electrode dislocation and breakage of the extension cable.

Table 2. (Continued)

Author, year	N	Diagnosis	Outcome/improvement (Before/after DBS)	Mean follow up (in months)	Complications	
					Subsequent to DBS programming*	Surgical complications
Jeong et al. 2009 [50].	6	Cervical dystonia	• The TWSTRS total scores improved by 64.5%, 65.5%, 75.8%, and 76.0% at 3, 6, 12 months, and at the last available follow-up after surgery, respectively.	19	Gait disturbance, difficulty in speaking and swallowing.	None reported
Cacciola et al. 2010 [51].	10	Cervical dystonia	• TWSTRS was improved by 68%.	37	None reported	Localized infection and lead breakage
Ghang et al. 2010 [52].	11	Meige syndrome	• Total BFMDRS improved by 74.5% and 85.5% at 12 months and 24 months.	24	Dysarthria, difficulty swallowing, fatigue, depression and general weakness	No major complications
Lyons et al. 2010 [53].	3	Meige syndrome	• Mean BFM improved by 82% at 12 month	48	None reported	None reported
Limotai et al. 2011 [54].	6	Meige syndrome	• UDRS improved 31.6% and 63.7% at 6 months and 12 months. • BFM scale improved 45.3% and 61.8% at 6 months and 12 months.	36	None reported	None reported
Reese et al. 2011 [55].	12	Meige syndrome	• The mean BFM improved by 45% and 53% at 4 months and 39 months	39	Dysarthria	Localized infection
Skogseid et al. 2012 [56].	8	Cervical dystonia	• TWSTRS improved by 70%. • Disability and pain scores improved by 91% and 92%, respectively.	30	Dysesthesias and motor changes	Edema surrounding an electrode
Sarubbo et al. 2012 [57].	11	Segmental or multisegmental dystonia	• BFM motor score improved by 59% • BFM disability score improved by 57%	60	Dysarthria and paresthesia	Electrode migration
Walsh et al. 2013 [58].	10	Cervical dystonia	• TWSTRS improved by 47.6%.	92	Deterioration in handwriting, dysarthria	infection

Author, year	N	Diagnosis	Outcome/improvement (Before/after DBS)	Mean follow up (in months)	Complications	
					Subsequent to DBS programming*	Surgical complications
Witt et al. 2013 [59].	28	Cervical dystonia	• TWSTRS improved by 55.6%.	33	None reported	Hemorrhages, infection
Volkmann et al. 2014 [60].	62	Cervical dystonia	• TWSTRS improved by 26% in the neurostimulation group compare to 6% in in the sham-stimulation group (p=0.0024)	3	Dysarthria, dyskinesia, worsening of dystonia, depression, hand tremor, facial numbness, paraesthesia, and muscles stiffness	Device infection, electrode misplacement, electrode dislocation. hemiparesis

* In clinical practice, most of these complications can be alleviated with changes in the stimulation parameters.

Table 3. STN in Focal/segmental dystonia

Author. year	N	Diagnosis	Outcome/improvement	Mean follow up (in months	Complications	
					Subsequent to DBS programming*	Surgical complications
Chou et al. 2005 [61].	1	Cervical dystonia and essential tremor	DBS on/off: • TWSTRS motor and disability sections improved by 78% and 100% respectively.	6	Dysarthria	Lead infection
Kleiner-Fisman et al. 2007 [62].	4	Cervical dystonia	Before/after DBS: • Significant improvement were seen in motor (p=0.04), disability (p=0.02)and total TWSTRS scores (p=0.03)	12	None reported	None reported
Ostrem et al. 2011 [63].	9	Cervical dystonia	• Before/after DBS: TWSTRS improved by 36% at 12 months.	12	Depression, transient dyskinetic movements	None reported
Mills et al. 2014 [64].	8	Cervical dystonia	DBS on/off: • No effect on working memory or motor function.	0	None reported	None reported

* In clinical practice, most of these complications can be alleviated with changes

may be an alternate target in the setting of structural injury to the basal ganglia [88]. Neurodegeneration with brain iron accumulation (NBIA) syndromes have been noted to have marked improvement of dystonia over 15 months in up to 67% of patients in one multicentered study [89].

B. Patient Screening and Selection

Selecting the appropriate candidate for DBS surgery for dystonia may be challenging given the complex and heterogeneous nature of this group of disorders.

In 2006, the national institute for clinical excellence, the European federation of neurological societies (EFNS) and the movement disorder society established consensus recommendations that DBS should be considered for the treatment of dystonia:

- After failure of anticholinergic drugs, benzodiazepines and levodopa in generalized/segmental dystonia and after failure of botulinum injection toxin injection in cranial and cervical dystonia.
- Symptoms should be disabling enough to justify the surgical risk.

Prior to consideration for surgery, an unequivocal diagnosis of dystonia that is refractory to conservative medical therapies needs to be established. Bronte-Stewart et al. proposed inclusion and exclusion criteria for DBS in dystonia that will be reviewed in more detail in the following sections [90].

Medications

Treatment can be challenging and available medications may have unwanted adverse effects and/or inconsistent results.

The most commonly prescribed agent for the treatment of primary generalized dystonia is trihexyphenidyl; variable success has been observed with alternate anticholinergic agents. Adverse effects such as cognitive impairment, confusion, insomnia, blurred vision, dry mouth, constipation and urinary retention may preclude its use at high doses in some patients [91].

Early empiric studies of dopaminergic agents were inconclusive in the treatment of dystonia with the exception of patients with dopa-responsive dystonia (DRD). Side effects are mild and usually include nausea, drowsiness and dizziness [92-93]. Dopamine depleting agents such as tetrabenazine reduce focal and generalized dystonia symptoms especially when dynamic movements are present. It is the treatment of choice in medication-induced tardive dystonia as well as myoclonus-dystonia syndrome (DYT-11) [94, 95]. Side effects of tetrabenazine include transient acute dystonic reaction, drowsiness, insomnia, depression and akathisia, and may limit its use.

Botulinum toxin (BoNT) has revolutionized the treatment of dystonia and is now considered the treatment of choice for focal and segmental dystonia. BoNT is generally not applicable to patients with generalized dystonia because of the multitude of muscles involved. Adverse effects of the injections include weakness of injected muscles or weakness of nearby muscles, flu-like symptoms and site specific complications including pain and bruising, dry eye or dry mouth. The typical duration of BONT's therapeutic effect is approximately 12-16 weeks. Nevertheless, over time, some patients may develop a shortened therapeutic window requiring more frequent injection visits [96-101].

GABA receptor agonists such as baclofen and benzodiazepines are most often used as primary or adjuvant therapies. Baclofen is often used as an antispasmodic agent. Clonazepam is the most frequently used benzodiazepine. The potential for dependence and negative interaction with alcohol, in addition to the development of side effects of sedation, confusion, impaired coordination and depression, often limits its use in clinical practice [92].

There are no established guidelines for the approach to medical therapy in dystonia, thus the following recommendations are in the opinion of these authors. A trial of trihexyphendyl and levodopa at maximally tolerated doses in all patients with young onset focal and generalized dystonia should be attempted, with or without adjuvant muscle relaxants. In adults with focal or segmental dystonia, the patient must have tried at least two immunologically distinct preparations of BoNT formulations at adequate doses and a trial of trihexyphendyl prior to consideration for DBS surgery.

Age

The influence of age should be taken into consideration when evaluating a patient for DBS therapy. When controlling for duration of dystonia, Isaias et al. found that patients with primary generalized dystonia younger than 27 years of age achieved a similar degree of symptom relief earlier than the older cohort of patients who ultimately achieved optimal symptom control around 3 years after surgery [102]. An increased risk for post-operative complications such as infection, hardware complications and recurrence of symptoms on stimulation was reported in children younger than 11 years of age [103, 104]. There is limited information on the efficacy of DBS on the maturing brain, and consideration for surgery should be done on a case-by-case basis for children younger than seven years of age. Age at onset of dystonia had little influence on the benefit from DBS [90], but shorter duration of symptoms of less than 15 years is one of the main predictor factors for a good postoperative response at 1 and 3 years [105].

Dystonia Subtype

The phenomenology and etiology of dystonia needs to be taken into consideration when evaluating a patient for surgery as certain characteristics have been associated with better outcomes [106].

Variables such as 1) duration of dystonia prior to surgery 2) clinical pattern (phasic movements improve better than tonic postures) and 3) body distribution of dystonia (neck, trunk and limb dystonia response better than face, speech or swallowing) have been recognized to influence the degree of clinical improvement observed with DBS. The presence of fixed skeletal deformities or cervical myelopathy is often associated with poor outcomes and should be identified prior to consideration for DBS surgery. The impact of genetic status does not appear to influence the efficacy of DBS as DYT-1 positive or negative adults with primarily generalized dystonia achieved similar outcomes [25, 28, 39, 107, 108].

Primary generalized and focal/segmental dystonias have normal brain magnetic resonance imaging and are likely to have the best outcome, especially in patients who are younger with a short disease duration and a less severe dystonia.

Patients with myoclonus dystonia, tardive dystonia and writer's cramp generally have a good response that sometimes even compares to the benefit observed in patients with primary dystonia. DBS for patients with secondary dystonia should be carefully considered on a case by case basis as it is generally ineffective and the available data to support its use is scant. Those dystonia syndromes with "functional" impairment in basal ganglia circuitry rather than injury to the basal ganglia tend to improve with DBS surgery.

Pre-Operative Evaluations

Neuroimaging is often obtained when identifying the etiology of dystonia, thus no additional intracranial imaging is required prior to surgery. In patients with severe cervical dystonia, a cervical spine MRI is useful to identify spinal cord pathology such as myelopathy or radiculopathy as this may contribute to pain and additional disability that is not expected to improve with DBS therapy. In case of myelopathy, spinal surgery may be required prior to consideration for DBS [108].

Preoperative neuropsychiatric testing is recommended in all patients being considered for DBS therapy. Though dystonia affects a younger population, subtle cognitive dysfunction affecting nonverbal reasoning, executive dysfunction as well as an increased risk for psychiatric symptoms has been reported in up to 91% of patients with cervical dystonia in one study [109]. Cervical dystonia patients also exhibit deficits with visuospatial function, impaired semantic fluency, deficits in shifting, impaired in complex movement planning and motor dexterity . Co-morbid depression, anxiety (especially social phobia and panic disorder) and obsessive compulsive disorder (OCD) are often present in this population and may been to be treated prior to consideration for DBS [37].

Though GPi DBS does not generally contribute to significant adverse effect on cognition, any form of brain surgery potentially carries a risk of unwanted cognitive effects. It is reasonable to consider pre and post implantation neurocognitive testing, including a battery of tests that assesses global cognitive function, nonverbal reasoning/cognitive efficiency, frontal executive function as well as a specific evaluation for depression and anxiety [110].

C. Programming

After DBS implantation, patients may notice a transient improvement of symptoms often referred to as the microlesion effect. It is generally recommended to schedule the first programming visit 4 weeks after implantation of the DBS electrodes to allow time for healing. The approach to evaluating and treating patients with DBS in dystonia varies among practitioners; and we here recommend a stepwise approach to programming (Figure 2) [111].

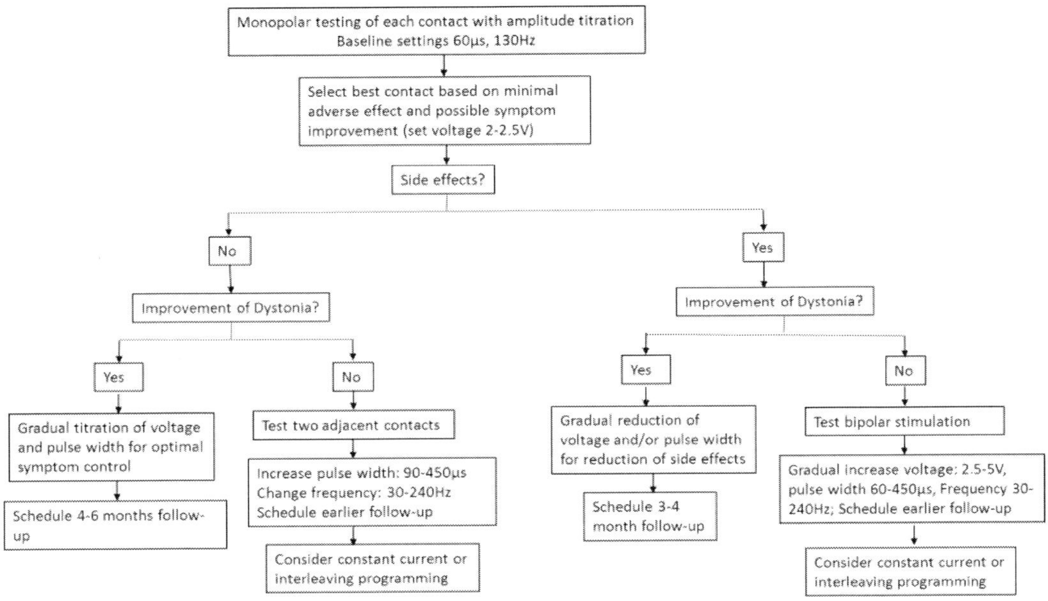

Figure 2: stepwise approach to programming in patients with dystonia

During the first programming visit, a detailed evaluation of stimulation thresholds at each electrode is recommended; this is often referred to as a "monopolar map" or "monopolar review." The monopolar configuration sets the battery (i.e. case) as positive and the electrode as negative. Mapping of each electrode consists of testing each individual contact to maximally tolerated voltages (typically 4-5V) utilizing the monopolar configuration with a standard pulse width (60-90μs) and frequency (130Hz) [112]. The immediate benefits of stimulation may not be observed at the initial programming session in dystonia (especially with stimulation of the GPi), therefore evaluation of each contact for maximally tolerated voltages is primarily obtained for spatial orientation of the lead location based on thresholds of side effects. (Figure 2)

Once the monopolar map is obtained, the contact with the highest thresholds for side effects should be selected with stimulation parameters set at a moderate amplitude (2-2.5V) using a standard pulse width and frequency at the end of the first visit. The Medtronic® Activa SC, PC and RC batteries offer the opportunity for the patient to adjust the stimulation parameters at home within pre-specified limits designated by the physician. Those patients that demonstrate compliance and aptitude for manipulating settings with their home programmer are allowed for further self-managed gentle titration of stimulation before the next visit.

A second programming visit should be scheduled approximately 2-3 months after activating the device in order to evaluate the initial response to stimulation. Indeed, the benefit of DBS on dystonia requires weeks to months to become visible in contrast to Parkinson's disease or essential tremor where benefits can be observed in a few days, if not instantly during the programming visit. Further adjustments of amplitude, pulse width and frequency settings can be performed to provide additional symptom control and reduction of side effects. It is important to note that the optimal degree of symptom relief may not be observed for up to 12 months or longer [48].

The final settings for each patient are selected through gradual titration of stimulation parameters through the best contacts typically utilizing the monopolar configuration. In a 5 year study of 60 patients with GPi DBS, beneficial effects of stimulation were noted over a broad range of settings utilizing a mean voltage of 3.5V with pulse width range of 150-240μs and frequency range of 130-180Hz, while another study reported good clinical response in patients using a pulse width as high as 450μs [39, 113]. In general, the GPi target requires higher stimulations to provide optimal symptom control in dystonia. We suggest first optimizing amplitude to a goal of 3.5-5V while utilizing standard pulse width (60-90μs) and frequency (130Hz) parameters prior to adjustment of the latter two parameters.

The role of low frequency stimulation (30-60Hz) in both GPi and STN stimulation has been reported with varied degrees of efficacy [114-116]. Low frequency stimulation is generally not recommended in the initial approach to programming. This programming strategy may be considered in patients with poor response to standard stimulation parameters or those who experience side effects with standard settings.

When there is suboptimal response but no side effect from monopolar stimulation, additional contacts can be added to create double monopolar settings in order to deliver a higher intensity of stimulation to the region. The most common side effects to stimulation include dysarthria, paraesthesias, transient worsening of dystonia, dizziness, weakness, blepharospasm, and balance disturbance. Most of the side effects are mild and can resolve by adjusting the stimulation settings. If side effects are the limiting factor in obtaining an optimal response in the monopolar configuration, bipolar configuration will narrow the field of electrical stimulation and minimize spread of stimulation to surrounding structures. When there is persistent limitations with achieving optimal symptom control due to side effects, interleaving programs can be considered. Interleaving allows for the delivery of rapidly alternating stimulation through two separate contacts [117]. Constant current stimulation has also been reported as an alternative programming strategy when side effects limit the use of standard settings [118].

There are a few unique considerations to be aware of when managing GPI DBS for dystonia. The beneficial effects of stimulation are often delayed for months or even years [60, 64]. Patients should thus be counseled appropriately and closely monitored over the first few years. Patients with focal and segmental dystonia have been observed to develop DBS induced parkinsonism with chronic stimulation, specifically bradykinesia in the unaffected limb and hypokinetic gait disorder with freezing. In the majority of cases, adjustment of stimulation parameters can minimize these side effects [52, 71-73].

STN DBS is considered experimental in the treatment of dystonia. Good clinical responses were noted with a pulse width of 60μs without the need for further increase. This observation may in part be related to frequent DSB STN side effects when using a higher pulse width. STN stimulation in dystonia has been associated with stimulation induced dyskinesia, which is mild and can often improve with adjustment of stimulation parameters [36, 63].

CONCLUSION

Dystonia is a rare and disabling disorder that is challenging to diagnose and treat. Categorization of dystonia phenotype by duration of symptoms, age of onset and regions affected can help in selecting appropriate candidates for DBS. GPi DBS should be considered for the treatment of primary generalized or segmental dystonia including cervical dystonia that is refractory to medications and botulinum toxin therapy. The efficacy of DBS for dystonic tremor, myoclonus dystonia and other secondary dystonia is considered experimental, though small studies at various targets are promising. These include GPi DBS for myoclonus-dystonia and tardive dystonia, and Vo DBS for writer's cramp. STN as a target for dystonia remains under investigation and there are currently no specific indications for its use. The effects of stimulation on dystonia are delayed by several months to even a year. Therefore a structured approach to programming is important in the treatment of patients with dystonia.

REFERENCES

[1] Patel, N; Jankovic, J; Hallett, M. Sensory aspects of movement disorders. *Lancet Neurol.*, 2014 Jan, 13(1), 100-12

[2] Albanese, A; Bhatia, K; Bressman, SB; Delong, MR; et al. Phenomenology and classification of dystonia: A consensus update. *Mov Disord.*, 2013 Jun 15, 28(7), 863-73

[3] Balint, B; Bhatia, KP. Dystonia: an update on phenomenology; classification; pathogenesis and treatment. *Curr Opin Neurol.*, 2014, 27, 468-76.

[4] Defazio, G; Abbruzzese, G; Livrea, P; Berardelli, A. Epidemiology of primary dystonia. *Lancet Neurol.*, 2004 Nov, 3(11), 673-8.

[5] Risch, N; de Leon, D; Ozelius, L; Kramer, P; Almasy, L; Singer, B; Fahn, S; Breakefield, X; Bressman, S. Genetic analysis of idiopathic torsion dystonia in Ashkenazi Jews and their recent descent from a small founder population. *Nat Genet.*, 1995 Feb, 9(2), 152-9.

[6] Hendrix, CM; Vitek, JL. Toward a network model of dystonia. *Ann N Y Acad Sci.*, 2012 Aug, 1265, 46-55

[7] Quartarone, A; Hallett, M. Emerging concepts in the physiological basis of dystonia. *Mov Disord.*, 2013, 28(7), 958-67.

[8] Charlesworth, G; Bhatia, KP. Primary and secondary dystonic syndromes: an update. *Curr Opin Neurol.*, 2013 Aug, 26(4), 406-12.

[9] Bressman, SB. Dystonia genotypes, phenotypes, and classification. *Adv Neurol.*, 2004, 94, 101-7.

[10] Greene, P; Kang, UJ; Fahn, S. Spread of symptoms in idiopathic torsion dystonia. *Mov Disord.*, 1995 Mar, 10(2), 143-52.

[11] Fasano, A; Bove, F; Lang, AE. The treatment of dystonic tremor: a systematic review. *J Neurol Neurosurg Psychiatry.* 2014 Jul, 85(7), 759-69.

[12] Gironell, A; Kulisevsky, J. Diagnosis and Management of Essential Tremor and Dystonic Tremor. *Ther Adv Neurol Disord.*, 2009 Jul, 2(4), 215–222

[13] Chuang, C; Fahn, S; Frucht, SJ. The natural history and treatment of acquired hemidystonia: report of 33 cases and review of the literature. *J Neurol Neurosurg Psychiatry.* 2002 Jan, 72(1), 59-67.

[14] Lee, WW; Jeon, BS. Clinical spectrum of dopa-responsive dystonia and related disorders. *Curr Neurol Neurosci Rep.*, 2014 Jul, 14(7), 461.

[15] Mundinger, F. New stereotactic treatment of spasmodic torticollis with a brain stimulation system. *Med Klin.*, 1977, 72(46), 1982-6.

[16] Stavrinou, LC; Boviatsis, EJ; Leonardos, A; Panourias, IG; Sakas, DE. Current concepts on the mechanisms of dystonia and the beneficial effects of deep brain stimulation. *Cent Eur Neurosurg.*, 2011, 72(3), 144-8.

[17] Hammond, C; Ammari, R; Bioulac, B; Garcia, L. Latest view on the mechanism of action of deep brain stimulation. *Mov Disord.*, 2008 Nov, 15, 23(15), 2111-21

[18] De Carvalho Aguiar, PM; Ozelius, LJ. Classification and genetics of dystonia. *Lancet Neurol.*, 2002 Sep, 1(5), 316-25

[19] Klein, C. Genetics in dystonia. *Parkinsonism Relat Disord.*, 2014 Jan, 20 Suppl 1, S137-42.

[20] Lohmann, K; Klein, C. Genetics of dystonia: what's known? What's new? What's next?. *Mov Disord.*, 2013 Jun 15, 28(7), 899-905.

[21] Krauss, JK; Loher, TJ; Weigel, R; Capelle, HH et al. Chronic stimulation of the globus pallidus internus for treatment of non-dYT1 generalized dystonia and choreoathetosis: 2-year follow up. *J Neurosurg.*, 2003 Apr, 98(4), 785-92.

[22] Yianni, J; Bain, P; Giladi, N; Auca, M; Gregory, R; et al. Globus pallidus internus deep brain stimulation for dystonic conditions: a prospective audit. *Mov Disord.*, 2003 Apr, 18(4), 436-42.

[23] Coubes, P; Cif, L; El Fertit, H; Hemm, S; Vayssiere, N; Serrat, S; Picot, MC; Tuffery, S; Claustres, M; Echenne, B; Frerebeau, P. Electrical stimulation of the globus pallidus internus in patients with primary generalized dystonia: long-term results. *J Neurosurg.*, 2004 Aug, 101(2), 189-94

[24] Bittar, RG; Yianni, J; Wang, S; Liu, X; Nandi, D et al. Deep brain stimulation for generalised dystonia and spasmodic torticollis. *J Clin Neurosci.*, 2005 Jan, 12(1), 12-6.

[25] Vidailhet, M; Vercueil, L; Houeto, JL; Krystkowiak, P; Benabid, AL; Cornu, P;. Bilateral deep-brain stimulation of the globus pallidus in primary generalized dystonia. *N Engl J Med.*, 2005 Feb 3, 352(5), 459-67.

[26] Hälbig, TD; Gruber, D; Kopp, UA; Schneider, GH; et al. Pallidal stimulation in dystonia: effects on cognition; mood; and quality of life. *J Neurol Neurosurg Psychiatry.*, 2005 Dec, 76(12), 1713-6.

[27] Kupsch, A; Benecke, R; Müller, J; Trottenberg, T; Schneider, GH; Poewe, W; Eisner, W et al. Pallidal deep-brain stimulation in primary generalized or segmental dystonia. *N Engl J Med.*, 2006 Nov 9, 355(19), 1978-90

[28] Egidi, M; Franzini, A; Marras, C; Cavallo, M; Mondani, M et al. A survey of Italian cases of dystonia treated by deep brain stimulation. *J Neurosurg Sci.*, 2007 Dec, 51(4), 153-8.

[29] Vidailhet, M; Vercueil, L; Houeto, JL; Krystkowiak, P; Lagrange, C; Yelnik, J; et al. Bilateral, pallidal, deep-brain stimulation in primary generalised dystonia: a prospective 3 year follow-up study. *Lancet Neurol.*, 2007 Mar, 6(3), 223-9.

[30] Mueller, J; Skogseid, IM; Benecke, R; Kupsch, A; Trottenberg, T; Poewe, W; et al. Pallidal deep brain stimulation improves quality of life in segmental and generalized dystonia: results from a prospective; randomized sham-controlled trial. *Mov Disord.*, 2008 Jan, 23(1), 131-4.

[31] Mehrkens, JH; Bötzel, K; Steude, U; Zeitler, K; Schnitzler, A; et al. Long-term efficacy and safety of chronic globus pallidus internus stimulation in different types of primarydystonia. *Stereotact Funct Neurosurg.*, 2009, 87(1), 8-17

[32] Isaias, IU; Alterman, RL; Tagliati, M. Deep brain stimulation for primary generalized dystonia: long-term outcomes. *Arch Neurol.*, 2009 Apr, 66(4), 465-70

[33] Cif, L; Vasques, X; Gonzalez, V; Ravel, P; Biolsi, B; et al. Long-term follow-up of DYT1 dystonia patients treated by deep brain stimulation: an open-label study. *Mov Disord.*, 2010 Feb15, 25(3), 289-99

[34] Valldeoriola, F; Regidor, I; Mínguez-Castellanos, A; Lezcano, E; García-Ruiz, P; et al. Efficacy and safety of pallidal stimulation in primary dystonia: results of the Spanish multicentric study. *J Neurol Neurosurg Psychiatry.* 2010 Jan, 81(1), 65-9

[35] Volkmann, J; Wolters, A; Kupsch, A; Müller, J; Kühn, AA; Schneider, GH; et al. Pallidal deep brain stimulation in patients with primary generalised or segmental dystonia: 5-year follow-up of a randomised trial. *Lancet Neurol.*, 2012 Dec, 11(12), 1029-38.

[36] Schjerling, L; Hjermind, LE; Jespersen, B; Madsen, FF; et al. A randomized double-blind crossover trial comparing subthalamic and pallidal deep brain stimulation for dystonia. *J Neurosurg.*, 2013 Dec, 119(6), 1537-45.

[37] Jahanshahi, M; Torkamani, M; Beigi, M; Wilkinson, L; et al. Pallidal stimulation for primary generalised dystonia: effect on cognition; mood and quality of life. *J Neurol.*, 2014 Jan, 261(1), 164-73.

[38] Miri, S; Ghoreyshi, E; Shahidi, GA; Parvaresh, M; et al. Deep brain stimulation of globus pallidus internus for DYT1 positive primary generalized dystonia. *Med J Islam Repub Iran.*, 2014 Mar 1, 28, 18.

[39] Sobstyl, M; Kmieć, T; Ząbek, M; Szczałuba, K; Mossakowski, Z. Long-term outcomes of bilateral pallidal stimulation for primary generalised dystonia. *Clin Neurol Neurosurg.*, 2014 Nov, 126, 82-7

[40] Coubes, P; Roubertie, A; Vayssiere, N; Hemm, S; Echenne, B. Treatment of DYT1-generalised dystonia by stimulation of the internal globus pallidus. *Lancet.*, 2000 Jun 24, 355(9222), 2220-1.

[41] Vercueil, L1; Pollak, P; Fraix, V; Caputo, E; Moro, E; Benazzouz, A; et al. Deep brain stimulation in the treatment of severe dystonia. *J Neurol.*, 2001 Aug, 248(8), 695-700.

[42] Kleiner-Fisman, G; Liang, GS; Moberg, PJ; Ruocco, AC; et al. Subthalamic nucleus deep brain stimulation for severe idiopathic dystonia: impact on severity, neuropsychological status, and quality of life. *J Neurosurg.*, 2007 Jul, 107(1), 29-36.

[43] Sun, B; Chen, S; Zhan, S; Le, W; Krahl, SE. Subthalamic nucleus stimulation for primary dystonia and tardive dystonia. *Acta Neurochir Suppl.*, 2007, 97(Pt 2), 207-14.

[44] Bereznai, B; Steude, U; Seelos, K; Bötzel, K. Chronic high-frequency globus pallidus internus stimulation in different types of dystonia: a clinical, video, and MRI report of six patients presenting with segmental, cervical, and generalized dystonia. *Mov Disord.*, 2002 Jan, 17(1), 138-44.

[45] Ostrem, JL; Marks, WJ; Jr; Volz, MM; Heath, SL; Starr, PA. Pallidal deep brain stimulation in patients with cranial-cervical dystonia (Meige syndrome). *Mov Disord.*, 2007 Oct 15, 22(13), 1885-91.

[46] Kiss, ZH; Doig-Beyaert, K; Eliasziw, M; Tsui, J; Haffenden, A; et al. The Canadian multicentre study of deep brain stimulation for cervical dystonia. *Brain.* 2007 Nov, 130(11), 2879-86

[47] Hung, SW; Hamani, C; Lozano, AM; Poon, YY; Piboolnurak, et al. Long-term outcome of bilateral pallidal deep brain stimulation for primary cervical dystonia. *Neurology.*, 2007 Feb 6, 68(6), 457-9.

[48] Sensi, M; Cavallo, MA; Quatrale, R; Sarubbo, S; et al. Pallidal stimulation for segmental dystonia: long term follow up of 11 consecutive patients *Mov Disord.*, 2009 Sep 15, 24(12), 1829-35.

[49] Mehrkens, JH; Bötzel, K; Steude, U; Zeitler, K; et al. Long-term efficacy and safety of chronic globus pallidus internus stimulation in different types of primarydystonia. *Stereotact Funct Neurosurg.*, 2009, 87(1), 8-17

[50] Jeong, SG; Lee, MK; Kang, JY; Jun, SM; et al. Pallidal deep brain stimulation in primary cervical dystonia with phasic type: clinical outcome and postoperative course. *J Korean Neurosurg Soc.*, 2009 Oct, 46(4), 346-50

[51] Cacciola, F; Farah, JO; Eldridge, PR; Byrne, P; Varma, TK. Bilateral deep brain stimulation for cervical dystonia: long-term outcome in a series of 10 patients. *Neurosurgery.*, 2010 Oct, 67(4), 957-63

[52] Ghang, JY; Lee, MK; Jun, SM; Ghang, CG. Outcome of pallidal deep brain stimulation in meige syndrome. *J Korean Neurosurg Soc.*, 2010 Aug, 48(2), 134-8.

[53] Lyons, MK; Birch, BD; Hillman, RA; Boucher, OK; Evidente, VG. Long-term follow-up of deep brain stimulation for Meige syndrome. *Neurosurg Focus.*, 2010 Aug, 29(2), E5

[54] Limotai, N; Go, C; Oyama, G; Hwynn, N; Zesiewicz, T; et al. Mixed results for GPi-DBS in the treatment of cranio-facial and cranio-cervical dystonia symptoms. *J Neurol.*, 2011 Nov, 258(11), 2069-74

[55] Reese, R; Gruber, D; Schoenecker, T; Bäzner, H; et al. Long-term clinical outcome in meige syndrome treated with internal pallidum deep brain stimulation. *Mov Disord.*, 2011 Mar, 26(4), 691-8

[56] Skogseid, IM; Ramm-Pettersen, J; Volkmann, J; et al. Good long-term efficacy of pallidal stimulation in cervical dystonia: a prospective; observer-blinded study. *Eur J Neurol.*, 2012 Apr, 19(4), 610-5

[57] Sarubbo, S; Latini, F; Quatrale, R; Sensi, M; et al. Five-year follow-up of 10 patients treated with globus pallidus internus deep brain stimulation for segmental or multisegmental dystonia. *Stereotact Funct Neurosurg.*, 2012, 90(2), 84-91

[58] Walsh, RA; Sidiropoulos, C; Lozano, AM; Hodaie, M; Poon, YY; et al. Bilateral pallidal stimulation in cervical dystonia: blinded evidence of benefit beyond 5 years. *Brain.*, 2013 Mar, 136(3), 761-9

[59] Witt, JL; Moro, E; Ash, RS; Hamani, C; Starr, PA; Lozano, AM; et al. Predictive factors of outcome in primary cervical dystonia following pallidal deep brain stimulation. *Mov Disord.*, 2013 Sep, 28(10), 1451-5

[60] Volkmann, J; Mueller, J; Deuschl, G; Kühn, AA; Krauss, JK; Poewe, W; et al. Pallidal neurostimulation in patients with medication-refractory cervical dystonia: a randomised; sham-controlled trial. *Lancet Neurol.*, 2014 Sep, 13(9), 875-84

[61] Chou, KL; Hurtig, HI; Jaggi, JL; Baltuch, GH. Bilateral subthalamic nucleus deep brain stimulation in a patient with cervical dystonia and essential tremor *Mov Disord.*, 2005 Mar, 20(3), 377-80

[62] Kleiner-Fisman, G; Liang, GS; Moberg, PJ; Ruocco, AC; et al. Subthalamic nucleus deep brain stimulation for severe idiopathic dystonia: impact on severity, neuropsychological status, and quality of life. *J Neurosurg.*, 2007 Jul, 107(1), 29-36.

[63] Ostrem, JL; Racine, CA; Glass, GA; Grace, JK; et al. Subthalamic nucleus deep brain stimulation in primary cervical dystonia. *Neurology.*, 2011 Mar 8, 76(10), 870-8.

[64] Mills, KA; Markun, LC; San Luciano, M; Rizk, R; et al. Effect of subthalamic nucleus deep brain stimulation on dual-task cognitive and motor performance in isolateddystonia. *J Neurol Neurosurg Psychiatry.* 2014 Jul, 10.

[65] Cohen, LG; Hallett, M. Hand cramps: clinical features and electromyographic patterns in a focal dystonia. *Neurology.*, 1988 Jul, 38(7), 1005-12.

[66] Goto, S; Shimazu, H; Matsuzaki, K; Tamura, T; et al. Thalamic Vo-complex vs pallidal deep brain stimulation for focal hand dystonia. *Neurology.*, 2008 Apr 15, 70(16 Pt 2), 1500-1

[67] Goto, S; Tsuiki, H; Soyama, N; Okamura, A; et al. Stereotactic selective Vo-complex thalamotomy in a patient with dystonic writer's cramp. *Neurology.*, 1997 Oct, 49(4), 1173-4.

[68] Fukaya, C; Katayama, Y; Kano, T; Nagaoka, T; et al. Thalamic deep brain stimulation for writer's cramp. *J Neurosurg.*, 2007 Nov, 107(5), 977-82.

[69] Asahi, T; Koh, M; Kashiwazaki, D; Kuroda, S. Stereotactic neurosurgery for writer's cramp: report of two cases with an overview of the literature. *Stereotact Funct Neurosurg.*, 2014, 92(6), 405-11.

[70] Tolosa, ES; Klawans, HL. Meiges disease: a clinical form of facial convulsion; bilateral and medial. *Arch Neurol.*, 1979 Oct, 36(10), 635-7

[71] Berman, BD; Starr, PA; Marks, WJ; Jr. Ostrem, JL. Induction of bradykinesia with pallidal deep brain stimulation in patients with cranial-cervical dystonia. *Stereotact Funct Neurosurg.*, 2009, 87(1), 37-44

[72] Zauber, SE; Watson, N; Comella, CL; Bakay, RA; Metman, LV. Stimulation-induced parkinsonism after posteroventral deep brain stimulation of the globus pallidus internus for craniocervical dystonia. *J Neurosurg.*, 2009 Feb, 110(2), 229-33

[73] Schrader, C; Capelle, HH; Kinfe, TM; Blahak, C; et al. GPi-DBS may induce a hypokinetic gait disorder with freezing of gait in patients with dystonia. *Neurology.*, 2011 Aug 2, 77(5), 483-8

[74] Kinugawa, K; Vidailhet, M; Clot, F; Apartis, E; Grabli, D; Roze, E. Myoclonus-dystonia: an update *Mov Disord.*, 2009 Mar 15, 24(4), 479-89.

[75] Azoulay-Zyss, J; Roze, E; Welter, ML; Navarro, S; Yelnik, J; et al. Bilateral deep brain stimulation of the pallidum for myoclonus-dystonia due to ε-sarcoglycan mutations: a pilot study. *Arch Neurol.*, 2011 Jan, 68(1), 94-8

[76] Gruber, D; Kühn, AA; Schoenecker, T; Kivi, A; Trottenberg, T; et al. Pallidal and thalamic deep brain stimulation in myoclonus-dystonia. *Mov Disord.*, 2010 Aug 15, 25(11), 1733-43

[77] Trottenberg, T; Meissner, W; Kabus, C; Arnold, G; et al. Neurostimulation of the ventral intermediate thalamic nucleus in inherited myoclonus-dystonia syndrome. *Mov Disord.*, 2001 Jul, 16(4), 769-71.

[78] Kuncel, AM; Turner, DA; Ozelius, LJ; Greene, PE; Grill, WM; Stacy, MA. Myoclonus and tremor response to thalamic deep brain stimulation parameters in a patient with inherited myoclonus-dystonia syndrome. *Clin Neurol Neurosurg.*, 2009 Apr, 111(3), 303-6

[79] Kim, JH; Na, YC; Lee, WH; Chang, WS; Jung, HH; Chang, JW. Bilateral globus pallidus interna deep-brain stimulation in a patient with myoclonus-dystonia: a case report. *Neuromodulation.*, 2014 Dec, 17(8), 724-8

[80] Sidiropoulos, C; Mestre, T; Hutchison, W; Moro, E. Bilateral pallidal stimulation for sargoglycan epsilon negative myoclonus. *Parkinsonism Relat Disord.*, 2014 Aug, 20(8), 915-8.

[81] Rughani, AI; Lozano, AM. Surgical treatment of myoclonus dystonia syndrome. *Mov Disord.*, 2013 Mar, 28(3), 282-7.

[82] Morishita, T; Foote, KD; Haq, IU; Zeilman, P; Jacobson, CE; et al. Should we consider Vim thalamic deep brain stimulation for select cases of severe refractory dystonic tremor. *Stereotact Funct Neurosurg.*, 2010, 88(2), 98-104.

[83] Hedera, P; Phibbs, FT; Dolhun, R; Charles, PD; et al. Surgical targets for dystonic tremor: considerations between the globus pallidus and ventral intermediate thalamic nucleus. *Parkinsonism Relat Disord.*, 2013 Jul, 19(7), 684-6.

[84] Keen, JR; Przekop, A; Olaya, JE; Zouros, A; et al. Deep brain stimulation for the treatment of childhood dystonic cerebral palsy. *J Neurosurg Pediatr.*, 2014 Dec, 14(6), 585-93.

[85] Aniello, MS; Martino, D; Petruzzella, V; Eleopra, R; et al. Bilateral striatal necrosis; dystonia and multiple mitochondrial DNA deletions: case study and effect of deep brain stimulation. *Mov Disord.*, 2008 Jan, 23(1), 114-8.

[86] Cif, L; Biolsi, B; Gavarini, S; Saux, A; Robles, SG; et al. Antero-ventral internal pallidum stimulation improves behavioral disorders in Lesch-Nyhan disease. *Mov Disord.*, 2007 Oct, 31, 22(14), 2126-9.

[87] Wadia, PM; Lim, SY; Lozano, AM; Adams, JR; et al. Bilateral pallidal stimulation for x-linked dystonia parkinsonism. *Arch Neurol.*, 2010 Aug, 67(8), 1012-5

[88] Ghika, J; Villemure, JG; Miklossy, J; Temperli, P; et al. Postanoxic generalized dystonia improved by bilateral Voa thalamic deep brain stimulation. *Neurology.*, 2002 Jan 22, 58(2), 311-3.

[89] Timmermann, L; Pauls, KA; Wieland, K; Jech, R; Kurlemann, G; et al. Dystonia in neurodegeneration with brain iron accumulation: outcome of bilateral pallidal stimulation. *Brain.*, 2010 Mar, 133(Pt 3), 701-12

[90] Bronte-Stewart, H; Taira, T; Valldeoriola, F; Merello, M; et al. Inclusion and exclusion criteria for DBS in dystonia. *Mov Disord.*, 2011 Jun, 26 Suppl 1, S5-16.

[91] Cloud, LJ; Jinnah, HA. Treatment strategies for dystonia. *Expert Opin Pharmacother.*, 2010 Jan, 11(1), 5-15

[92] Jankovic, J. Medical treatment of dystonia. *Mov Disord.*, 2013 Jun 15, 28(7), 1001-12

[93] Fletcher, NA; Thompson, PD; Scadding, JW; Marsden, CD. Successful treatment of childhood onset symptomatic dystonia with levodopa. *J Neurol Neurosurg Psychiatry.* 1993 Aug, 56(8), 865-7.

[94] Jankovic, J; Clarence-Smith, K. Tetrabenazine for the treatment of chorea and other hyperkinetic movement disorders. *Expert Rev Neurother.*, 2011 Nov, 11(11), 1509-23.

[95] Luciano, AY; Jinnah, HA; Pfeiffer, RF; et al. Treatment of myoclonus-dystonia syndrome with tetrabenazine. *Parkinsonism Relat Disord.*, 2014 Dec, 20(12), 1423-6

[96] Hallett, M; Benecke, R; Blitzer, A; Comella, CL. Treatment of focal dystonias with botulinum neurotoxin. *Toxicon.*, 2009 Oct, 54(5), 628-33

[97] Simpson, DM; Blitzer, A; Brashear, A; Comella, C; Dubinsky, R; et al. Assessment: Botulinum neurotoxin for the treatment of movement disorders (an evidence-based review), report of the Therapeutics and Technology Assessment Subcommittee of the American Academy of Neurology. *Neurology.*, 2008 May 6, 70(19), 1699-706.

[98] Ramirez-Castaneda, J; Jankovic, J; Comella, C; et al. Diffusion; spread; and migration of botulinum toxin. *Mov Disord.*, 2013 Nov, 28(13), 1775-83

[99] Baizabal-Carvallo, JF; Jankovic, J; Feld, J. Flu-like symptoms and associated immunological response following therapy with botulinum toxins. *Neurotox Res.*, 2013 Aug, 24(2), 298-306.

[100] Evidente, VG; Pappert, EJ. Botulinum toxin therapy for cervical dystonia: the science of dosing. *Tremor Other Hyperkinet Mov* (N Y). 2014 Nov 12, 4, 273

[101] Ferreira, JJ; Colosimo, C; Bhidayasiri, R; Marti, MJ. Factors influencing secondary non-response to botulinum toxin type A injections in cervical dystonia. *Parkinsonism Relat Disord.*, 2015 Feb, 21(2), 111-5

[102] Isaias, IU; Volkmann, J; Kupsch, A; Burgunder, JM; Ostrem, JL; et al. Factors predicting protracted improvement after pallidal DBS for primary dystonia: the role of age and disease duration. *J Neurol.*, 2011 Aug, 258(8), 1469-76

[103] Air, EL; Ostrem, JL; Sanger, TD; Starr, PA. Deep brain stimulation in children: experience and technical pearls. *J Neurosurg Pediatr.*, 2011 Dec, 8(6), 566-74.

[104] Miyagi, Y; Koike, Y. Tolerance of early pallidal stimulation in pediatric generalized dystonia. *J Neurosurg Pediatr.*, 2013 Nov, 12(5), 476-82

[105] Vidailhet, M; Jutras, MF; Roze, E; Grabli D. Deep brain stimulation for dystonia. *Handb Clin Neurol.*, 2013, 116, 167-87

[106] Holloway, KL; Baron, MS; Brown, R; Cifu, DX; et al. Deep brain stimulation for dystonia: a meta-analysis. *Neuromodulation.*, 2006 Oct, 9(4), 253-61

[107] Anheim, M; Vercueil, L; Fraix, V; Chabardès, S ; et al. Early stimulation of DYT1 primary generalized dystonia prevents from its secondary irreversible complications. *Mov Disord.*, 2008 Nov 15, 23(15), 2261-3.

[108] Guettard, E; Ricard, D; Roze, E; Elbaz, A; Anheim, M; et al. Risk factors for spinal cord lesions in dystonic cerebral palsy and generalised dystonia. *J Neurol Neurosurg Psychiatry.*, 2012 Feb, 83(2), 159-63

[109] Gündel, H; Wolf, A; Xidara, V; Busch, R; Ceballos-Baumann, AO. Social phobia in spasmodic torticollis. *J Neurol Neurosurg Psychiatry*, 2001 Oct, 71(4), 499-504.

[110] Jahanshahi, M; Czernecki, V; Zurowski, AM. Neuropsychological, neuropsychiatric, and quality of life issues in DBS for dystonia. *Mov Disord.*, 2011 Jun, 26 Suppl 1, S63-78.

[111] Ondo, WG; Bronte-Stewart, H. DBS Study Group. The North American survey of placement and adjustment strategies for deep brain stimulation. *Stereotact Funct Neurosurg.*, 2005, 83(4), 142-7.

[112] Kupsch, A; Tagliati, M; Vidailhet, M; Aziz, T; Krack, P; Moro, E; Krauss, JK. Early postoperative management of DBS in dystonia: programming, response to stimulation, adverse events, medication changes, evaluations, and troubleshooting. *Mov Disord.*, 2011 Jun, 26 Suppl 1, S37-53

[113] FitzGerald, JJ; Rosendal, F; de Pennington, N; Joint, C; Forrow, B; et al. Long-term outcome of deep brain stimulation in generalised dystonia: a series of 60 cases. *J Neurol Neurosurg Psychiatry.* 2014 Dec, 85(12), 1371-6

[114] Alterman, RL; Miravite, J; Weisz, D; Shils, JL; et al. Sixty hertz pallidal deep brain stimulation for primary torsion dystonia. *Neurology.*, 2007 Aug 14, 69(7), 681-8.

[115] Kupsch, A; Kuehn, A; Klaffke, S; Meissner, W; et al. *J Neurol.*, 2003 Feb, 250 Suppl 1, I47-52.

[116] Ostrem, JL; Markun, LC; Glass, GA; Racine, CA; et al. Effect of frequency on subthalamic nucleus deep brain stimulation in primary dystonia. *Parkinsonism Relat Disord.*, 2014 Apr, 20(4), 432-8

[117] Miocinovic, S; Khemani, P; Whiddon, R; Zeilman, P; et al. Outcomes, management, and potential mechanisms of interleaving deep brain stimulation settings. *Parkinsonism Relat Disord.*, 2014 Dec, 20(12), 1434-7.

[118] Lettieri, C; Rinaldo, S; Devigili, G; Pisa, F; Mucchiut, M; et al. Clinical outcome of deep brain stimulation for dystonia: constant-current or constant-voltage stimulation? A non-randomized study. Eur *J Neurol.*, 2014 Jul 10

In: Deep Brain Stimulation
Editor: Raja Mehanna

ISBN: 978-1-63483-282-3

Chapter 9

DEEP BRAIN STIMULATION IN OTHER NEUROLOGICAL AND PSYCHIATRIC CONDITIONS

William Ondo, MD
University of Texas Health Science Center at Houston, Houston, Texas, US

ABSTRACT

Deep brain stimulation (DBS) in the sub-thalamic nucleus, globus pallidus internus, and thalamus are accepted treatments for movement disorders, including tremor, Parkinson's disease, and dystonia. DBS has also been implanted into these and other brain locations for a variety of other neurologic and psychiatric conditions. There is very good evidence supporting efficacy for obsessive compulsive disorder and Tourette's syndrome. There is good evidence supporting use for depression, seizures and tardive dyskinesia. There is less evidence supporting DBS for dementia, restless legs syndrome, post-traumatic stress disorder, and anorexia nervosa. This chapter will explore current knowledge of DBS for these indications, emphasizing clinical data and practical considerations. It is important to note that only Parkinson's disease, essential tremor, dystonia and obsessive compulsive disorders are currently approved indications by European and US regulatory agencies.

INTRODUCTION

Neuropsychiatric disorders remain full of management challenges. In most cases the exact pathophysiology and precise brain anatomy is not elucidated, which hinders the development of rational therapy. Pharmacologic treatments exist for depression, dementia, obsessive-compulsive disorders, Tourette's syndrome, anxiety disorders and restless legs syndrome, but the anatomic substrate for these drugs is often speculative. The neuroanatomy of seizure disorders is better understood but epilepsy is still not adequately managed.

Surgical management of psychiatric disorders has a long but checkered history, and special caution and restraint is now required due to past practices. This being said, the marked consequence of severe psychiatric disease often warrants very aggressive treatment options, even when efficacy data is not definitive.

Deep brain stimulation (DBS) has been widely used for more than 20 years, mostly to treat movement disorders including Parkinson's disease, tremor, and dystonia. The mechanism of action is discussed in detail elsewhere, but the device can deliver a very focal electrical discharge that alters intrinsic circuitry. Importantly, this effect is reversible, simply by deactivating the device, and the targeted anatomy can be adjusted to some extent.

This chapter will discuss the use of DBS in a number of neuropsychiatric conditions. It will concentrate mostly of human efficacy data, specific side effects associated with locations, and future directions.

Among all the conditions detailed below, only obsessive compulsive disorders are currently approved DBS indications by European and US regulatory agencies.

TOURETTE'S SYNDROME

Tourette's syndrome (TS) is defined by multiple motor tics and at least one vocal tic, with an onset before 21, without any other identified culpable etiology. Tics are partially suppressible movements that vary in complexity, arise out of a normal background, are sometimes associated with an urge and may be suggestible. Tic disorders that do not meet the criteria for TS are not felt to be intrinsically different than those seen in TS. Up to 10% of boys demonstrate tics at some point, usually mild. The mean age of onset is 7 and they generally improve during the late teens. The pathophysiology is poorly understood but increased dopamine sensitivity is suggested, and pathophysiology in parallel thalamocorticalstriatal pathways has been suggested. Tics are variably associated with obsessive compulsive features (OCD), attention deficit problems (ADD), impulsivity, and oppositional behavior. Therefore treatment plan needs to determine the overall major morbidities. Pharmacological treatment of tics includes dopamine antagonists, tetrabenazine, α2 agonists, and topiramate. DBS treatment for TS has generated tremendous interest despite a modest number of published cases [1]. In fact there are more published reviews than original efficacy data publications. Most original publications are case reports or small series but some partially controlled data (usually blindly activating/deactivating the DBS) exist.

DBS for TS has unique considerations. Most cases of TS are pediatric with developing, and sometimes physically growing brains. Unlike most DBS indications, tics generally improve as the patient ages. Co-morbidities including OCD, ADD and other behavioral issues should also impact patient selection. Therefore DBS is appropriately reserved for the most severe and refractory cases, typically older patients, in whom spontaneous improvement is thought unlikely. Overall, DBS seems to reduce tics by about 50% [2]. One meta-analysis reported generally good outcomes, somewhat superior to those reported in depression and OCD [3]. However, numerous DBS targets have been used to treat tics, making a global assessment difficult. The most commonly reported target for DBS for tics are adjacent regions of the medial thalamus: centromedian nucleus (CM)/centromedian-parafascicular complex (CM-PF) / ventral-oral internal thalamic nucleus (VOI) / substantia periventricularis (SP) [Table] [2, 4-8]. The exact reported anatomy in individual series can vary (CM-SP, CM-PF-VOI, CM-VOI-SP, etc.). Procedures are bilateral and DBS settings are generally similar to those used for Parkinson's disease or tremor, but often require increased power over time. Published results have reported a tic reduction of 40-90%, although most patients in these series continue to require tic medications. Most report continued benefit for at least 12-24 months. Several medial thalamic series also report improvement in OCD, depression, and anxiety [4, 5].

Table.

Condition	Target	Quality data*	Comment
Tourette's (tics)	MT - centromedian nucleus (CM)	+++	Numerous reports overlap these specific sites, may also improve mood, anxiety and OCD
	MT -centromedian-parafascicular complex (CM-PF)		
	MT- ventral-oral internal thalamic nucleus (VOI)		
	MT- substantia periventricularis (SP)		
	Globus Pallidus Internus posteroventral (GPi-PV)	+++	No sham trials but blindly compared to MT
	Globus Pallidus Internus anteromedial (GPi-AM)		
	Anterior Limb Int Capsule – Nucleus Accumbens (ALIC-NA)	+	Probably less effective than MT or GPi for tics
	Globus Pallidus Externus (GPe)	+	Case report
	Sub-thalamic nucleus (STN)	+	One subject with PD and tics
Obsessive-Compulsive Disorder	Anterior Limb Int Capsule – Nucleus Accumbens (ALIC-NA)	++++	Approved by European and US regulatory agencies
	Nucleus Accumbens (NA)	+++	Single cross-over trial N=14
	Sub-thalamic nucleus (STN)	+++	Single cross-over trial, N=16
	ventral capsule/ventral striatum VC/VS	++	A 6 subject trial, no efficacy statistics
Dementia	Nucleus Basalis of Meynert (NBM)	+	Low frequency stim.
	Fornix	+	Single 6 pt. series
	Entorhinal cortex	+	Case implanted for epilepsy
	pedunculopontine nucleus	+	Case implanted for epilepsy

Table. (Continued)

Condition	Target	Quality data*	Comment
Depression	Ventral striatum/ventral capsule (VS/VC)	+ --	Negative controlled trial
	subcallosal cingulate white matter/singulate cortex (SCC)	++	Multiple open label series
	nucleus accumbens (NA)	++	
	Medial forebrain bundle (MFB)	++	A single 7 pt series
	lateral habenula (LH)	+	case

+ any case report, ++ open label case series, +++ any controlled or blinded trial, ++++ approved by some regulatory agency, --- negative controlled trial

A couple of controlled trials, usually randomized to DBS "on" or DBS "off," also show benefit. One cross-over trial blindly assessed seven subjects s/p CM-VOI-SP thalamic implantation randomized to 3 months of activated versus 3 months of deactivated leads. Although the trial design suffered from many limitations, they found superior tic suppression with DBS activated, with a tic reduction of 41.1 +/- 5.4% versus 25.6 +/- 12.8%, P = 0.046 [8]. Another five subject cross-over trial compared CM-PF DBS in 4 conditions: bilateral off, left side activated, right side activated, and bilateral active, and found significant improvement in the bilateral group using video tic counts [7]. As with all DBS studies, true blinding can be problematic.

The second most reported target is the Globus Pallidus Internus (GPi), although most of these are case reports [2, 9-12]. Both the posteroventral GPi, the same site as dystonia, and the anteromedial GPi [13] have been targeted. Reported reduction in tics ranged from 0-95%, and improved concurrent OCD was also reported.

Several reports that targeted the anterior limb of the internal capsule (ALIC) and/or the nucleus accumbens (NA) reported mixed results that tended to be inferior to the medial thalamus or GPi [14-16]. This target is also use for idiopathic OCD and has been adjunctively targeted with medial thalamic DBS in subjects with tics and OCD. Other reported targets include the globus pallidus externus (GPe) [17], and the sub-thalamic nucleus (STN) [18].

There are a few reports comparing different sites in a small number of tic subjects. One report of 5 total subjects modestly favored the anteromedial GPi over the ventromedial GPi [12]. A single case had better control with medial thalamus compared to ALIC-NA. One case had similar tic improvement with only GPi activated, only medial thalamus activated, and in combination [19]. Mood, however, improved more with the medial thalamus DBS. Another dual placement report found that the posteroventral GPi tended to reduce tics more than the CM-PF thalamus in three subjects [20]. Combination stimulation did not further improve tics. Clearly additional data is needed to determine optimal placement for tics and associated conditions.

There are some specific potential safety issues concerning DBS in the TS population. First this is mostly a pediatric condition, which generally improves with age, so case series mostly report late adolescent and young adult patients, who have a fully developed brain size.

The age is still younger than other indications. Neuropsychiatric cognitive evaluations have been performed in some series. One thalamic implantation study of 5 males (age 28.2±7.5 y) reported some worsened verbal fluency, visual immediate memory, and reaction time, with improvement in mood and anxiety [21]. The majority of DBS studies in TS have not reported cognitive worsening but methodology and level of scrutiny vary [22]. One group reported significantly more infections in their 39 subjects with TS compared to 233 subjects implanted for other indications [23].

Overall there is compelling data to support the efficacy of DBS for severe refractory tics. Recent guidelines for patient selection and targeting are reported [1]. However, this indication has not been approved by US and European regulatory agencies and cannot be formally recommended at this time. Many issues including optimal target and effect on associated conditions remain unresolved.

Obsessive Compulsive Disorder

OCD is a common condition characterized by intrusive and repetitive thoughts and repetitive highly patterned behavior or mental acts aimed at reducing anxiety. Treatments include cognitive behavioral therapy and serotonergic reuptake inhibitors, often supplemented with anti-psychotic medications, but are still often inadequate. The consequences of severe OCD have justified attempts at numerous brain ablation procedures since the 1950s.

More recently, OCD has become the best studied psychiatric indication for DBS, and this indication is actually approved by the U.S. Food and Drug Agency under a Humanitarian Device Exemption, and by European agencies. When considering DBS, strict inclusion criteria are proposed, including severe OCD defined by a Yale-Brown Obsessive Compulsive Scale (Y-BOCS) >30, failure of combination medical therapy (at least three different medications) and cognitive behavioral therapy, and the absence of other Axis I psychiatric disease or other neurological disease, with the possible exception of tics.

Two recent meta-analyses of clinical trials have been published [24, 25]. Controlled trials show efficacy when placed in the anterior limb of the internal capsule (ALIC) [26-28], the nucleus accumbens (NA) [29], the sub-thalamic nucleus (STN) [30], and the ventral capsule/ventral striatum (VC/VS) [27]. These still represent a small number of subjects so comparing the efficacy among different sites is problematic. The most commonly performed site is the ALIC, which connects non-motor fibers from the prefrontal cortex to the dorsi-medial thalamus and other subcortical sites. Of note, the ALIC and NA are contiguous and can both be stimulated with a single electrode. A site with the inferior lead in the NA but passing through the ALIC is commonly employed (X: 13-14 mm lateral to midline, Y: 3.5 mm anterior to the anterior commissure, Z: at the inter-commissural plain) although this is variably reported in the literature as implantation into the ALIC, the NA, or both. No identifiable and reproducible microelectrode recording (MER) has been reported to assist targeting this site, however, some operative macro stimulation effects are reported, including a contralateral "smile" (not facial dystonia), giddiness and panic/anxiety [31]. The "smile" is thought to predict a good response. The time to maximal efficacy for this, and other sites for OCD, is usually delayed, complicating adjustment sessions, since there is little immediate response. Higher pulse width, higher frequencies and greater overall power settings tend to be used for OCD, except if the STN is targeted, resulting in reduced battery life [31]. In controlled trials, the Y-BOCS improved 25-40% compared to sham surgery. The most common site specific adverse events include mania and depression. However, formal testing of cognition, general anxiety, and depression in OCD subjects with DBS has generally showed neither improvement nor worsening [24].

The VC/VS is also adjacent to the NA, and has been specifically targeted by several groups. Only a 6 subject controlled trial (4 randomized to active treatment) has been reported but open label data up to 36 months follow-up also reports a 30-40% improvement in Y-BOCS. Hypomania is also reported in this location.

One controlled trial and several other open label studies targeted the STN for OCD. The single controlled cross-over trial reported a 30% improvement in the device activated arm. A single group has also reported open label benefit of OCD with implantation of the inferior thalamic peduncle [32].

Ablative procedures for OCD are also still performed. One open label series reported similar efficacy between ablative capsulotomy and ALIC DBS [33]. Both also normalize altered metabolic brain functioning in OCD: reduced superior frontal and supplementary motor cortex activity, and increased subgenual anterior cingulate, occipital cortex (cuneus), and posterior cerebellum activity, although lesioning actually resulted in more robust metabolic changes than DBS. Non-invasive capsulotomies, mostly gamma knife procedures are also reported [31].

Overall there is good efficacy data (30-40% reduction in Y-BOCS) for multiple DBS implantation sites, most commonly the ALIC. These are reserved for the most severe and refractory cases, are usually done bilaterally, require high pulse width/ frequency, and have a delayed peak response.

DEPRESSION

Major depressive disorder is one of the leading causes of disability in developed nations, affecting up to 4% of the population. Medicines that increase synaptic serotonin, norepinephrine, and dopamine, electroconvulsive therapy and psychotherapy often improve symptoms; but are not always satisfactory. Refractory depression has been reported to respond to DBS of the subcallosal cingulate white matter (SCC)/subgenual cingulate cortex/Brodmann area 25, the internal capsule, the nucleus accumbens, the medial forebrain bundle, and the inferior thalamic peduncle [34-36].

The SCC was initially targeted based on functional imaging abnormalities that changed with successful pharmacologic treatment of depression [37, 38]. A number of open label series support SCC implantation, although controlled trials are still lacking. The exact coordinates, and sometimes nomenclature, vary slightly among groups. Most report a response rate (>50% reduction in depression scales) in 40-65% of subjects, and remission rates (Hamilton depression 17 scale < 7) of up to 40% [39-41]. One meta-analysis of this target in a total of 66 subjects reported a 40% response rate at 12 months [39]. The results are relatively rapid but in one large series tended to lessen over time, from 1 month to 12 months [42]. All aspects of depression seem to improve equally. A single randomized cross-over study of DBS deactivation after successful treatment tended to show modestly better results in those maintained on DBS in five subjects [43]. Other cognitive testing results after SCC DBS are generally unchanged [44]. Using tractography analysis of SCC DBS, researchers found that DBS depression responders showed activation of pathways from 1.medial frontal cortex via forceps minor and uncinate fasciculus; 2. rostral and dorsal cingulate cortex via the cingulum bundle; and 3. the subcortical nuclei [35]. One group reported that longer pulse widths (270-450 μs) improved results [45]. Additional trials of this target are ongoing.

Open label trials of DBS to the NA have shown moderate benefit. Anhedonia seemed to improve most [46, 47]. One group also targeted the caudate subsequently in cases that were unresponsive to NA placement, but reported no additional benefit [48].

Stimulation at the VC/VS markedly improved depression scales (40% remission rate) in one long term open label report [49]. However, a subsequent 30 subject, 4 month sham controlled trial did not significantly improve depression (response rates were 20% with DBS and 14% with sham). [Dougherty-presented 2012]. Similar to when used for OCD, stimulation at this site may cause anxiety.

One group reported that 6 of 7 depression subjects markedly improved after DBS into the medial forebrain bundle, specifically targeting the supero-lateral branch [50]. Response was rapid and maintained. Vision and eye movement abnormalities presented in all patients but responded to adjustments. The lateral habenular complex and inferior thalamic peduncle (for concurrent depression and OCD) have also been reported to benefit patients [51, 52].

To date, there is no positive controlled data supporting the use of DBS for depression, although some of the open label data is fairly impressive. The large placebo response seen in depression trials, and surgical trials, mandates that additional controlled trials be done.

DEMENTIA

Current pharmacologic treatments of dementia, especially Alzheimer's disease, are markedly inadequate. Thus, treatment of dementia and improvement of memory without overt dementia are two of the most discussed possibilities for DBS. Much animal data (usually rodents) has been generated and several human trials are ongoing, but very little human clinical data has yet been published. In animals, a number of sites within the Papez Circuit have improved some aspect of cognition, although direct stimulation into the hippocampus reduces memory formation [53]. Specifically, animal studies show increased learning with DBS into the anterior nucleus of the thalamus [53], the CA1 region (midline thalamus) [54], and the central thalamic nuclei (intralaminar) [53].

In humans, the only reported targets have been the fornix [53, 55], and the Nucleus Basalis of Meynert (NBM) [56, 57]. The entorhinal cortex [58], and pedunculopontine nucleus [59] have been reported to improve some features of cognition when implanted for other indications, usually epilepsy. The fornix is part of the Papez Circuit and connects the hippocampus and hypothalamus. Human clinical data from high frequency stimulation of the fornix is fairly modest. In an open label series, Laxton et al. implanted bilateral leads targeting 2 mm anterior to the fornix, parallel to the hypothalamus with the most ventral contact 2 mm above the dorsal surface of the optic tract, 5 mm from midline [55]. Overall, the 6 subjects showed only slowing in cognitive decline compared to historic controls. Only 1 of 6 subjects had actual improvement on the Alzheimer's Disease Assessment Scale-Cognitive

Subscale (ADAS-Cog) at 12 months. Functional imaging showed more impressive increased temporoparietal cortical glucose utilization [55, 60]. Increased glucose utilization was also seen in primary motor and sensory cortex and cerebellum, but was decreased in some frontal areas. Side effects specific to this site included déjà vu feelings and an unpleasant warmness.

The NBM, which sends cholinergic fibers diffusely through the brain, degenerates in Alzheimer's disease and other dementias. A number of animal studies report improved cognition from NBM DBS [53]. A human trial is ongoing, but currently only a couple of case reports exist. A single published case of PD dementia showed marked cognitive improvement with low frequency (20-25 Hz) bilateral stimulation of the NBM. The patient was also implanted into the STN [56]. At this point, DBS for dementia must be considered highly investigational.

Seizures

DBS for refractory epilepsy has been used since the 1970s and more than 10 different anatomic sites are beneficial in case reports or open label series [61, 62] .The more commonly reported areas include the anterior thalamic nucleus (ATN), the caudate nucleus, the subthalamic nucleus (STN), the cerebellum (multiple sites but usually midline cortex), the centromedian nucleus of the thalamus (CMT), and the hippocampus [63, 64]. Other areas have been less frequently chosen. A recent Cochrane analysis reported good evidence of benefit for the anterior thalamic nuclei and moderate evidence supporting the hippocampus, but inconclusive evidence for all other sites [65]. Device settings depend on the location but unlike most other indications, stimulation may be pulsatile (on for minutes, then off for minutes) rather than continuous.

Numerous open label trials support DBS of the ATN, which is a complex relay station and part of the Papez circuit [61]. The SANTE study was a 109 subject randomized bilateral ATN DBS placement trial that remains one of the largest DBS trials for any indication [66]. During the three month controlled portion, subjects were randomized 1:1 to activation at 5 V, 145Hz, 90μsec,on for 1 minute and off for 5 minutes; or to not being activated. Additional settings were allowed in the open label portion. The results were mixed. After excluding one outlier, the total seizure frequency was significantly reduced (p=0.04). This was powered mostly by relatively more robust efficacy in the final month. A temporal lobe seizure origin predicted a better response compared to a frontal/parietal origin, which was similar to sham. Quality of life and seizure impact scales did not improve over placebo. Patients in the active group reported more depression and memory loss as adverse events, although assessed cognition and moods scales were not significantly different. Open label, long term efficacy was good, with the sham randomized group quickly equaling improvement with the original stimulation group [67].

A single group has reported excellent short and long term results with both high and low frequency stimulation of the CMT in generalized seizures, including Lennox-Gastaut syndrome [68]. Partial complex seizure response was less robust. A small seven subject cross-over trial (65 Hz frequency) of CMT DBS failed to demonstrate efficacy, although there was a modest trend [61].

Many small open label series report robust improvement with various locations in and adjacent to the hippocampus, most commonly the posterior portion [61, 69, 70]. Both unilateral and bilateral implantations are done depending on the postulated seizure locus. Some, but not all, report greater benefit if the MRI is normal. One trial that activated the second side if unilateral DBS was not satisfactory did not show further benefit [69]. One partially controlled 4 subject cross-over trial found a non-significant 15% reduction in seizure frequency compared to sham [71]. Another 2 subject cross-over trial found a 33% reduction when activated but no change in quality of life [72]. No large scale controlled trial has been attempted around the hippocampus.

Several other sites have also been implanted for seizures. The cerebellar cortex inhibits deep cerebellar nuclei, which send generally inhibitory connections diffusely through the brain. Cooper first implanted the cerebellar cortex, and several open label, mostly older, reports show benefit [61]. Several older large series report benefit of low frequency caudate stimulation [73]. No controlled trials were attempted nor has any literature on this site been published in the last 10 years. Multiple small series also advocate the STN, at continuous typical high frequency settings. Again no controlled trial has been attempted. Other implanted locations include the locus coeruleus, mammillary bodies, and corpus callosum [61].

Response neurostimulation or closed loop stimulation consists of multiple cortical electrodes placed over an electroencephalogram (EEG) identified seizure locus, which are programmed to fire after detecting a seizure. Therefore this is not "deep" brain stimulation. Nevertheless a controlled trial reported significant reduction compared to an inactive device (38% vs 17% reduction) [74]. Long term open label efficacy was maintained and adverse events were minimal.

Given the pathophysiology of seizures, DBS is an enticing treatment option. Currently only placement the ATN is supported by a large, well designed trial, but this has not yet been approved by European or US regulatory agencies.

TARDIVE DYSKINESIA

Tardive dyskinesia is an involuntary movement caused by exposure to dopamine blocking agents, most commonly psychiatric and anti-nausea mediations. Most commonly these are stereotypic (repetitive, patterned but not rhythmic enough to be tremor) movements effecting the lower face and feet. Other phenotypes include whole body extension dystonia (commonly seen in younger males), and midline pain. The movement does not resolve upon discontinuation of the offending agent, and often transiently worsens. It may persist or very gradually diminish over years. Risk factors for TD include older age, female sex, and duration of treatment. Although current psychiatric medications tend to have less dopamine antagonism, use of these drugs has increased so that the incidence of TD has remained stable, despite better recognition. Tetrabenazine effectively treats TD but has numerous potential side effects.

Tardive dystonia cases, which tend to be more severe than stereotype cases are most commonly operated upon. DBS targeting the GPi markedly improves TD, usually 75-85%, in a number of open label studies [75, 76], and by 61% in one 10 patient controlled trial [77]. This is arguably the most robust response of any dystonia cause [78]. Improvement is rapid, probably faster than idiopathic dystonia, and persists for as long as the stimulation continues [79-81]. Overall GPi DBS can be considered for refractory tardive dystonia. Fewer cases of tardive stereotype are reported.

Restless Legs Syndrome

Restless legs syndrome is a common sensory motor disorder manifest by the urge to move the legs with or without any additional sensation, transient improvement of symptoms with movement, worsening of symptoms with immobility, and onset or worsening of symptoms in the evening. It affects about 10% of Caucasians and justifies treatment in 2-3% of the population. There is a strong genetic component but the pathophysiology is not clear. Dopaminergic systems are mostly implicated by the robust response to dopamine agonists. Pathology shows reduced iron throughout the CNS but no neurodegeneration and no pathological association with Parkinson's disease.

DBS and lesioning of the GPi have been reported to improve RLS symptoms in patients when used to treat Parkinson's disease (PD) and dystonia [82, 83]. DBS of the sub-thalamic nucleus (STN) has been reported to both improve and worsen RLS in PD patients [84-86], and DBS of the ventralis intermedius nucleus (VIM) did not improve concurrent RLS in patients when used to treat essential tremor [87]. Many of the VIM implanted subjects did have idiopathic RLS as defined by a young age of onset and positive family history of RLS.

A single case of bilateral GPi DBS reported improvement in idiopathic RLS symptoms in a severely refractory subject who failed multiple therapeutic agents [88]. Anecdotally, response to GPi DBS for idiopathic RLS is mixed.

Other Miscellaneous Uses

Based on animal data and a few case reports, DBS has been proposed for several other neuropsychiatric conditions. Several anatomic sites are proposed for the treatment of addiction, although there is no published human efficacy data [89]. Based on animal results, DBS into the basolateral amygdala is currently being evaluated for post-traumatic stress disorder [90]. Bilateral DBS (N=2) and ablation (N=6) of the NA have been reported to improved anorexia nervosa [91]. Mood, anxiety, and cognitive benefits were also reported at one year in this small, open label series.

Conclusion

In general, DBS for psychiatric and epilepsy is not nearly as established as DBS used for movement disorders. In most cases multiple placement targets exist, some based on theoretic/rational targets, others on empiric or serendipitous experience. Only a few large well controlled trials exist, which is very problematic given the large placebo response in surgical trials. However, dramatic results are sometimes reported and additional targets and indications for DBS will no doubt continue to propagate.

REFERENCES

[1] Schrock, L; Mink, J; Woods, D; Porta, M; Servello, D; Visser-Vandewalle, V; et al. Tourette Syndrome Deep Brain Stimulation: A Review and Updated Recommendations. *Movement Disorders*, 2015,(in press).

[2] Rotsides, J; Mammis, A. The use of deep brain stimulation in Tourette's syndrome. *Neurosurg Focus*, 2013, 35, E4.

[3] Nangunoori, R; Tomycz, ND; Quigley, M; Oh, MY; Whiting, DM. Deep brain stimulation for psychiatric diseases: a pooled analysis of published studies employing disease-specific standardized outcome scales. *Stereotact Funct Neurosurg*, 2013, 91, 345-54.

[4] Savica, R; Stead, M; Mack, KJ; Lee, KH; Klassen, BT. Deep brain stimulation in tourette syndrome: a description of 3 patients with excellent outcome. *Mayo Clinic proceedings*, 2012, 87, 59-62.

[5] Servello, D; Sassi, M; Brambilla, A; Defendi, S; Porta, M. Long-term, post-deep brain stimulation management of a series of 36 patients affected with refractory gilles de la tourette syndrome. *Neuromodulation: journal of the International Neuromodulation Society*, 2010, 13, 187-94.

[6] Porta, M; Brambilla, A; Cavanna, AE; Servello, D; Sassi, M; Rickards, H; et al. Thalamic deep brain stimulation for treatment-refractory Tourette syndrome: two-year outcome. *Neurology*, 2009, 73, 1375-80.

[7] Maciunas, RJ; Maddux, BN; Riley, DE; Whitney, CM; Schoenberg, MR; Ogrocki, PJ; et al. Prospective randomized double-blind trial of bilateral thalamic deep brain stimulation in adults with Tourette syndrome. *J Neurosurg*, 2007, 107, 1004-14.

[8] Ackermans, L; Duits, A; van der Linden, C; Tijssen, M; Schruers, K; Temel, Y; et al. Double-blind clinical trial of thalamic stimulation in patients with Tourette syndrome. *Brain*, 2011, 134, 832-44.

[9] Cannon, E; Silburn, P; Coyne, T; O'Maley, K; Crawford, JD; Sachdev, PS. Deep brain stimulation of anteromedial globus pallidus interna for severe Tourette's syndrome. *Am J Psychiatry*, 2012, 169, 860-6.

[10] Dehning, S; Leitner, B; Schennach, R; Muller, N; Botzel, K; Obermeier, M; et al. Functional outcome and quality of life in Tourette's syndrome after deep brain stimulation of the posteroventrolateral globus pallidus internus: long-term follow-up. *The world journal of biological psychiatry : the official journal of the World Federation of Societies of Biological Psychiatry*, 2014, 15, 66-75.

[11] Shahed, J; Poysky, J; Kenney, C; Simpson, R; Jankovic, J. GPi deep brain stimulation for Tourette syndrome improves tics and psychiatric comorbidities. *Neurology*, 2007, 68, 159-60.

[12] Martinez-Fernandez, R; Zrinzo, L; Aviles-Olmos, I; Hariz, M; Martinez-Torres, I; Joyce, E; et al. Deep brain stimulation for Gilles de la Tourette syndrome: a case series targeting subregions of the globus pallidus internus. *Mov Disord*, 2011, 26, 1922-30.

[13] Sachdev, PS; Mohan, A; Cannon, E; Crawford, JD; Silberstein, P; Cook, R; et al. Deep brain stimulation of the antero-medial globus pallidus interna for Tourette syndrome. *PloS one*, 2014, 9, e104926.

[14] Burdick, A; Foote, KD; Goodman, W; Ward, HE; Ricciuti, N; Murphy, T; et al. Lack of benefit of accumbens/capsular deep brain stimulation in a patient with both tics and obsessive-compulsive disorder. *Neurocase*, 2010, 16, 321-30.

[15] Flaherty, AW; Williams, ZM; Amirnovin, R; Kasper, E; Rauch, SL; Cosgrove, GR; et al. Deep brain stimulation of the anterior internal capsule for the treatment of Tourette syndrome: technical case report. *Neurosurgery*, 2005, 57, E403, discussion E.

[16] Neuner, I; Halfter, S; Wollenweber, F; Podoll, K; Schneider, F. Nucleus accumbens deep brain stimulation did not prevent suicide attempt in tourette syndrome. *Biol Psychiatry*, 2010, 68, e19-20.

[17] Piedimonte, F; Andreani, JC; Piedimonte, L; Graff, P; Bacaro, V; Micheli, F; et al. Behavioral and motor improvement after deep brain stimulation of the globus pallidus externus in a case of Tourette's syndrome. *Neuromodulation: journal of the International Neuromodulation Society*, 2013, 16, 55-8, discussion 8.

[18] Martinez-Torres, I; Hariz, MI; Zrinzo, L; Foltynie, T; Limousin, P. Improvement of tics after subthalamic nucleus deep brain stimulation. *Neurology*, 2009, 72, 1787-9.

[19] Houeto, JL; Karachi, C; Mallet, L; Pillon, B; Yelnik, J; Mesnage, V; et al. Tourette's syndrome and deep brain stimulation. *J Neurol Neurosurg Psychiatry*, 2005, 76, 992-5.

[20] Welter, ML; Mallet, L; Houeto, JL; Karachi, C; Czernecki; Cornu. P; et al. Internal pallidal and thalamic stimulation in patients with Tourette syndrome. *Arch Neurol*, 2008, 65, 952-7.

[21] Schoenberg, MR; Maddux, BN; Riley, DE; Whitney, CM; Ogrocki, PK; Gould, D; et al. Five-Months-Postoperative Neuropsychological Outcome From a Pilot Prospective Randomized Clinical Trial of Thalamic Deep Brain Stimulation for Tourette Syndrome. *Neuromodulation: journal of the International Neuromodulation Society*, 2014.

[22] Bergfeld, IO; Mantione, M; Hoogendoorn, ML; Denys, D. Cognitive functioning in psychiatric disorders following deep brain stimulation. *Brain Stimul*, 2013, 6, 532-7.

[23] Servello, D; Sassi, M; Gaeta, M; Ricci, C; Porta, M. Tourette syndrome (TS) bears a higher rate of inflammatory complications at the implanted hardware in deep brain stimulation (DBS). *Acta Neurochir (Wien)*, 2011, 153, 629-32.

[24] Kisely, S; Hall, K; Siskind, D; Frater, J; Olson, S; Crompton, D. Deep brain stimulation for obsessive-compulsive disorder: a systematic review and meta-analysis. *Psychological medicine*, 2014, 44, 3533-42.

[25] Kohl, S; Schonherr, DM; Luigjes, J; Denys, D; Mueller, UJ; Lenartz, D; et al. Deep brain stimulation for treatment-refractory obsessive compulsive disorder: a systematic review. *BMC psychiatry*, 2014, 14, 214.

[26] Abelson, JL; Curtis, GC; Sagher, O; Albucher, RC; Harrigan, M; Taylor, SF, et al. Deep brain stimulation for refractory obsessive-compulsive disorder. *Biol Psychiatry*, 2005, 57, 510-6.

[27] Goodman, WK; Foote, KD; Greenberg, BD; Ricciuti, N; Bauer, R; Ward, H; et al. Deep brain stimulation for intractable obsessive compulsive disorder: pilot study using a blinded, staggered-onset design. *Biol Psychiatry*, 2010, 67, 535-42.

[28] Nuttin, BJ; Gabriels, LA; Cosyns, PR; Meyerson, BA; Andreewitch, S; Sunaert, SG; et al. Long-term electrical capsular stimulation in patients with obsessive-compulsive disorder. *Neurosurgery*, 2003, 52, 1263-72, discussion 72-4.

[29] Denys, D; Mantione, M; Figee, M; van den Munckhof, P; Koerselman, F; Westenberg, H; et al. Deep brain stimulation of the nucleus accumbens for treatment-refractory obsessive-compulsive disorder. *Arch Gen Psychiatry*, 2010, 67, 1061-8.

[30] Mallet, L; Polosan, M; Jaafari, N; Baup, N; Welter, ML; Fontaine, D; et al. Subthalamic nucleus stimulation in severe obsessive-compulsive disorder. *N Engl J Med*, 2008, 359, 2121-34.

[31] Tierney, TS; Abd-El-Barr, MM; Stanford, AD; Foote, KD; Okun, MS. Deep brain stimulation and ablation for obsessive compulsive disorder: evolution of contemporary indications, targets and techniques. *Int J Neurosci*, 2014, 124, 394-402.

[32] Jimenez, F; Nicolini, H; Lozano, AM; Piedimonte, F; Salin, R; Velasco, F. Electrical stimulation of the inferior thalamic peduncle in the treatment of major depression and obsessive compulsive disorders. *World Neurosurg*, 2013, 80, S30 e17-25.

[33] Suetens, K; Nuttin, B; Gabriels, L; Van Laere, K. Differences in Metabolic Network Modulation Between Capsulotomy and Deep-Brain Stimulation for Refractory Obsessive-Compulsive Disorder. *Journal of nuclear medicine : official publication, Society of Nuclear Medicine*, 2014, 55, 951-9.

[34] Schlaepfer, TE; Bewernick, BH; Kayser, S; Hurlemann, R; Coenen, VA. Deep brain stimulation of the human reward system for major depression--rationale, outcomes and outlook. *Neuropsychopharmacology*, 2014, 39, 1303-14.

[35] Riva-Posse, P; Choi, KS; Holtzheimer, PE; McIntyre, CC; Gross, RE; Chaturvedi, A; et al. Defining Critical White Matter Pathways Mediating Successful Subcallosal Cingulate Deep Brain Stimulation for Treatment-Resistant Depression. *Biol Psychiatry*, 2014.

[36] Morishita, T; Fayad, SM; Higuchi, MA; Nestor, KA; Foote, KD. Deep brain stimulation for treatment-resistant depression: systematic review of clinical outcomes. *Neurotherapeutics*, 2014, 11, 475-84.

[37] Mayberg, HS; Lozano, AM; Voon, V; McNeely, HE; Seminowicz, D; Hamani, C; et al. Deep brain stimulation for treatment-resistant depression. *Neuron*, 2005, 45, 651-60.

[38] Seminowicz, DA; Mayberg, HS; McIntosh, AR; Goldapple, K; Kennedy, S; Segal, Z; et al. Limbic-frontal circuitry in major depression: a path modeling metanalysis. *Neuroimage*, 2004, 22, 409-18.

[39] Berlim, MT; McGirr, A; Van den Eynde, F; Fleck, MP; Giacobbe, P. Effectiveness and acceptability of deep brain stimulation (DBS) of the subgenual cingulate cortex for treatment-resistant depression: a systematic review and exploratory meta-analysis. *Journal of affective disorders*, 2014, 159, 31-8.

[40] Bogod, NM; Sinden, M; Woo, C; Defreitas, VG; Torres, IJ; Howard, AK; et al. Long-term neuropsychological safety of subgenual cingulate gyrus deep brain stimulation for treatment-resistant depression. *The Journal of neuropsychiatry and clinical neurosciences*, 2014, 26, 126-33.

[41] Delaloye, S; Holtzheimer, PE. Deep brain stimulation in the treatment of depression. *Dialogues in clinical neuroscience*, 2014, 16, 83-91.

[42] Lozano, AM; Giacobbe, P; Hamani, C; Rizvi, SJ; Kennedy, SH; Kolivakis, TT; et al. A multicenter pilot study of subcallosal cingulate area deep brain stimulation for treatment-resistant depression. *J Neurosurg*, 2012, 116, 315-22.

[43] Puigdemont, D; Portella, M; Perez-Egea, R; Molet, J; Gironell, A; de Diego-Adelino, J; et al. A randomized double-blind crossover trial of deep brain stimulation of the

subcallosal cingulate gyrus in patients with treatment-resistant depression: a pilot study of relapse prevention. *Journal of psychiatry & neuroscience : JPN*, 2015, 40, 130295.

[44] Moreines, JL; McClintock, SM; Kelley, ME; Holtzheimer, PE; Mayberg, HS. Neuropsychological function before and after subcallosal cingulate deep brain stimulation in patients with treatment-resistant depression. *Depression and anxiety*, 2014, 31, 690-8.

[45] Ramasubbu, R; Anderson, S; Haffenden, A; Chavda, S; Kiss, ZH. Double-blind optimization of subcallosal cingulate deep brain stimulation for treatment-resistant depression: a pilot study. *Journal of psychiatry & neuroscience* : *JPN*, 2013, 38, 325-32.

[46] Bewernick, BH; Kayser, S; Sturm, V; Schlaepfer, TE. Long-term effects of nucleus accumbens deep brain stimulation in treatment-resistant depression: evidence for sustained efficacy. *Neuropsychopharmacology*, 2012, 37, 1975-85.

[47] Schlaepfer, TE; Cohen, MX; Frick, C; Kosel, M; Brodesser, D; Axmacher, N; et al. Deep brain stimulation to reward circuitry alleviates anhedonia in refractory major depression. *Neuropsychopharmacology*, 2008, 33, 368-77.

[48] Millet, B; Jaafari, N; Polosan, M; Baup, N; Giordana, B; Haegelen, C; et al. Limbic versus cognitive target for deep brain stimulation in treatment-resistant depression: accumbens more promising than caudate. *Eur Neuropsychopharmacol*, 2014, 24, 1229-39.

[49] Malone DA; Jr. Dougherty, DD; Rezai, AR; Carpenter, LL; Friehs, GM; Eskandar, EN; et al. Deep brain stimulation of the ventral capsule/ventral striatum for treatment-resistant depression. *Biol Psychiatry*, 2009, 65, 267-75.

[50] Schlaepfer, TE; Bewernick, BH; Kayser, S; Madler, B; Coenen, VA. Rapid effects of deep brain stimulation for treatment-resistant major depression. *Biol Psychiatry*, 2013, 73, 1204-12.

[51] Jimenez, F; Velasco, F; Salin-Pascual, R; Velasco, M; Nicolini, H; Velasco, AL; et al. Neuromodulation of the inferior thalamic peduncle for major depression and obsessive compulsive disorder. *Acta neurochirurgica Supplement*, 2007, 97, 393-8.

[52] Sartorius, A; Kiening, KL; Kirsch, P; von Gall, CC; Haberkorn, U; Unterberg, AW; et al. Remission of major depression under deep brain stimulation of the lateral habenula in a therapy-refractory patient. *Biol Psychiatry*, 2010, 67, e9-e11.

[53] Hardenacke, K; Shubina, E; Buhrle, CP; Zapf, A; Lenartz, D; Klosterkotter, J; et al. Deep brain stimulation as a tool for improving cognitive functioning in Alzheimer's dementia: a systematic review. *Frontiers in psychiatry*, 2013, 4, 159.

[54] Arrieta-Cruz, I; Pavlides, C; Pasinetti, GM. Deep Brain Stimulation in Midline Thalamic Region Facilitates Synaptic Transmission and Shortterm Memory in a Mouse Model of Alzheimer's Disease. *Translational neuroscience*, 2010, 1, 188-94.

[55] Laxton, AW; Tang-Wai, DF; McAndrews, MP; Zumsteg, D; Wennberg, R; Keren, R; et al. A phase I trial of deep brain stimulation of memory circuits in Alzheimer's disease. *Ann Neurol*, 2010, 68, 521-34.

[56] Hardenacke, K; Kuhn, J; Lenartz, D; Maarouf, M; Mai, JK; Bartsch, C; et al. Stimulate or degenerate: deep brain stimulation of the nucleus basalis Meynert in Alzheimer dementia. *World Neurosurg*, 2013, 80, S27 e35-43.

[57] Barnikol, TT; Pawelczyk, NB; Barnikol, UB; Kuhn, J; Lenartz, D; Sturm, V; et al. Changes in apraxia after deep brain stimulation of the nucleus basalis Meynert in a patient with Parkinson dementia syndrome. *Mov Disord*, 2010, 25, 1519-20.
[58] Suthana, N; Fried, I. Deep brain stimulation for enhancement of learning and memory. *Neuroimage*, 2014, 85 Pt 3, 996-1002.
[59] Stefani, A; Pierantozzi, M; Ceravolo, R; Brusa, L; Galati, S; Stanzione, P. Deep brain stimulation of pedunculopontine tegmental nucleus (PPTg) promotes cognitive and metabolic changes: a target-specific effect or response to a low-frequency pattern of stimulation? *Clin EEG Neurosci*, 2010, 41, 82-6.
[60] Smith, GS; Laxton, AW; Tang-Wai, DF; McAndrews, MP; Diaconescu, AO; Workman, CI; et al. Increased cerebral metabolism after 1 year of deep brain stimulation in Alzheimer disease. *Arch Neurol*, 2012, 69, 1141-8.
[61] Fisher, RS. Deep brain stimulation for epilepsy. *Handbook of clinical neurology*, 2013, 116, 217-34.
[62] Rahman, M; Abd-El-Barr, MM; Vedam-Mai, V; Foote, KD ; Murad, GJ; Okun, MS; et al. Disrupting abnormal electrical activity with deep brain stimulation: is epilepsy the next frontier? *Neurosurg Focus*, 2010, 29, E7.
[63] Lega, BC; Halpern, CH; Jaggi, JL; Baltuch, GH. Deep brain stimulation in the treatment of refractory epilepsy: update on current data and future directions. *Neurobiol Dis*, 2010, 38, 354-60.
[64] Laxpati, NG; Kasoff, WS; Gross, RE. Deep brain stimulation for the treatment of epilepsy: circuits, targets, and trials. *Neurotherapeutics*, 2014, 11, 508-26.
[65] Sprengers, M; Vonck, K; Carrette, E; Marson, AG; Boon, P. Deep brain and cortical stimulation for epilepsy. *The Cochrane database of systematic reviews*, 2014, 6, CD008497.
[66] Fisher, R; Salanova, V; Witt, T; Worth, R; Henry, T; Gross, R; et al. Electrical stimulation of the anterior nucleus of thalamus for treatment of refractory epilepsy. *Epilepsia*, 2010, 51, 899-908.
[67] Salanova, V; Witt, T; Worth, R; Henry, TR; Gross, RE; Nazzaro, JM; et al. Long-term efficacy and safety of thalamic stimulation for drug-resistant partial epilepsy. *Neurology*, 2015.
[68] Velasco, AL; Velasco, F; Jimenez, F; Velasco, M; Castro, G; Carrillo-Ruiz, JD; et al. Neuromodulation of the centromedian thalamic nuclei in the treatment of generalized seizures and the improvement of the quality of life in patients with Lennox-Gastaut syndrome. *Epilepsia*, 2006, 47, 1203-12.
[69] Cukiert, A; Cukiert, CM; Burattini, JA; Lima, AM. Seizure outcome after hippocampal deep brain stimulation in a prospective cohort of patients with refractory temporal lobe epilepsy. *Seizure*, 2014, 23, 6-9.
[70] Vonck, K; Sprengers, M; Carrette, E; Dauwe, I; Miatton, M; Meurs, A; et al. A decade of experience with deep brain stimulation for patients with refractory medial temporal lobe epilepsy. *International journal of neural systems*, 2013, 23, 1250034.
[71] Tellez-Zenteno, JF; McLachlan, RS; Parrent, A; Kubu, CS; Wiebe, S. Hippocampal electrical stimulation in mesial temporal lobe epilepsy. *Neurology*, 2006, 66, 1490-4.
[72] McLachlan, RS; Pigott, S; Tellez-Zenteno, JF; Wiebe, S; Parrent, A. Bilateral hippocampal stimulation for intractable temporal lobe epilepsy: impact on seizures and memory. *Epilepsia*, 2010, 51, 304-7.

[73] Chkhenkeli, SA; Sramka, M; Lortkipanidze, GS; Rakviashvili, TN; Bregvadze, E; Magalashvili, GE; et al. Electrophysiological effects and clinical results of direct brain stimulation for intractable epilepsy. *Clin Neurol Neurosurg*, 2004, 106, 318-29.

[74] Morrell, MJ. Responsive cortical stimulation for the treatment of medically intractable partial epilepsy. *Neurology*, 2011, 77, 1295-304.

[75] Shaikh, AG; Mewes, K; DeLong, MR; Gross, RE; Triche, SD; Jinnah, HA; et al. Temporal profile of improvement of tardive dystonia after globus pallidus deep brain stimulation. *Parkinsonism Relat Disord*, 2015, 21, 116-9.

[76] Mentzel, CL; Tenback, DE; Tijssen, MA; Visser-Vandewalle, VE; van Harten, PN. Efficacy and safety of deep brain stimulation in patients with medication-induced tardive dyskinesia and/or dystonia: a systematic review. *The Journal of clinical psychiatry*, 2012, 73, 1434-8.

[77] Damier, P; Thobois, S; Witjas, T; Cuny, E; Derost, P; Raoul, S; et al. Bilateral deep brain stimulation of the globus pallidus to treat tardive dyskinesia. *Arch Gen Psychiatry*, 2007, 64, 170-6.

[78] Andrews, C; Aviles-Olmos, I; Hariz, M; Foltynie, T. Which patients with dystonia benefit from deep brain stimulation? A metaregression of individual patient outcomes. *J Neurol Neurosurg Psychiatry*, 2010, 81, 1383-9.

[79] Boulogne, S; Danaila, T; Polo, G; Broussolle, E; Thobois, S. Relapse of tardive dystonia after globus pallidus deep-brain stimulation discontinuation. *J Neurol*, 2014, 261, 1636-7.

[80] Chang, EF; Schrock, LE; Starr, PA; Ostrem, JL. Long-term benefit sustained after bilateral pallidal deep brain stimulation in patients with refractory tardive dystonia. *Stereotact Funct Neurosurg*, 2010, 88, 304-10.

[81] Gruber, D; Trottenberg, T; Kivi, A; Schoenecker, T; Kopp, UA; Hoffmann, KT; et al. Long-term effects of pallidal deep brain stimulation in tardive dystonia. *Neurology*, 2009, 73, 53-8.

[82] Okun, MS; Fernandez, HH; Foote, KD. Deep brain stimulation of the GPi treats restless legs syndrome associated with dystonia. *Mov Disord*, 2005, 20, 500-1.

[83] Rye, DB; DeLong, MR. Amelioration of sensory limb discomfort of restless legs syndrome by pallidotomy. *Ann Neurol*, 1999, 46, 800-1.

[84] Chahine, LM; Ahmed, A; Sun, Z. Effects of STN DBS for Parkinson's disease on restless legs syndrome and other sleep-related measures. *Parkinsonism & Related Disorders*, 2011,17, 208-11.

[85] Driver-Dunckley, E; Evidente, VG; Adler, CH; Hillman, R; Hernandez, J; Fletcher, G; et al. Restless legs syndrome in Parkinson's disease patients may improve with subthalamic stimulation. *Mov Disord*, 2006, 21, 1287-9.

[86] Kedia, S; Moro, E; Tagliati, M; Lang, AE; Kumar, R. Emergence of restless legs syndrome during subthalamic stimulation for Parkinson disease. *Neurology*, 2004, 63, 2410-2.

[87] Ondo, W. VIM deep brain stimulation does not improve pre-existing restless legs syndrome in patients with essential tremor. *Parkinsonism Relat Disord*, 2006, 12, 113-4.

[88] Ondo, WG; Jankovic, J; Simpson, R; Jimenez-Shahed, J. Globus pallidus deep brain stimulation for refractory idiopathic restless legs syndrome. *Sleep medicine*, 2012, 13, 1202-4.

[89] Luigjes, J; van den Brink, W; Feenstra, M; van den Munckhof, P; Schuurman, PR; Schippers, R; et al. Deep brain stimulation in addiction: a review of potential brain targets. *Mol Psychiatry*, 2012, 17, 572-83.

[90] Koek, RJ; Langevin, JP; Krahl, SE; Kosoyan, HJ; Schwartz, HN; Chen, JW; et al. Deep brain stimulation of the basolateral amygdala for treatment-refractory combat post-traumatic stress disorder (PTSD): study protocol for a pilot randomized controlled trial with blinded, staggered onset of stimulation. *Trials*, 2014, 15, 356.

[91] Wang, J; Chang, C; Geng, N; Wang, X; Gao, G. Treatment of intractable anorexia nervosa with inactivation of the nucleus accumbens using stereotactic surgery. *Stereotact Funct Neurosurg*, 2013, 91, 364-72.

In: Deep Brain Stimulation
Editor: Raja Mehanna

ISBN: 978-1-63483-282-3

Chapter 10

TROUBLESHOOTING IN DBS

Aparna Wagle Shukla, MD[1], Alberto Riccardo Bona, MD[1] and Roger Walz, MD[1,2]
[1]University of Florida, Gainesville, Florida, US
[2]University of Santa Catarina, Brazil

ABSTRACT

Previous chapters detailed the physiology of basal ganglia and deep brain stimulation, as well as the available evidence and programming algorithms in Parkinson's disease, essential tremor and dystonia. A successful DBS outcome is dependent on many interrelated factors such as appropriate selection of candidates, disease characteristics, accurate lead placement, expertise in DBS programming and knowledge and experience to manage DBS related complications. DBS related complications are broadly categorized into those related to the surgical procedure, those stemming from the DBS device and those seen in relation to stimulation itself. With an increasing experience in DBS, most complications in each of these categories can be managed with reasonable satisfaction if a systematic approach is followed.

INTRODUCTION

Deep brain stimulation (DBS) therapy is an established, widely applied, FDA approved treatment for essential tremor, Parkinson's disease, dystonia and obsessive compulsive disorder. Recently, there has been increasing numbers of successful reports of DBS in Tourette's syndrome, but this is not yet an FDA approved indication. DBS in these movement disorders has been found to reduce motor disability and improve quality of life [1-5]. There is emerging new research to show DBS applications in major depressive disorders, obsessive-compulsive disorders [6], Alzheimer´s disease [7], aggressiveness [8], addiction [9, 10], obesity [11], anorexia nervosa [12] and epilepsy [13], but these are not approved FDA approved indications. A successful DBS outcome in these conditions is dependent on many interrelated factors such as appropriate selection of candidates, disease characteristics, accurate lead placement, expertise in DBS programming and knowledge and experience to manage DBS related complications. In the initial part of this chapter, we will review general facts related to DBS programming in essential tremor, Parkinson's disease, dystonia, obsessive compulsive disorder and Tourette's syndrome. DBS programming for essential tremor, Parkinson's disease and dystonia has already been covered in previous chapters. However, different centers have different plans and algorithms and we here present our way of programming at the University of Florida in Gainesville, to offer our readers a variety of approaches to DBS programming throughout this book. It has to be noted that no single approach presented in this book has been proven better than the others, and our readers will be able to choose the one that suits them the most. Subsequently, we will discuss complications observed around the time of surgery and the complications related to the device itself (the lead, the lead connector and the neurostimulator). Finally we will discuss complications arising from stimulation of the anatomical target used in each of these conditions with disease specific comments if applicable.

Introduction to Programming

Introduction to Programming in Essential Tremor

Pharmacological treatment is the first line therapy for essential tremor. Propranolol, primidone, alprazolam, atenolol, gabapentin and topiramate have shown an established efficacy in reducing both limb and head tremors [14]. About 50% of essential tremor patients do not respond to pharmacologic treatments and these patients are offered DBS of the ventralis intermedius nucleus (VIM, Figure 1) of the thalamus [15]. DBS is mostly focused towards control of arm tremor since this is the most common disabling symptom in essential tremor patients. Studies indicate that there is significant improvement of the contralateral limb tremor on clinical exam, during writing tests, pouring tests, and activities of daily living questionnaires [14, 15]. Several long-term studies (7 years follow-up) have demonstrated improvement of arm tremors in the range of 50% to 90%. There are also improvements seen in head and voice tremor but these are more pronounced with bilateral VIM stimulation [15]. In our retrospective analysis of essential tremor patients, we found that a more vertical AC-PC angle of the DBS lead trajectory was associated with greater suppression of head tremor [16].

An important concern related to VIM DBS in essential tremor is the possible loss of surgical efficacy over time. In a small case series, brain atrophy and disease progression were suspected to contribute towards emergence of unexpected stimulation induced side-effects and loss of efficacy with chronic DBS [17]. The worsening of tremor is related to tolerance (the brain's loss of responsiveness to the VIM DBS) [3, 18] according to some authors, or to disease progression according to others [19, 20]. In a retrospective analysis of data conducted at our center, we found that tolerance to DBS was probably over-reported in the literature. A work-up for tolerance versus disease progression should include: examining the trend in off stimulation scores, imaging guided lead locations, and checking for thresholds during programming sessions which may elicit clinical benefits and side effects [21].

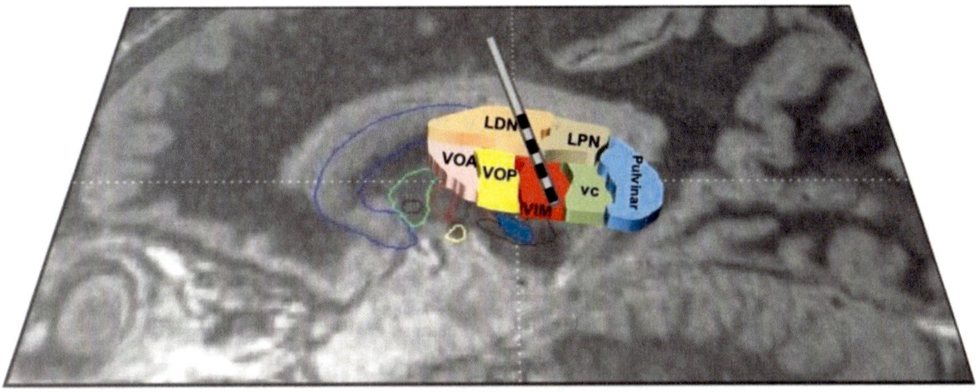

Figure 1. DBS implantation into VIM nucleus in thalamus. The optimal location for DBS lead is 2mm anterior to the border of ventralis caudalis nucleus.

Although the reported benefit in multiple sclerosis and post-traumatic related tremor are less dramatic than in essential tremor and these are not FDA approved indications, DBS is offered as a potential therapy and the programming approach in these cases are similar to that applied in essential tremor cases [15].

General Considerations for Programming

DBS programming in essential tremor is initiated about 3-4 weeks after the placement of electrode once the microlesion effects begin to fade. Microlesion effects are referred to initial benefits related to trauma of the DBS lead implantation in the targeted region and not those arising from therapeutic stimulation of the target. Prior to proceeding with DBS programming, the bedside programming professional should be aware of the lead type and the configuration to implement an appropriate treatment. We routinely obtain a postoperative imaging, usually a CT brain co-registered with a preoperative MRI scan. These scans are helpful in identifying lead configuration (which refers to the size of the contacts and the distance between them) and in confirming lead location. Once the lead placement is confirmed with imaging, lead type and lead configuration is determined, impedance at each of the contacts is recorded to verify the integrity of the electrical system and also to provide a baseline for future reference. The impedances that fall outside the designated normal range for that particular DBS device are interpreted either as a short circuit (excessively low impedance) or as an open circuit (excessively high impedance).

The clinical response to DBS depends on several factors such as disease characteristics, DBS lead position, stimulation parameters, and individual patient profile. In general, electrical stimulation is likely to activate large myelinated fibers before activation of small axons or cell bodies, axons that are near the cathode before those near the anode, and axons oriented parallel to the electrode before those oriented transversely [22, 23]. Each electrode is tested in a monopolar configuration (electrode contact is negative and neurostimulator case is positive) using pulse width, frequency and voltage considered standard for programming in essential tremor. Each electrode is tested with a pulse width of 60 to 90 μs, a frequency of 130 to 160 Hz, and the voltage is gradually increased in increments of 0.5 V until adverse effects are elicited (objective or subjective). The stimulation parameters used across multiple studies with follow-up as long as six years have shown a stimulation voltage in the range of 2.4 to 4.4 V, frequency in the range of 143 to 173 Hz and pulse width in the range of 67 to 138 μs [15]. Once the threshold for side effects is noted, each electrode contact is tested in a monopolar setting for efficacy where the programmer employs voltage 0.5-1.0V below these side-effects thresholds. Once the monopolar setting that shows complete suppression of tremor is identified, the voltage is gradually reduced to the lowest level necessary to maintain clinical benefits. If DBS lead is well-positioned, the clinical benefits are seen with voltages well below the thresholds that induce side effects [24]. The electrode contact with lowest threshold for inducing clinical benefits of greatest magnitude and the largest therapeutic width is finally selected for chronic stimulation. If single monopolar stimulation is not adequate for suppression of tremors, double monopolar stimulation of electrodes is employed. In these cases, negative polarity is assigned to the two contacts selected for stimulation and the neurostimulator case is assigned positive polarity. If stimulation-induced side effects are elicited at lower voltages, bipolar configuration is considered even though monopolar stimulation usually requires a lower stimulation intensity to achieve the same clinical benefit. In these cases, the most effective contact selected in the previous monopolar evaluation is assigned negative polarity and the adjacent contact is assigned positive polarity. If tremor continues to remain uncontrolled, a reversal of polarity or alternate bipolar configurations is explored.

During initial DBS programing, patients are seen every month for the first six months and then they are followed on an annual basis for clinical performance and troubleshooting. Although the need for continuation of tremor suppressing medications is not well studied, many patients after DBS surgery may continue oral medications in order to achieve effective tremor control. In our retrospective analysis of 69 essential tremor patients, we found there was a near complete elimination of tremor suppressing medications in patients with bilateral VIM DBS, while about 40% of unilateral VIM DBS continued their medications at 36 months follow-up [25]. In order to conserve battery life, some programmers suggests turning off DBS device while asleep during the night. Interestingly, some of our patients have reported a better stimulation response the following day after turning off the device the previous night. This observation will require further investigation. If tremor are not controlled due to stimulation-related side-effects and alternate stimulation parameters are not able to provide relief, repositioning of DBS lead is reconsidered [26, 27].

Introduction to Programming in Parkinson's Disease

Pharmacological treatment is the first line therapy for treatment of motor symptoms in Parkinson disease. Monoamine oxidase type B inhibitors, amantadine, anticholinergics, beta blockers, or dopamine agonists are used for treatment of mild symptoms. These medications may also be combined with levodopa which is the most effective medication for treatment of motor symptoms [28] Several randomized clinical studies have demonstrated the effectiveness of DBS surgery for control of Parkinson's disease symptoms. Although VIM DBS has shown effectiveness in control of Parkinson's disease tremors, globus pallidus internus (GPi) and subthalamic nucleus (STN, Figure 2) are now considered standard targets for control of motor symptoms in Parkinson disease [29]. DBS has demonstrated improvement of bradykinesia, rigidity, tremor, off-medication painful dystonia and levodopa-induced dyskinesia. DBS effectiveness is maximal for those motor symptoms that show response to levodopa treatment. Cognitive, autonomic and neuropsychiatric symptoms are not expected to show improvement with DBS therapy [30].

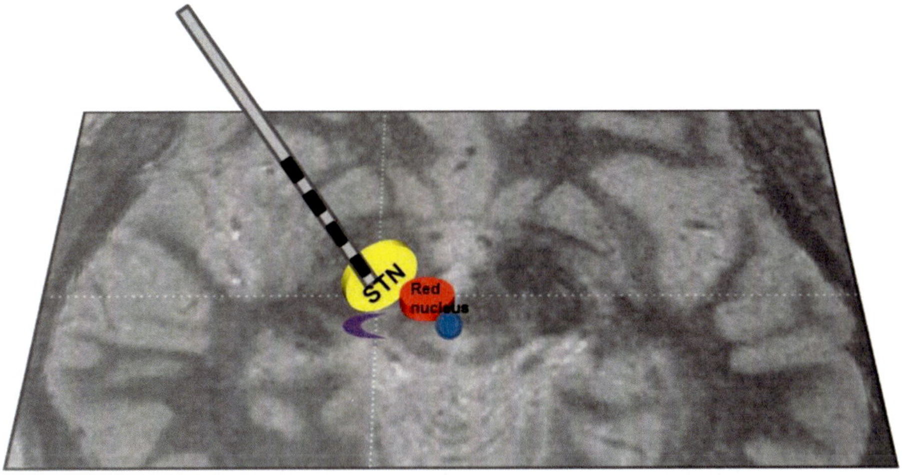

Figure 2. DBS implantation into subthalamic nucleus. The optimal location for DBS lead is in the dorsolateral part of nucleus If the lead is too lateral it will stimulate the internal capsule and if too medial it will stimulate the red nucleus.

General Considerations for Programming

The initial steps for programming DBS in Parkinson's disease are similar to those in Essential tremor. DBS programming is initiated about 3-4 weeks after the electrode placement surgery when the microlesion effects disappear. Lead type and lead configuration is determined and lead placement is confirmed by neuroimaging analysis. Impedances are recorded to confirm the intactness of the electrical system. DBS programming is performed usually in the morning with patients presenting in an off-medication state after an overnight medication washout. Occasionally inpatient programming is recommended if off-medication symptoms are intolerably severe or there is a lack of family support for outpatient management. Alternately, patients are allowed to present in on-medication state and they are examined once the medications effects show signs of wearing off (suboptimal on-medication). Rigidity and tremors are usually alleviated within seconds to minutes of STN or GPi stimulation. Rigidity does not require much patient participation. In contrast bradykinesia responds with a variable time delay, sometimes influenced by fatigue, patient comfort, and training. Tremor is evaluated with patient in a relaxed sitting position and hand and arms placed over the thigh in a resting position. Ideally standardized motor tasks of the Unified Parkinson's Disease Rating Scale motor scale are recommended for exam. Each electrode is tested in a monopolar configuration using standard pulse width (60 to 90μs for STN and 90μs to 120μs for GPi) and frequency (130 to 160 Hz) [24]. Voltage is gradually increased in increments of 0.5 V until the occurrence of a persistent adverse effect (objective or subjective) is noted. Once the threshold for side effects are defined, the programmer tests efficacy of stimulation at each contact in a monopolar setting using a voltage 0.5-1.0 V below the voltage causing stimulation induced side-effects. The clinical benefit of stimulating at each electrode contact (using contacts 0 to 3 as negative and case as positive) is recorded in details. If no benefit is recorded under the threshold voltage that induces side effects, testing is discontinued and the next contact is selected [24]. If single monopolar setting does not suppress the symptoms completely using tolerable voltages it is possible to test with bipolar stimulation. Sometimes double monopolar stimulation is employed in which the two contacts (or even three contacts) selected during monopolar evaluation are used. Polarity may be reversed or other bipolar configurations can be explored if necessary. DBS programming should be focused on one side at a time. Although each side stimulation is expected to induce contralateral benefits, it is also important to acknowledge the ipsilateral effects of stimulation.

In most individuals, optimum programing settings are accomplished within three to six months of surgery. In cases with STN DBS, dopaminergic medication doses are gradually reduced as the programming parameters become established. For evaluation of DBS effects on levodopa induced dyskinesia, patients are administered their dopaminergic doses once the off-medication state programming is completed. Levodopa induced dyskinesia may not emerge immediately after the first dose, sometimes requiring cumulative effects of two or three doses which is generally seen in the afternoons. Sometimes dorsal GPi stimulation may be observed to induce dyskinesia that can be confused with medication related dyskinesia. In these cases, if stimulation contact is shifted ventrally, dyskinesias are expected to be suppressed, however caution needs to be exercised since bradykinesia may inadvertently worsen. The best electrode combination is a configuration that adequately improves off-medication parkinsonism, reasonably suppresses on-medication dyskinesia and yet does not worsen on-medication parkinsonism. A similar challenge may arise in some STN DBS cases where stimulation induced dyskinesia are found to be related to a DBS lead well-located in the motor territory. In these circumstances, a gradual reduction of stimulation voltage is recommended to achieve balance between control of parkinsonism and control of dyskinesias.

Introduction to Programming in Dystonia

Pharmacological agents such as anticholinergic medications, benzodiazepines, and baclofen and botulinum toxin injections are the first line therapy for treatment of dystonia [31, 32]. Despite multiple pharmacological options, many patients with generalized dystonia and some with focal dystonia experience inadequate symptom relief, at which time surgical interventions are considered. DBS of the GPi target is an effective and established surgical treatment for dystonia (Figure 3) although a wide range (21-95%) of clinical outcomes has been reported across studies and these outcomes are poorly predictable in individual patients [33]. Selection of candidates for DBS is based on the presence of disabling symptoms that persist despite optimal medical management in unequivocally diagnosed primary or secondary dystonia. The exact physiological mechanisms underpinning these effects are not clear. DBS in dystonia is more likely to improve the mobile aspects of clinical syndrome (tremor, chorea, choreodystonia, and myoclonus) than tonic or fixed aspects of dystonia. Fixed deformities and arthrosis secondary to dystonia and nondystonic neurologic symptoms such as spasticity or cognitive dysfunction do not respond to DBS. Other important factors impacting clinical outcomes are inaccurate lead placement, suboptimal DBS programming and poor medication management while interval exacerbation of dystonia is usually related to technical failure or device malfunction.

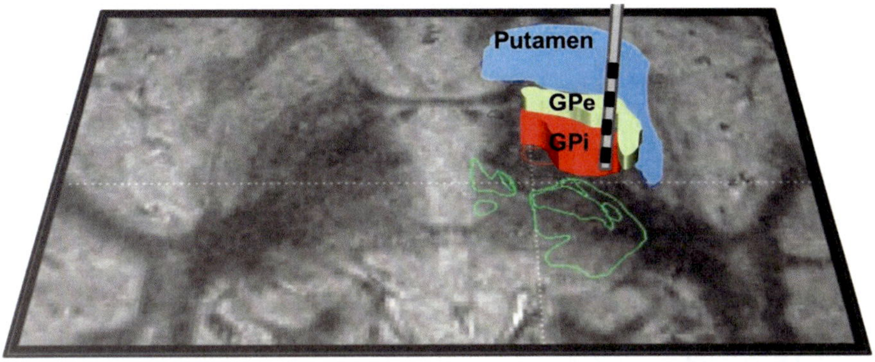

Figure 3. DBS implantation into Globus pallidus interna. The optimal location for DBS lead is in the postero-ventro-lateral part of nucleus. If the lead is too medial it will stimulate the internal capsule and if too lateral it will be outside the target.

General Considerations for Programming

DBS programming in dystonia is initiated about 3-4 weeks after the placement of electrode even though unlike essential tremor and Parkinson's disease, there are no benefits related to the microlesion effects. Patients are scheduled every month for programming. During these visits, withholding of medications as followed in Parkinson's disease is not implemented in order to avoid the discomfort related to dystonic symptoms.

Once the impedances are determined, the first step in programming is to identify the thresholds for each of the lead contacts. Thresholds are referred to the lowest stimulation amplitude that induces side effects at each of the contact. Most programmers tend to choose active stimulation contact in the ventral region of the GPi located just above the optic tract. This practice has evolved from initial primate studies that found the sensorimotor territory of the GPi is located in the ventral and posterior region which when stimulated controls dyskinesias in many patients [34, 35]. Although some have argued that the upper limb symptoms respond to anterodorsal stimulation and lower limb symptoms improve on posteroventral stimulation [36, 37]. Over the years many DBS programmers have now published on the choice of electrode contact that provides the best clinical outcome. In their experience out of contacts 0, 1, 2, and 3 (0 as most ventral), contacts 1 and 2 are the most frequently chosen contacts. Majority of patients need double monopolar stimulation or sometimes even triple monopolar stimulation [38]. One important challenge while programming in dystonia is the lack of immediate clinical effects in response to acute stimulation. If there is no acute benefit with stimulation, more chronic stimulation for 1–2 days is pursued. In these cases, higher stimulation voltages, frequencies and pulse widths maybe required for control of symptoms. Some investigators have also advocated the use of lower frequencies for symptomatic relief of dystonia although the pulse widths used in these patients is notably long. We made similar observations at our center in generalized dystonia where the frequency used was 60-90 Hz but the pulse widths were 180-220 μsec. It is noteworthy that higher frequency and higher pulse widths result in frequent neurostimulator replacement surgeries almost every 12 to 18 months [2, 39]. This may pose a lifelong medical burden in children. Rechargeable batteries in these circumstances are a good option.

Although stimulation parameters are important, in a large series of patients, lead location and quality of stimulation parameters have been found to have greater effects on control of dystonia symptoms than the amount of stimulation delivered [40].

The clinical improvement in dystonia in response to DBS may characteristically evolve over several months. For example, at our center we have observed improvement in dystonia emerging as late as nine months after surgery. The clinical response should be carefully documented preferably on a video using systematic clinical scales such as Burke-Fahn-Marsden Dystonia Rating Scale, Unified Dystonia Rating Scale for generalized dystonias and the Toronto Western Spasmodic Torticollis Rating Scale for cervical dystonias. Most DBS groups have observed that there is about 50-60% overall reduction in medication dosages [33]. These medications should be tapered or withdrawn only when the clinical benefits related to DBS begin to show effects.

Programming in Obsessive-Compulsive Disorder

Obsessive-compulsive disorder is characterized by recurrent, undesirable intrusive, anxious thoughts (obsessions) and repetitive intentional repetitive behaviors (compulsions) designed to neutralize both the cognitive intrusions and associated anxiety. Pharmacotherapy and psychotherapy are the first line treatment for obsessive-compulsive disorders however 40% to 60% of the patients continue to experience symptoms despite adequate medical management [41]. DBS is used when first line therapy fails in treatment of obsessive-compulsive disorder symptoms [4]. In 1999, Nuttin et al. targeted the anterior limb of the internal capsule and successfully treated obsessive-compulsive disorder symptoms in six patients [42]. These results generated great enthusiasm for this treatment. Multiple studies followed including some of which were double blind randomized controlled studies. Obsessive-compulsive disorder is conceptualized as a disorder of the cortico-striatothalamo-cortical circuitry which are parallel, segregated circuits. These include (1) projections from the sensorimotor cortex via the putamen modulating sensorimotor function; (2) projections from the limbic cortex (medial orbitofrontal complex [OFC], cingulate, anterior temporal, parahippocampal, and insular cortex) via the nucleus accumbens modulating affective symptoms such as anxiety; (3) projections from anterior and lateral OFC via the ventromedial caudate considered to modulate context-related function and response inhibition, on a more complex level mediating obsessional symptoms; and (4) projections from dorsolateral prefrontal cortex via the dorsolateral caudate, modulating executive functions or mediating compulsions of obsessive-compulsive disorder [43].

In the light of these proposed circuits that are implicated in mediating obsessive-compulsive disorder symptoms, the main DBS targets investigated for treatment of obsessive-compulsive disorder include the anterior limb of the internal capsule (ALIC) [44, 45], the ventral caudate (VC)/ventral striatum(VS) [46, 47], the subthalamic nucleus (STN)[41, 48, 49] the inferior thalamic peduncle (ITP) [50, 51], and the nucleus accumbens (NAc) [52-54]. These structures have also been noted to improve the obsessive-compulsive disorder symptoms that are comorbid in other DBS indications (e.g., Parkinson's disease) [41, 48]. In 2009, the FDA granted a limited humanitarian device exemption for the use of DBS targeting the ALIC, VC/VS or NAc as a treatment for medication refractory obsessive-compulsive disorder., STN and ITP are not yet approved targets for DBS in OCD. Currently, neurosurgical procedures for the treatment of obsessive-compulsive disorder aim to modulate a pathway in the aberrant circuit rather than addressing a single area that could be responsible for etiology [55].

General Considerations for Programming

The first step in DBS programming is identification of lead configuration and confirmation of lead location. In earlier studies, DBS leads with larger distances between contacts and larger contact sizes (e.g., Medtronic model 3391) were mainly used for VC/VS stimulation [46, 56], in more recent VC/VS cases [48], DBS lead with relatively smaller configuration (i.e., Medtronic model 3389) has been used. A smaller lead configuration lead is usually preferred for smaller targets such as the STN. Once the lead location is confirmed, it is important to record impedances at each of the four contacts on the lead to establish the integrity of the electrical system.

Currently there is no consensus on the best approach to acute and long-term DBS programming in obsessive-compulsive disorder. In the beginning threshold levels at each of the active contacts are determined. Thresholds in the context of obsessive-compulsive disorder refer to the amount of voltage required to induce a mood change. While the voltage (amplitude) is gradually increased at each of the contacts, the frequency and pulse width are intentionally kept constant. Voltage levels are important for mood assessments, higher levels are associated with mood aggravation, and lower levels are associated with positive mood changes [57]. It is noteworthy that favorable responses may not always be encountered in the acute phase of stimulation and that side effects such as worsening of anxiety emerging at high voltages may only be transient. Once the threshold levels are determined, the programmer selects the contacts or a contact that provides benefits at low stimulation voltage and side effects at high stimulation voltage.

The programming professional then proceeds with adjustment of pulse width and frequency based stimulation parameters. Across studies, the programming parameters have shown high incidence of variability and are particularly influenced by the target of stimulation. For example, the pulse widths used for stimulation of ALIC, VC/VS and ITP have ranged from 90-450 μsec but for STN they are usually low in the range of 60 μsec. It should also be noted that higher pulse widths greater than 210 μsec have been found to induce physiologic responses such as nausea, cold sensation, fear, and panic response [57]. Most studies have tended to empirically apply high-frequency stimulation in obsessive-compulsive disorder based on the authors experience in other movement disorders such as essential tremor. In essential tremor, low-frequency (<60 Hz) stimulation was found to increase tremor, whereas high-frequency stimulation has been found to suppress it [58, 59]. No specific pattern has been observed in obsessive-compulsive disorder and the frequencies used across targets have remained in the range of 100-130 Hz.

The frequency of programming visits is another important consideration while controlling obsessive-compulsive disorder symptoms. Earlier studies found that symptoms may improve as early as the first week of stimulation. However, recent double blinded studies with VC/VS stimulation found approximately two-thirds of the contacts did not demonstrate any acute beneficial effects [57]. It is therefore reasonable to schedule frequent follow-ups in earlier phases of programming. Most centers follow the patient every month for stimulation adjustment in the first six months after surgery although more data is needed.

In the following sections, we will focus on the anatomical site of stimulation and its influence on DBS programming obsessive-compulsive disorder.

Anterior limb of the internal capsule (ALIC), nucleus accumbens (NAc), and ventral caudate (VC)/ventral striatum (VS)

The ALIC is an important structure in the obsessive-compulsive disorder circuitry carrying the frontopontine fibers, thalamic peduncles, and possibly the medial forebrain bundle [60, 61]. The results of gamma capsulotomy have suggested that the more ventral portion of the ALIC seems to be associated with greater benefits [46, 60] Since the ALIC and VC/VS are relatively large DBS targets, most studies have used DBS leads with larger configuration to cover wider target areas [42,46,56] compared to the usual 3389 and 3387 models. These large configuration DBS leads are the Medtronic model 3391(Medtronic, Minneapolis, MN, USA) (diameter = 1.27 mm, each contact length = 3 mm, inter-electrode spacing edge to edge = 4 mm) and the model 3887 (diameter = 1.3 mm, each contact length = 3 mm, inter-electrode spacing edge to edge = 4 mm). In cases of VC/VS stimulation with 3391 leads, the most ventral contact (0) stimulates the ventromedial region of the NAc, and the middle contacts (1 and 2) stimulates the ventral portion of the ALIC, which is also a target similar that used in ventral capsulotomy. Recently, relatively smaller electrodes with closer intercontact distances have been used to stimulate the NAc and the ventral capsule [52, 62, 63]. In the modified VC/VS trajectory located posterior to the original VC/VS trajectory, the most ventral contact is located close to the border between the NAc and nucleus basalis. Most experts find that the location of active contact contributes significantly to the final outcome [54, 56].

Many investigators have noted that intraoperative test stimulation of the ALIC region induces mirthful laughter [64-66]. This intraoperative phenomenon has been proposed to predict favorable outcomes in obsessive-compulsive disorder DBS [65]. The smile induced by electrical stimulation is observed contralateral to the side of the stimulation which then spreads rapidly to the ipsilateral side. This phenomenon is not a simple motor response caused by internal capsule stimulation as there is a euphoric sensation frequently accompanying the smile. Thus during the initial programming visits, it is helpful to use this contact that induced intraoperative smile response for guidance.

Most centers recommend bilateral implantation of DBS leads. Bilateral independent programming of the devices is necessary to obtain maximal benefits. Although the active contacts on DBS leads in obsessive-compulsive disorder may be selected symmetrically, the lead location may be slightly different between the left and right sides. Some investigators have advocated the use of unilateral stimulation [52, 63, 67] as in their experience, the clinical benefits seen with right unilateral stimulation were not the same as the left side stimulation. Many subsequent observations have not supported this laterality concept.

The benefits mediated through NAc stimulation in obsessive-compulsive disorder is likely related to reward processing and behavioral addiction [62]. An alternate explanation is the spread of the electric current to the ventral capsule. The NAc has two different areas, the shell and the core), and these two regions are assumed to have two different functions [68]. The shell region probably has more dense μ receptors related to the reward mechanism [43]. It remains unclear whether it is more advantageous to target the shell or the core of the NAc.

Subthalamic nucleus (STN) and inferior thalamic peduncle (ITP)

Multiple studies have targeted the STN for treatment of obsessive-compulsive disorder since it has distinct limbic and associative territories, in addition to the motor territory [49, 69]. Unlike other obsessive-compulsive disorder targets, STN seems to require relatively lower charge densities for stimulation. During programming, voltage adjustment is typically performed with a fixed frequency (130 Hz) and pulse width (60 μ sec) [49].

ITP has been explored only in few cases so far. The ITP lies adjacent to the fornix and the hypothalamus, and stimulation of this region has potential to induce side effects. Although the ITP is a relatively small target, high voltage stimulation maybe required to address the obsessive-compulsive disorder symptoms. Jimenez-Ponce et al. applied bipolar stimulation as a strategy to concentrate the electrical current within a small area and to avoid the spread of current and development of side effects [51].

Programming in Tourette's Syndrome

Gilles de la Tourette syndrome is a childhood-onset movement disorder characterized by multiple motor tics and one or more phonic tics, lasting longer than one year. With the rising popularity of DBS in the modern era and expansion of indications into neuropsychiatry, it is not surprising that DBS is offered to patients with medication refractory Tourette's syndrome [5,70]. However, Tourette's syndrome had not been approved by US or European agencies as an indication for DBS and DBS cannot be formally recommended in these patients. In milder forms, psychobehavioral therapies such as relaxation training, cognitive behavioral therapy, habit reversal training, and comprehensive behavioral intervention are used for control. Pharmacological treatment is used for patients with moderate to severe Tourette's syndrome. Standard medications include a2-adrenergic agonists, typical and atypical neuroleptics, benzodiazepines [71], tetrabenazine and sometimes botulinum toxin injections are used for the muscle groups involved in disabling tics. A small subset of patients with potentially life-threatening tics or self-injurious behavior ("malignant Tourette's syndrome") do not respond to these treatments [72]. For these subjects, Vandewalle et al. in 1999 experimentally targeted the ventral oral internus (Voi) and center median parafascicular (CMPf) nuclei of the thalamus with DBS [73]. The rationale to modulate (or ablate) these areas stemmed from the concept of a dysfunctional cortico-striato-thalamocortical circuitry involving the frontal associative and limbic territories of the basal ganglia and the thalamus. An increased excitation of the cortex and a decreased inhibition of the thalamus result in a failure to suppress, or, in other words, result in increased exhibition of involuntary movements. Since this first report, there have been more than 120 patients reported worldwide who have received DBS therapy for Tourette's syndrome. Most studies have been open label case reports or small series and only four studies with randomized controlled design have been published so far [74-77]. Most studies, including blinded ones, reported more than 50-70% reduction in tics at one year follow-up.

Numerous anatomical targets have been identified for DBS in Tourette's syndrome. These include the medial thalamus (eg, centromedian nucleus–parafascicular complex [CM-Pf]) [73, 78, 79, 80], GPi [74, 81-83, 84], and the ALIC/NAc [85-88]. Globus pallidus externus (GPe) [89], and STN are additional targets [69] but have been tried in only one or two studies. The most commonly used target is the CM-Pf with 70 cases reported in literature.

Some investigators favor a motor target such as the sensorimotor pallidum which is the main basal ganglia output towards the thalamus and the motor cortex in the motor circuitry. So far 31 cases of pallidal DBS have been reported, some targeting the anteromedial GPi (n=14) and some targeting the posteroventral GPi (n=16) [5].

Most studies have observed about 50-70% reduction in tics with GPi DBS and medial thalamus DBS. While these two targets have shown similar efficacy, stimulation of ALIC/NAc has shown mixed results. In one series of Tourette's syndrome patients(n=4), three initially underwent thalamic DBS which was supplemented with additional targeting of the ALIC/NAc but only one out of these three patients noticed any improvement in tics. The fourth patient with stimulation of ALIC/NAc remained dissatisfied since there was no improvement [90].

General Guidelines for Programming

DBS leads with larger distances between contacts and larger contact sizes (e.g., Medtronic model 3391) are mainly used. In many studies double monopolar stimulation was found to be effective although in some all 4 contacts on the quadripolar electrode (tetrapolar) were required for stimulation suggesting that the volume of tissue activation needed is sometimes much greater than the area intended in the beginning.

The first step in programming is to identify the threshold levels at each of the active contacts. The amount of voltage at each contact is gradually increased with frequency and pulse width kept constant. At optimal voltages, the patient reports alleviation of anxiety and tension. These are temporary benefits that serve as clinical guides for further programming. The voltages are then titrated upwards to identify the upper threshold limits that induce acute stimulation related side effects. Most studies have found that, regardless of the target selected, higher pulse widths, usually stimulating the larger neural elements, and increased frequencies are effective parameters for programming. The pulse widths reported by most studies have ranged from 90-210 μsec whereas the frequency of stimulation has been observed to range from 100-185 Hz. During the initial programming visits, the motor tics related to Tourette's syndrome may not necessarily be controlled. However with selection of optimal contact, stimulation settings and with the use of these settings for chronic stimulation, there is a gradual reduction in the frequency of motor tics.

Tourette's syndrome is accompanied by several nonmotor comorbidities such as anxiety disorder and obsessive-compulsive disorder. The phenotypic variability of Tourette's and the variations in the expressions of comorbidities are important considerations when programming these patients. Whether the limbic and associative circuitry is targeted or the motor circuitry is targeted, there is significant variation in the amount of current delivered across individuals and even between brain sides of the same patient. Since there are multiple factors that contribute towards clinical outcomes, currently there is no consensus on programming guidelines and the time course of outcomes [45, 91, 92].

TROUBLESHOOTING COMPLICATIONS

The number of patients undergoing DBS has shown a significant increase over the past two decades and thus newer complications are expected to emerge in increasing proportions.

In the following section, we will describe the potential problems encountered with DBS related to surgery, devices (hardware), or stimulation itself. Additional variables that may negatively affect DBS effectiveness including unrealistic patient expectations, inadequate patient selection, tolerance development or disease progression will not be discussed in this chapter.

Complications from Surgery

DBS surgery may result in infection, clinical complications (pneumonia and venous thrombo-embolism), transient confusion state, seizures, intra-cranial hemorrhage, transient and permanent neurologic deficit or even death. According to an expert consensus on DBS [93]: 1) advanced age and multiple comorbidities add to surgical risks but these should not exclude someone from consideration; 2) the experience of the surgical team is a key factor in lowering the risk of surgical complications; 3) there is a critical need for prospective standardized reporting of complications. We reviewed 31 studies on DBS related complications published between January 2001 and August 2014 that included on an average at least 40 patients. There were 9 multicenter prospective studies (n = 40 - 299 patients) [1,94-101]one multicenter retrospective study (n =1183 patients)[102] and 21 retrospective series of individual centers (n = 45 – 728 patients) [103-123]. In 27 studies all patients (n = 40 – 728 patients) were implanted with bilateral DBS (simultaneous or staged procedures) and the remaining four studies (n = 191 – 1183 patients) included patients with unilateral as well as bilateral DBS (50 to 70% were bilateral). There was one retrospective study [120] that included complications related to ablative and DBS surgeries combined, but we considered only the DBS related complications in the present analysis (n = 115 patients).

DBS surgery-related complications are discussed below and summarized in the table 1.

Deaths

According to six prospective multicenter clinical trials that included nearly 504 bilateral DBS surgeries (simultaneous or staged), the mortality rate was found to be null [1, 96-98, 100, 101]. In three prospective multicenter clinical trials the mortality was 0.7% (of 299 patients) [95], 2.6% (of 76 patients) [94] and 0.8% (of 121 patients) [99]. Taken together, the mortality rate was 0.61% among the 1138 pooled patients of these prospective multicenter clinical trials. In one retrospective European multicenter study (n = 1183) the incidence of deaths related to DBS-surgery was 0.4% [102]. The recent retrospective analysis of US based Thomson Reuters Market Scan national database identified 1757 DBS surgeries between 2000 and 2009 for Parkinson's disease and they reported an overall mortality of 0.3%. In this study, 34% (n = 590) patients underwent unilateral DBS implantation, 31% had bilateral implants (n = 551), 7% (n = 122) with staged implantation and remainder 28% (n = 494) with indeterminate implantation [124].

When we examined mortality among retrospective studies conducted by 21 individual centers, the mortality rate was clearly described by only 20 studies. Sixteen centers (n = 3205 patients) reported no deaths [103-123] and in four centers (n = 304 patients) the mortality ranged between 1 to 4.4% [103-123]. The overall mortality was 0.20% among the 3509 pooled patients of the retrospective studies. Among the 19 deaths described in the reviewed studies, 8 were caused by intracranial hemorrhage, 6 were related to pneumonia, 2 pulmonary embolism, 1 hepatic insufficiency and 1 was caused by acute progression of encephalitis in a multiple sclerosis patient. In single center retrospective analysis of 115 bilateral DBS implants, 8.6% patients were reported to either die or be transferred to a rehabilitation or skilled nursing facility without specifying the exact mortality rate [120]. In comparison to prospective studies, mortality reported by retrospective national data base study or by most single center studies has been slightly lower. This may in part be related to methodological issues inherent to retrospective analysis.

Intracranial Hemorrhage (ICH) and Ischemic Stroke

Intracranial hemorrhage in relation to DBS may be symptomatic or asymptomatic (Figure 4). Although post-operative neuroimaging is required to confirm symptomatic hemorrhage or identify sub-clinical hemorrhage, in several centers the imaging was reportedly done in only symptomatic patients. In multicenter studies, the incidence of asymptomatic ICH was reportedly seen between 0 and 2.6% (mean 1.3%) [1, 94-102] and symptomatic ICH seen between 0 and 4.2% (mean 1.7%) [1, 94-102].

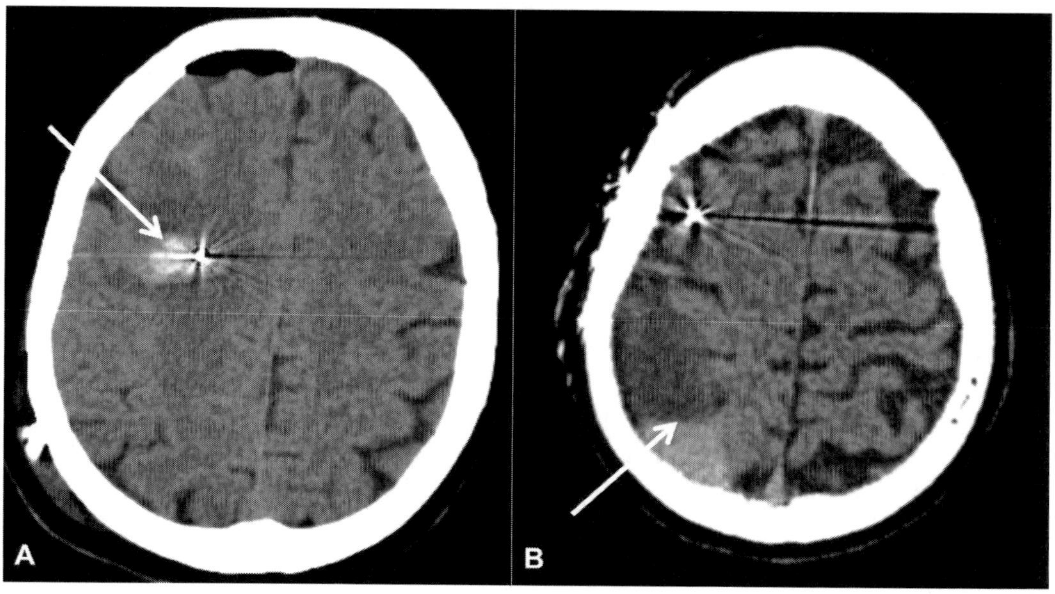

Figure 4. A: Right frontal hemorrhage occurring during DBS lead implantation. This patient developed mild drowsiness and left hemibody weakness during lead placement procedure; post-operative CT-scan showed a right subcortical frontal hemorrhage. Patient was managed conservatively with good recovery after 4 weeks.

B: Right fronto-parietal subdural hematoma. This patient presented at 4 weeks follow-up after DBS surgery complaining of mild right sided headache and postural instability. CT head revealed a right hemispheric chronic subdural hematoma.

Table 1. Complications related to DBS surgery

Surgery-related complications	Multicenter studies incidence (%)	References	Single Center studies incidence (%)	References
Deaths	None	[1, 96-98, 100, 101]	none	[103-123]
	0.7, 2.6 and 0.8	[95]	1 to 4.4	[103-123]
	0.4	[102]	N.A.	N.A.
Intracranial Hemorrhage (ICH)				
Asymptomatic ICH	0 to 2.6 (mean 1.3)	[1, 94-102]	0 to 34 (mean 5.0)	[104,105,107-116,122,123]
Symptomatic ICH	0 to 4.2 (mean 1.7)	[1, 94-102]	0 to 8.9 (mean 2.2)	[104-120,123]
Permanent neurologic deficit	0 to 2.8 (mean 0.8)	[94-98, 101, 102]	0 to 4.1 (mean 1.1)	[104-120,123]
Deep cerebral venous thrombosis	0.1	[102]	0.5 and 0.9	[112,116]
Seizures	0 to 3.1 (mean 1.6)	[94, 96-98, 100-102]	0.7 to 6.5 (mean 2.1)	[108,111,112,115-118,121]
Transoperative Vasovagal reaction	Non-reported	N.A.	1.1 and 3.7	[115,117]
Sterile seroma	1.4 to 5.2 (mean 3.0)	[94, 96, 101]	Non-reported	N.A.
Venous thromboembolism	0.1 to 0.7	[101]	0 to 2.5	[109]
Pneumonia	1.3 and 4	[94, 95, 102]	Non-reported	N.A.
Peri/postoperative confusion/delirium	0 to 5.2 (mean 1.9)	[1, 94-96, 98, 100, 101]	2.3 to 24 (mean 12.4)	[106-108,113,115-119]
Sub-optimal lead placement	1.2 and 1.3	[94, 101]	1.2 to 11 (6.5)	[106,111,115,121]

* The reference [102] was a retrospective multicenter study and all the others were prospective multicenter trials.

N.A. – Non-applicable

Permanent deficits were seen in up to 2.8% of patients (mean 0.8%) [94-98, 101, 102], although the incidences were higher in retrospective series. The incidence of asymptomatic ICH ranged between 0 to 34% (mean 5%) [104, 105, 107-116, 122, 123], symptomatic ICH ranged between 0 to 8.9% (2.2%) and permanent deficits were seen in up to 4.1% (mean 1.1%) [104-120, 123]. The incidence of ICH seemed to be higher when multiple electrode passes were used during the microelectrode recording (MER) [125, 126]. According to the DBS Study Group, the number of MER penetrations has been associated with increased incidence of ICH. Patients without ICH have a mean of 2.9 (± 1.8) penetrations, compared with 4.1 (± 2.0) among those who have ICH ($p < 0.05$) [101] Similarly another study has found a non-significant ($p = 0.21$) trend towards increased number of MER penetrations in those patients who develop ICH (median 3, IQ range 2-4), compared to those who do not (median 2, IQ range 1-3) [105]. Systemic hypertension has been another important risk factor associated with ICH [127]. Since the blood pressure levels are kept under control during and after surgery, a systematic examination of vascular changes will likely better explain the bleeding risk than recordings of hypertensive peaks [127].

In addition to ICH, it is possible to develop ischemic stroke in relation to DBS. Ischemic strokes have been reported by three retrospective series with an incidence ranging between 0.4% to 2.1% [104, 114, 115]. A direct injury to the perforating arteries, or a vasospasm induced by direct mechanical stimulation, edema, or electrical stimulation has been considered a potential explanation.

Prevention

1) Discontinuation of aspirin and nonsteroidal anti-inflammatory medications should be performed at least 1 week before surgery, and bleeding time should be obtained if the interval is shorter or the medical history is unreliable; 2) Patients who receive anticoagulation therapy with warfarin should be switched to heparin and heparin should be discontinued 6 hours prior to surgery; 3) Controlling blood pressure before, during and after surgery is important; 4) The procedure should be avoided in patients with respiratory condition that causes severe cough or sneezing in order to prevent sudden increase in intracranial pressure with consequent venous bleedings [103]; 5) During the MER, the use of lower number of electrode passes is recommended [103] ; 6) A meticulous use of neuroimaging should be performed for planning the trajectory and target verification in order to avoid unnecessary sulcal or ventricular incursions that may injure venous or arterial vessels.

Troubleshooting

ICH is suspected during surgery if: i) Blood is seen to flow out through the cannula; ii) There is deterioration in the level of consciousness; iii) Focal neurologic deficit develops; iv)Focal or secondarily generalized seizure is seen. In these cases medical management of the airway, ventilation, hemodynamic and intracranial pressure should be immediately implemented. A CT scan should be done as soon as possible to confirm diagnosis and the size of the hemorrhage. In rare cases of large intra-axial bleeding a decompression craniotomy to avoid brainstem herniation may be required [128]. If an ischemic stroke is found on the CT scan, the treatment is supportive. Management of ICH related seizures is discussed in the subsequent sections.

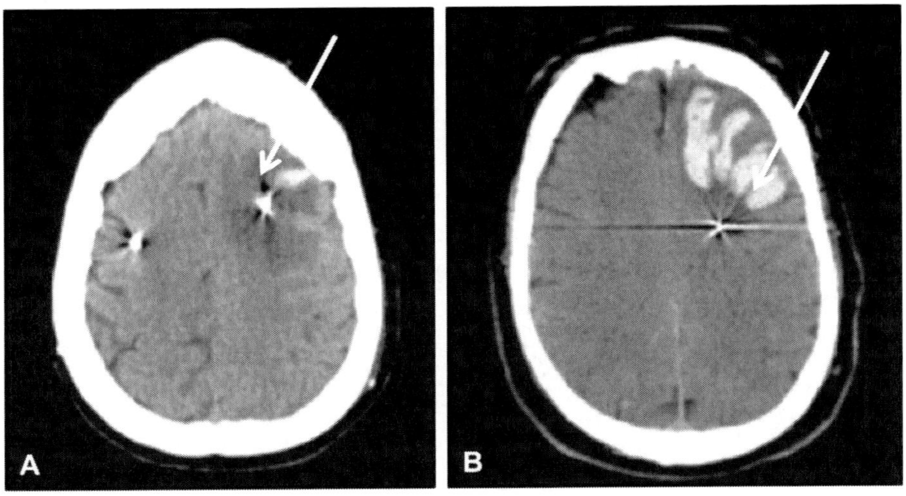

Figure 5. A: Left frontal cerebral venous thrombosis with subcortical edema and little hemorrhage. This patient developed altered mental status and right upper extremity weakness the day after DBS- lead placement. Post-operative CT-scan showed left subcortical edema associated with a little hemorrhage. Patient was managed conservatively with good recovery after 4 weeks.

B: Left frontal cerebral venous thrombosis associated with a subcortical hemorrhage.

This patient developed drowsiness and right hemibody weakness the day after DBS- lead placement. Post-operative CT-scan showed left subcortical hemorrhage. Patient was managed conservatively with good recovery after 8 weeks.

Delayed Deep Cerebral Venous Thrombosis or Hemorrhage

Cerebral venous thrombosis (CVT) results from a thrombus formed at the site of burr hole in the draining veins entering through the dura mater, or is related to injuries sustained during the surgical procedure (Figure 5). The incidence of CVT was 0.1% in one multicenter retrospective analysis [102] and was 0.5 to 0.9% when examined by two single center retrospective studies [112, 116].

Clinical manifestations of CVT includes severe headache, changes in the mental status, seizures or focal neurologic deficits [129]. MRI venography is useful in these cases demonstrating the thrombus in the draining vein and the dural system [130].

Prevention

Specific laboratory based screening tests before the surgery may facilitate confirmation of a suspected hypercoagulable state. During the surgery, a cautious surgical planning with gadolinium brain MRI and the placement of burr hole anterior to the coronal suture reduces the risk of venous thrombosis.

Troubleshooting

CVT may require anti-coagulation or thrombolytics to increase the chances for recanalization and to prevent the spread of a thrombus. A hematology consultation may be helpful for decision-making in these cases. If anticoagulation is prescribed, an international normalized ratio (INR)should be maintained between 2 and 3.5 for at least 3 months. In cases with evolving headache and papilledema, repeated lumbar punctures or lumboperitoneal shunt surgery may be needed [130]. Seizures should be treated with anti-epileptic drugs as discussed below [131].

Seizures

The presumed mechanisms for seizure in the context of DBS surgery includes either presence of a localized structural lesion or functional disturbance contributing towards the formation of an epileptogenic focus. In seven multicenter studies, the incidence of seizures, mostly secondary generalized convulsions, was found to range between 0 and 3.1% (mean 1.6%) [94, 96-98, 100-102]. When examining single center experience (n=8), a slightly higher incidence in the range 0.7 to 6.5% (mean 2.1%) was reported [108, 111, 112, 115-118, 121].

In a comprehensive retrospective analysis by Pouratina et al., [132] seizures were found to be significantly associated with older age, abnormal findings on postoperative neuroimaging and use of trans ventricular electrode trajectory. In a cohort of 22 patients with abnormal postoperative imaging, 6 (27.3%) developed seizures in comparison to only 1 (0.9%) of the 139 patients whom postoperative imaging was unremarkable (odds ratio 37.9, p = 0.0002). Some patients developed pneumoencephalus, however the size was not associated with the occurrence of a seizure. In 6 patients (86%), the seizures presented within 48 hours of surgery whereas in the remaining patient they presented once the hospitalization was over. Most patients (71%) with a single seizure were treated pharmacologically for about 1 to 4 weeks. Recurrent seizures were seen in only 2 patients (up to 4 seizures) and these remained seizure-free once they completed 4 and 8 months of treatment respectively.

Prevention

Prophylactic antiepileptic drug (AED) therapy is not recommended and an effort to minimize structural damage probably reduces the risk of seizures.

Troubleshooting

Parkinson's disease patients with DBS related seizures may have comorbidities requiring medications which may potentially interact with AED therapy. Although no class I evidence is available, considering the benign nature of DBS related seizures and the side effect profile of AEDs, a short-term monotherapy treatment (4 to 6 weeks) is the best approach. In the elderly patients gabapentin, lamotrigine, low dose topiramate, or levetiracetam, are the preferred AEDs [133].

Vasovagal Reaction and Hypotension

Vasovagal reaction with hypotension during the perioperative period has been reported in 1.1% and 3.7% of patients by two retrospective series [115, 117] Fenoy et al. described the vasovagal reaction in four patients who also developed other complications such as transient hemiparesis, a small ICH, air in the cavernous sinus and ischemic stroke respectively [115].

Troubleshooting

Hemodynamic support including atropine and adequate hydration should be provided by the anesthesiologist. Although vasovagal reaction is a benign complication, it may require additional specific treatment if associated with other complications.

Sterile seroma

Sometimes surgical injury may cause an accumulation of sterile serum in a circumscribed tissue area that is usually absorbed gradually. The incidence of seroma has been reported in 1.4 to 5.2% (mean 1.4%) of patients in three multicenter trials [94, 96, 101].

Troubleshooting

If the seroma is not spontaneously absorbed over days or weeks, it should be drained by a needle puncture. If an infection is suspected, the fluid should be sent for direct analysis and culture.

Venous Thromboembolism (VTE)

The venous thromboembolism (VTE) related to surgeries may be influenced by several variables including age, duration of immobilization, and presence of thrombogenic risk factors such as cancer or auto-immune diseases. Surgeries in awake patients are associated with lower incidence of VTE compared to DBS surgeries performed under general anesthesia. VTE and pulmonary embolism is a clinical challenge and the diagnosis should be suspected in patients with sudden onset of dyspnea, tachypnea, pleuritic chest pain, cough, and hemoptysis. The incidence of pulmonary embolism in bilateral DBS was 0.1% in a prospective multicenter trial [101] and 0.7% in a retrospective multicenter trial [102]. Bauman et al. [109] found a non-significant trend (p=0.11) for higher incidence of VTE among patients who did not receive prophylactic heparin. These patients underwent bilateral DBS surgeries (in 77.5%) involving MER, and most patients had Parkinson's disease (79%). None of the patients treated with mechanical plus heparin prophylaxis (n = 133) developed clinically detected VTE in comparison to 3 events (2.5% of cases, one deep vein thrombosis and 2 with pulmonary embolism) in the group of patients treated with mechanical prophylaxis only (n = 121) [109].

Prevention

Decision on mechanical prophylaxis with and without heparin should be based on the risk factor profile which includes duration of immobility, presence of general anesthesia, duration of surgery and other additional risk factors such as presence of hypercoagulable state. For lead implantation surgeries in awake patients, mechanical prophylaxis alone is probably sufficient. However, for the pulse generator implantation requiring general anesthesia, mechanical plus heparin prophylaxis are indicated.

Troubleshooting

Initial VTE or pulmonary embolism treatment requires subcutaneous low molecular weight heparin therapy followed by oral warfarin to achieve a goal INR (2.0 - 3.0). This can be increased to approximately 2.5 - 3.5 if another episode of PE occurs. For patients with significant bleeding risk, an inferior vena cava filter may be an alternative [134].

Pneumonia

Swallowing difficulties that are common in Parkinson's disease patients increase the risk of post-operative aspiration pneumonia. The incidence of aspiration pneumonia after DBS implant was 1.3% and 4% in two prospective multicenter trials [94, 95] and 4% in a retrospective multicenter trial [102].

Prevention

Aspiration risk may be reduced by the use of mechanical swallowing techniques, including changing the consistency of food, or alternatively teaching chin-down swallowing technique. Another recently used approach for aspiration prevention has been expiratory muscle strength training [135] At our center, subjects at increased risk of aspiration pneumonia are not allowed oral intake after the DBS surgery until they are reevaluated for swallowing performance.

Troubleshooting

Pneumonias in Parkinson's disease may either be community acquired or hospital acquired. Antibiotic choices should be dictated by culture, as well as by the clinical setting and knowledge on local bacterial resistance [135]. An infectious diseases consultation is often appropriate in these cases.

Peri and Postoperative Confusion and Delirium

The incidence of reversible psychiatric symptoms such as anxiety, psychosis, mania and confusional state related to DBS-surgery has been in the range 0 to 5.2% (mean 1.9%) according to seven prospective multicenter studies [1, 94-96, 98, 100, 101] and 2.3 to 24% (mean 12.4) in nine retrospective series [106-108, 113, 115-119]. In a retrospective analysis of 59 patients who underwent bilateral STN DBS surgery, Carlson et al. [136] reported delirium in 22% of patients following the DBS implant, and 10% following the second surgery (placement of neurostimulator and lead extension). Most studies have been found to be related to DBS in Parkinson's disease. Delirium in these studies was found to be associated with older age, history of hallucinations prior to surgery and delay in administration of Parkinson's disease medications after surgery. As a result, some DBS centers including ours prefer to perform staged DBS lead implantation instead of bilateral simultaneous implantation, although strictly speaking there are no published data favoring one technique over the other.

Prevention

Dopaminergic medications should be started as soon as possible after the DBS lead implantation surgery in Parkinson's disease. Avoid prolonged hospitalization and encourage close supervision by the caregiver.

Troubleshooting

In general, delirium following DBS surgery resolves relatively quickly in almost all patients. Often, gentle redirection by nursing staff, restarting the home medication schedule and close involvement of caregiver work effectively [136]. Sometimes, neuroimaging, blood analysis and urinalysis may be necessary to exclude an underlying neurological or medical complication. For benign hallucinations or confusion, observation is usually the best treatment and patients are discharged home if otherwise medically stable. Physical restraints are required only if there is a risk to physical safety. Dopaminergic blockers such as quetiapine are used only as a last resort to control extreme agitation [136].

Sub-Optimal Lead Placement

Sub-optimal lead implantation is a common cause of DBS failure and may be related to poor surgical technique, intra operative lead movement, frame shift, misinterpretation of MER data and brain shift [26]. The incidence of sub-optimal lead placement was reported to be 1.2 to 11% in four retrospective series [106, 111, 115, 121] but only 1.3 and 1.4% in two prospective multicenter trials [94, 101].

Prevention

1) Improving the surgical technique; 2) Confirming the DBS lead position by intra-operative fluoroscopy before and after the lead has been locked by a securing device; 3) Confirming the lead position post-operatively by head CT/MRI; [26] 4) Minimizing traction on brain while fixing the lead.

Troubleshooting

1) Test the intraoperative threshold at each electrode contact on the DBS lead with macrostimulation for benefits and side-effects before finally fixing the lead; 2) based on the intraoperative stimulation threshold findings, lead repositioning is sometimes necessary; 3) consider initiation of programming at one month; 4) follow the safety guidelines of device manufacturer to perform post-operative MRI; 5) use an image fusion software to determine the three-dimensional position of each electrode contact on the DBS lead using an appropriate image contrast; 6) based on clinical assessment, benefits, side effects and lead position decide whether electrode combination may provide the best result in the programming. Improper DBS effects related to a sub-optimally placed lead may be corrected by intracranial lead replacement [26].

Device-Related Complications

Infection

DBS surgery may be associated with superficial incisional infections, deep incisional infections and deep organ/space infections involving the DBS hardware implants (Figure 6). Infection of the implantable neurostimulator is one of the most common with most series reporting it in about 4-10% of the cases [137-139]. If the infection levels are noted to exceed the usual incidence, it is important to engage the hospital infectious disease committee. The committee works on identifying additional sources of infection within the hospital environment. If the infection involves the lead system, it may be necessary to remove the hardware since mere antibiotic course is often not effective. Importantly, if the hardware is left behind, it may serve as a constant nidus for infection and may evolve into major intracranial brain abscess or subdural empyema.

Prevention

In order to control the infection rates related to DBS surgery, every center is required to observe the following precautions. 1. It is important to follow strict aseptic surgical methods including the use of chlorhexidine at the surgical skin site [140] 2. Surgical incision for DBS is preferred to be curvilinear so it does not cross the lead anchoring device; 3. It is necessary to use prophylactic antibiotics for 2-3 days during the perioperative period. There is no consensus on the choice of antibiotics [138, 141] 4. Since, in theory, longer surgeries increase the risk of infection, it is important to control the duration of surgery without compromising on quality and adequate lead placement 5. Shaving of hair at the surgical skin site is still debated [142]. Some DBS centers do not shave the hair with low infection rates and those who advocate hair removal recommend use of hair clippers instead of a razor [143].

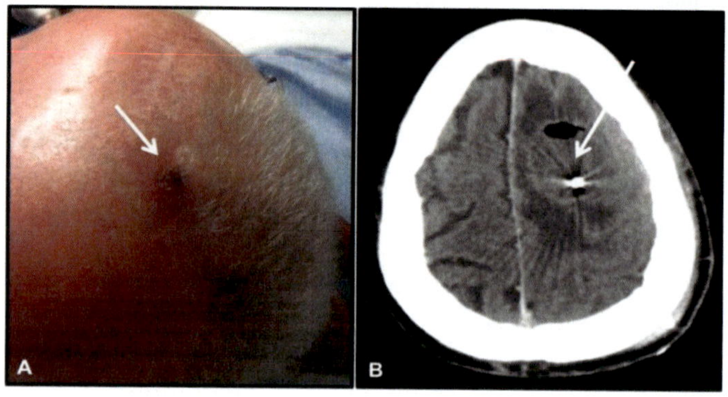

Figure 6. A: Parietal infection at the connector site.

This patient presented to clinic complaining of scalp tenderness and redness few weeks after DBS surgery. Afterwards the patient underwent DBS-lead ablation and explanation of the system.

B: Left frontal brain abscess with air and surrounding edema.

This patient presented to ER 12 days after DBS-lead placement because of drowsiness and right hemiparesis. CT-scan showed left frontal brain abscess with air and surrounding edema. Patient was operated right away and DBS-lead was explanted. Patient recovered well after 4 weeks of IV antibiotic therapy.

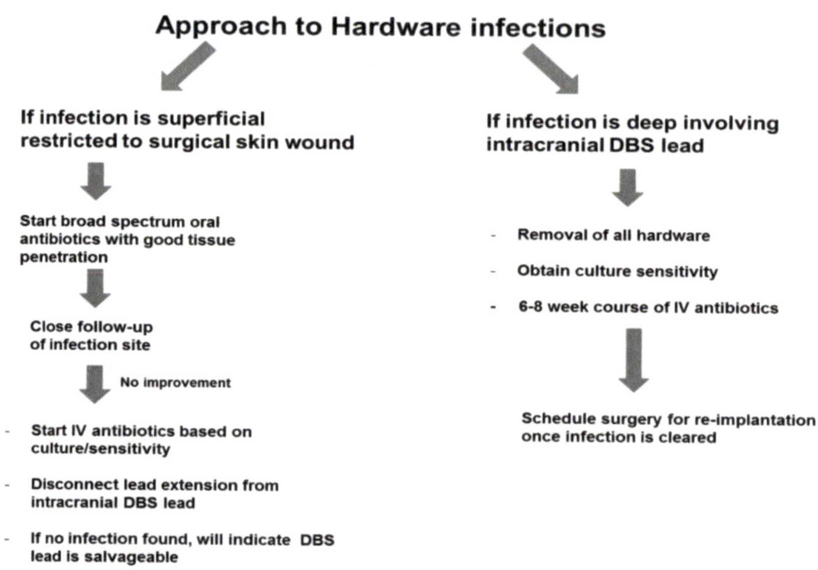

Figure 7. Approach to hardware infections.

Troubleshooting (Figure 7)

In cases of superficial skin infection at the surgical skin site such as one on the scalp (burr hole) or one over the chest wall (where the implantable neurostimulator is inserted), oral or IV antibiotics may suffice. In complicated cases, infections will require a close follow-up and infectious disease specialists will need to be consulted. Wound and blood cultures are valuable in guiding the appropriate antibiotic course. The antibiotic course is usually prolonged, lasting 6-8 weeks. If possible, the DBS lead system should be kept in place as removal of the hardware and discontinuation of DBS therapy can significantly impact the quality of life in these patients, but its removal will be necessary if the infection involves the lead. However, if the infection is restricted to the implantable neurostimulator in the chest wall and the lead connector is not involved, then only the neurostimulator hardware is removed and the DBS lead system is left behind. Once the infection resolves, the patient is scheduled for a reimplantation of the neurostimulator and/or lead (s).

Skin Erosion

Skin erosion related to the hardware can occur at multiple sites (Figure 8). The three common places are the burr hole site over the scalp, the site where the lead connector is attached to the DBS lead and the skin over the neurostimulator. These skins sites are susceptible to undergo erosion. This complication may occur several months after surgery thus considered a late occurring complication (incidence is about 3-6%) [137]. In the past few years, newer connectors and smaller neurostimulators have been used. Being less bulky, they are therefore less likely to contribute to skin erosion.

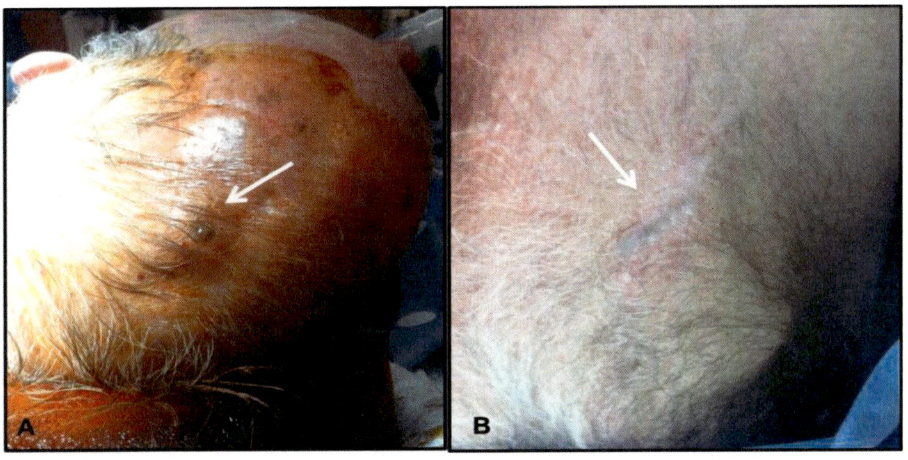

Figure 8. A: Threatening frontal scalp erosion at the lead-cap site (aseptic necrosis).

This patient presented to clinic about 4 months after DBS surgery showing a brown dead skin spot over frontal lead-cap without signs of infection. Eventually he underwent to frontal wound revision and primary closure.

B: Threatening chest skin erosion at the IPG site (aseptic necrosis).

This patient presented to clinic about 6 months after DBS surgery complaining of dark and tender skin over the chest at the IPG site; No signs of infection. Eventually he underwent chest wound revision and primary closure.

Prevention

Skin erosion is a preventable complication. The lead connector should be properly placed under the scalp into the deeper tissue plane and the galea should be properly closed. It is preferable to have one tunnel per neurostimulator system [112]. Skin above the burr hole site, the lead connector (behind the ear) and the neurostimulator should be frequently checked.

Troubleshooting

In cases of erosion over the burr hole site, a skin revision is adequate. Sometimes the burr-hole assembly ring and cap is replaced using bone cement and plate to lessen the pressure on the incision. In some centers, lead-cap counter sink is made at the site of burr hole so the protrusion above the scalp is minimal. The connector is placed into a trough drilled into the skull over the parietal region. Previously these troughs were not drilled and the connector was placed behind the ear which would often be a source of irritation for the patient. In cases of erosion over the connector, a new trough is drilled into the skull to relocate the connector (Figure 9). If the erosion occurs over the neurostimulator, a complete revision of the device is performed to relocate it to a deeper tissue plane in the chest [144].

Lead and Neurostimulator Migration

In rare instances, the DBS lead can migrate from its original intended position. The proposed mechanisms relate to inadequate fixation of lead to the skull which matters the most immediately after placement or when the leads are tunneled for placement of the IPG [141 145]. Additionally abnormal pressures, pulling or stretching of the lead system is important. In dystonia, there may be abnormal constant jerking movement of the head that drags the extension cable along with the implantable neurostimulator upwards [146]. Similar dragging may develop in children who have a skull growth after undergoing DBS [147]. With neurostimulator migration, the main reason for the change in subcutaneous position is related to inadequate securing of device at the time of implantation or when patients are obese.

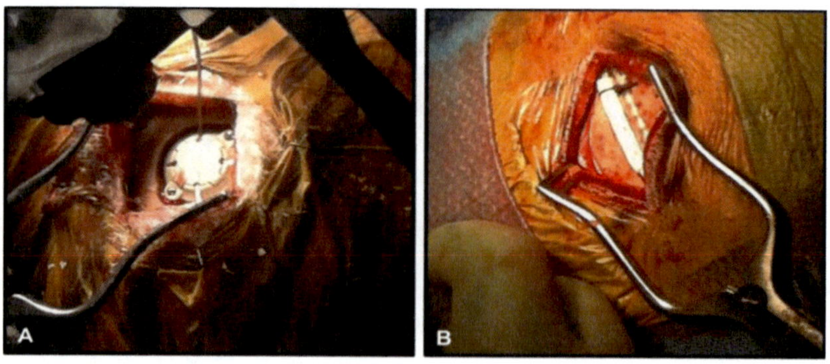

Figure 9. A: Lead-cap countersink.

This picture shows countersink drilled surrounding the burr hole to make lead-cap flush with the outer skull table. This technique aims to reduce risk of aseptic necrosis and eventual scalp erosion.

B: Parietal connector groove.

This picture shows connector groove drilled into parietal bone to connector flush with the outer skull table. This technique aims to reduce risk of aseptic necrosis and eventual scalp erosion.

Prevention

The DBS lead has to be secured carefully at the time of surgery. The burr-hole ring and cap should be anchored properly in the subgaleal space and, if using titanium microplate, caution should be exercised to prevent the lead from getting crushed [148]. When the microplate is used to compress the electrode against the skull, if the screws are not tightened sufficiently, there can be movement of the electrode. Once the lead is anchored, the extra lead wire should be wound around the cap in a loop to minimize any traction effects during pulling [146]. While these steps are followed, prior to closing the scalp incision, intraoperative fluoroscopy is necessary to ensure correct positioning of the DBS lead.

Troubleshooting

DBS lead location can be verified with postoperative radiology. Either a CT scan co-registered with preoperative MRI or at some centers a postoperative MRI scan is performed. If the lead is found to have minimally migrated for example in the dorsal direction, the DBS programmer uses this information to use deeper contacts for programming. If there is significant displacement, the lead is no longer programmable and a surgery to reposition the lead is necessary.

Pain, Discomfort and Neurostimulator Malfunction

Patients may complain of a nagging pain either along the DBS extension or over the neurostimulator. This issue is more likely in thin patients and those with dual channel neurostimulator where there is one tissue tunnel for both lead extensions (36%) rather than a single tunnel for each lead (11%).

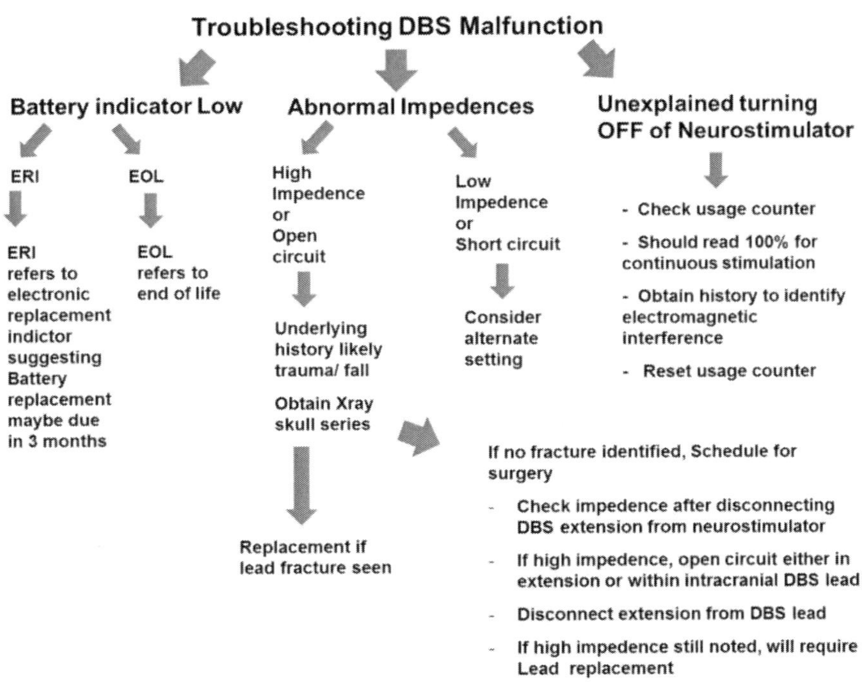

Figure 10. Troubleshooting DBS malfunction. Legend: EOL: end of life; ERI: electronic replacement indicator.

Neurostimulator battery life can range anywhere from 2-4 years. In patients with dystonia where higher voltages and pulse widths are used, battery replacement is required earlier in comparison to patients with essential tremor in whom DBS device maybe turned off every night. If the indicator on the programmer displays electronic replacement indicator or 'ERI', it often means the battery replacement is due in three months whereas end of life or 'EOL' indicates the need for immediate replacement (Figure 10). Neurostimulator malfunction has become rare with the advent newer generation devices. When present, patients will report a sudden loss of efficacy, or sudden "OFF," or a shocking sensation around the stimulator site [141].

Prevention

It may be beneficial to exercise the muscles in the neck region to improve their tolerance for the DBS extension. It might also be preferable to place the neurostimulator in the in the abdomen in thin individuals [149].

Troubleshooting

Topical application of capsaicin cream (0.025-0.075%) over the neurostimulator region was found useful in alleviating discomfort by one DBS group. The neurostimulator may require repositioning if initial simple measures fail [103]. In cases of 'ERI' or 'EOL', it is necessary to make arrangements for battery replacement. In neurostimulator malfunction, obtain history for electromagnetic interference.

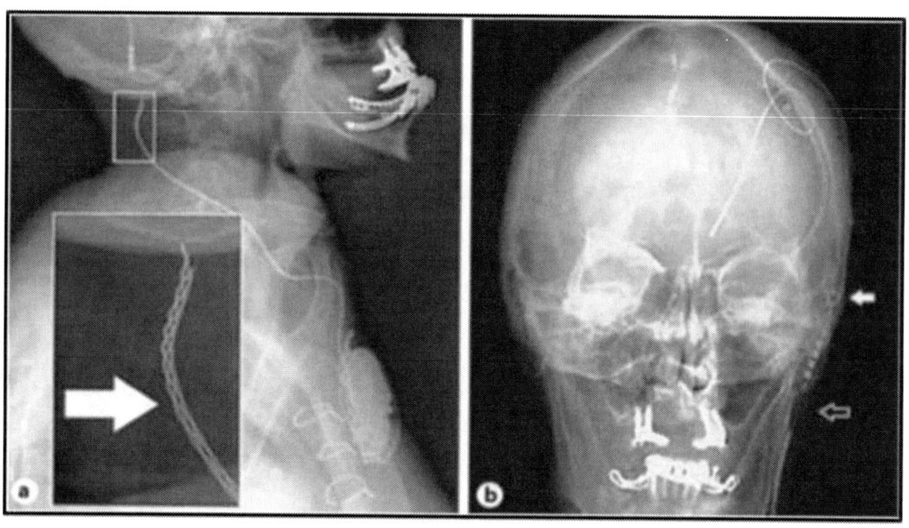

Figure 11. X-ray showing extension cable breakage right after connector in twiddler syndrome patient. This patient underwent to X-ray examination because of loss of DBS therapy benefit. a: On lateral Xray skull, the extension cable shows a severely twisted, braided pattern (inserted arrow) beneath the connector from which it has separated. b: AP skull radiograph showing the second instance of extension cable fracture. Note the braided extension cable beneath the break (open arrow) and the knotted coil in the cranial lead superior to the connector (solid arrow).

DBS Lead Break or Fracture

The common location for the DBS lead break or fracture is over the mastoid where the lead connector is connected to the DBS brain lead [145]. A common reason for DBS leads or wire to fracture is jerky movements of the head in cervical dystonia patients or head snap tics in Tourette's syndrome. The incidence of lead wire break is about 5.1% [137]. Sometimes, these fractures are symptomatic and patients report electric shock like sensations at the site of open circuit. Parkinson's disease patients may suffer from impulse control disorders and within this context trichotillomania and twiddler's syndrome are important [150] (Figure 11). In the twiddler's syndrome, the patient subconsciously spins the neurostimulator in the chest wall; as a result, the lead wire is brought under tension and may develop fracture [151, 152].

Prevention

Due to possibility of lead fracture some centers have begun to mount the DBS lead connector on the skull (parietal subgalea) and not over the mastoid.

Troubleshooting

In routine DBS programming, impedance at each electrode contact and current drain is checked. A low impedance and high current drain indicates a short circuit and high impedance and a low current drain indicates an open circuit [152]. If an open circuit is found, a plain X ray film series is performed to identify the site of fracture. In patients with twiddler's syndrome, when the neurostimulator is relocated, the contralateral side is selected; the device is placed under the pectoralis muscle fascia and sutured to the muscle. A Parsonnet pouch is used to prevent the lead wire break [153]. (Figure 10)

Stimulation-Related Side-Effects

The detailed mechanisms of action for DBS are still not known and are certainly multifaceted. The acute effects probably relate to the electrical modulation of the nuclei and network fibers that are anatomically related whereas long-term effects probably relate to adaptive neuroplasticity change. The same rationale may also apply to DBS induced side-effects. As discussed in the preceding sections, the acute effect of the lead impact (lesion effect) and the DBS threshold provides indirect information on DBS lead placement accuracy useful during the initial programming. If there are no benefits with acute stimulation for example as seen in dystonia and OCD, only the side-effects are used for programming. The anatomically based stimulation side effects of different targets are summarized in the table 2, 3 and 4.

Side Effects Related to Stimulation of VIM

When the lead placement is appropriate it is expected that tremor suppression can be obtained at voltage levels below the threshold for side-effects. The side-effects related to the electrical current spreading to the structures surrounding the VIM are summarized in the Table 2.

Muscle Contraction

Muscle contractions in the body parts or face contralateral to the side of stimulation are seen with current spreading to internal capsule fibers that are lateral and ventral to the VIM [15, 154].

Paresthesia

Current spreading to the Vc nucleus of thalamus (posterior to the VIM) or lemniscal pathway (ventral and posterior to the VIM), causes abnormal feelings including tingling and numbness on the side contralateral to brain stimulation [15, 155, 156].

Dysarthria

Dysarthria is caused by stimulation of internal capsule fibers (that are lateral and ventral to VIM) in relation to oropharynx muscles [15,157,158]. Dysarthria is more often seen with bilateral VIM stimulation in approximately 5-25% of patients [15, 159].

Ataxia and Balance Instability

Ataxia and balance difficulties results from current spreading to brachium conjunctivum (cerebellar fibers) that is ventral and medial to VIM [18, 157-160].The symptoms are more associated with bilateral VIM stimulation [15].

Mood Impairment and Suicide

Only two patients in essential tremor patients undergoing Vim DBS have reportedly committed suicide. One patient described by Borretzen et al. [161] was a 73 year old man, without prior history of psychiatric disease, and excellent tremor suppression. The second patient, reported by Burkhard and cols [162] was a 69 years old female with history of severe depression, who experienced a remarkable improvement of motor function followed VIM DBS surgery.

Troubleshooting of Side Effects Related VIM Stimulation

These side-effects may be reversed by adjusting the stimulation parameter settings [15] or by reduction in the stimulation levels (lower voltage and/pulse width), or by changing the electrode configuration to the bipolar mode. Patients with bilateral DBS showing a significant dysarthria or gait disturbance may consider the strategy to turn off one side when speaking or walking and turn on both sides when not engaged in walking and using both hands. In our experience, the use of a lower stimulation frequency can also alleviate gait and balance side effects.

Side Effects Related to Stimulation of STN

The side-effects related to the electrical current spreading to the structures surrounding the STN are summarized in Table 3.

Muscle Contraction

The dorsolateral aspect of the subthalamic nucleus borders the internal capsule. Patients may experience contralateral tightening or tonic contraction of muscles when the stimulation spreads to the internal capsule [27,163].

Table 2. Side-effects related to Vim-surrounding structures stimulation

Anatomic relation to the Vim[a]	Structure	Observed side-effects (usually seen on the contralateral side)
Lateral	Posterior limb of internal capsule	Muscle contractions, dysarthria, facial pulling
Medial	Medial part of Vim	Dysarthria
	Central median nucleus of thalamus	None
Anterior	Voa nucleus[b]	Sometimes reduces tremors with high voltages
	Vop nucleus[c] (posterior to Voa)	None
Posterior	Vc nucleus[d]	Paresthesia
Ventral	Internal capsule	Muscle contractions, dysarthria
	Medial lemniscus	Paresthesia
	Zona incerta	None
	Cerebellar fibers	Ataxia
Dorsal	Ventricle	None

[a] Vim Ventral intermedius nucleus VIM. Also called ventrolateral nucleus of thalamus.
[b] Voa Ventral anterior nucleus
[C] Vop Ventral posterior lateral nucleus of thalamus.
[d] Vc Ventralis caudalis nucleus

Troubleshooting

These muscle contractions can be controlled by reprogramming to a lower stimulation amplitude, changing the electrode configuration and, in worst situations, repositioning of DBS lead more medially should be considered.

Sensory Discomfort/Paresthesia

The medial meniscus is one of the main ascending sensory pathways and is located on the medial and ventroposterior aspect of STN. If the lead is malpositioned or the stimulation intensity are high enough to stimulate the medial lemniscus, paresthesia are experienced.

Troubleshooting

Adjustment of stimulation parameters or electrode configuration is required and usually sufficient to resolved this problem [27].

Dyskinesia

STN DBS can trigger immediate choreiform, ballistic, or dystonic movements that may resemble levodopa-induced dyskinesias [164, 165]. Stimulation of STN may induce dyskinesia which indicates the DBS lead is well positioned in the motor region of the STN. These dyskinesias may not necessarily be seen immediately after stimulation change is made and instead may develop hours later. DBS programmer and the patient should both be vigilant. Sometimes, these dyskinesias are seen in the operating room at the time of lead placement. Similar to any lesion effect, these dyskinesia resolve over weeks to months

[107,166]. The contact that produces dyskinesias is generally the most effective contact for the relief of akinetic–rigid symptoms. Since stimulation-induced dyskinesias are worsened by levodopa, initial programming should be performed before the morning medication dose. Low dosages of levodopa can be resumed if, after a few hours following programming, there is no appearance of dyskinesias.

Troubleshooting

In case of stimulation induced dyskinesia it is necessary to balance stimulation parameters or reduce the dopaminergic medication dose. If dyskinesia is related to lesion effect, it is necessary to wait.

Dysarthria/Dysphonia

Chronic stimulation with bilateral STN DBS has been found to worsen speech. The prevalence of speech disturbance has ranged from 4-17% [167]. Dysarthria is attributed to the spread of stimulation to the internal capsule, though some believe it is related to the stimulation of the zona incerta. In Parkinson's disease, speech impairment may be related to progression of disease.

Table 3. Side-effects related to stimulation of STN-surrounding anatomical structures

Anatomic relation to the STN [a]	Structure	Observed side-effects (usually seen on the contralateral side)
Lateral	Corticospinal fibers of the internal capsule	Muscle contractions
	Corticobulbar fibers of the internal capsule	Dysarthria and facial pulling
	Frontal eye field fibers of the internal capsule	Conjugated gaze deviation (contra-lateral)
Medial	Limbic STN	Personality changes, impulsivity, mood symptoms
	III Cranial nerve roots	Dizziness, dys-conjugated ipsilateral eye deviation, diplopia, eye lid open apraxia
	Red nucleus	Warm sensations, nausea and diaphoresis
Anterior and medial	Hypothalamus	Autonomic dysfunction (sweating, flushing)
Anterior and lateral	Corticospinal fibers of the internal capsule	Muscle contractions
	Corticobulbar fibers of the internal capsule	Dysarthria and facial pulling
Posterior	Medial lemniscus	Paresthesia
Ventral to STN	Substantia nigra	Mood symptoms, akinesia
	Internal capsule	Muscle contractions
Dorsal to STN	Zona incerta	None

[a] STN: Subthalamic nucleus.

Troubleshooting

A combined approach with adjustment of stimulation parameters (lower frequency might be particularly beneficial) and speech therapy may be helpful in these circumstances [168]. Since this complication is usually related to bilateral stimulation of STN, turning off one side on a temporary basis may also be needed to avoid this side effect during speaking. In Parkinson's disease patients, an increased dose of dopaminergic medications may be tried for treatment of post DBS dysarthria.

Gait Impairment/Postural Instability

In Parkinson's disease, these symptoms are related to nondopaminergic systems. STN DBS has shown mixed effects on gait and balance. Although many studies have observed improvement with STN DBS some have shown there is a decline in gait and postural stability[169][170-172] Long-term deterioration of axial symptoms after STN DBS has been attributed to the underlying disease progression and the effects of nondopaminergic pathways. Sometimes, there is medial spread of stimulation current involving the red nucleus and the cerebellar fibers causing truncal ataxia, and these complications can be resolved only with repositioning of the lead.

Troubleshooting

Physical and occupational therapy are often helpful in these circumstances. It is also important to adjust the stimulation parameters and medications for management of gait and postural impairment. As detailed in chapter 6, lower frequency of stimulation with concomitant increase in amplitude might be beneficial.

Abnormal Eye Movement/Diplopia

The overall incidence of severe eye movement disturbances in STN DBS appears to be low [160, 163]. The oculomotor nerve is anatomically located medial to the STN, and induces double vision (diplopia) or ipsilateral ocular deviation (dysconjugate gaze) when stimulated. These symptoms may not habituate therefore revision of the electrode position is necessary. In contrast, conjugate eye deviation reflects spread of stimulation current to the internal capsule and may improve with adjustment of stimulation parameters [163, 173]. Ipsilateral eye deviation has never been reported to occur in GPi DBS or Vim DBS.

Apraxia of Eyelid Opening

Several STN DBS studies in PD have reported eyelid opening apraxia in 1.8% to 30% of the patients [108, 112, 174]. Patients report difficulty in opening their eyes despite normal eyelid function. The underlying etiology is not well defined, but an association with blepharospasm and some response to Botulinum toxin injections suggests it may be some form of focal dystonia [175]. This complication may occur early after surgery, may either spontaneously improve, or may persist in the long term [108, 176].

Weight Gain

Weight gain has been reported in PD patients after DBS with an incidence of 6% to 100% after STN DBS [108, 177, 178], and 26% to 96% after GPi DBS [47]. It has not been reported after Vim DBS. The underlying reason for weight gain is not clear but there are several speculations such as1) improvement of dyskinesia with STN DBS results in lowering of energy expenditure 2) lowering of dopaminergic medication dose may increase the appetite for food intake 3) improvement in physical activities and normalization of metabolism 4) Stimulation of the appetite center in the hypothalamus located anterior to STN due to spread of electrical current. The extent of weight gain may be higher with STN DBS [179, 179, 180] than in GPi DBS [181].

Troubleshooting

Patients should be made aware, counseled on dietary habits and encouraged for physical activities.

Hypersexuality

There are suggestions that STN DBS, particularly in men with PD, results in increased excitation, increased frequency and increased satisfaction [182-184]. These complications have not been reported in women and the mechanism underlying this complication is not clear.

Troubleshooting

A reduction of dopaminergic medications, particularly the dose of dopamine agonists is recommended along with lowering of stimulation amplitude or selection of more dorsal contact. In one study, a trial of donepezil was found effective in control of these symptoms.

Neuropsychiatric Complications

In the immediate postoperative phase, transient confusion develops in 1-36% of cases and improves spontaneously over time Therefore, reassurance is enough.

Anxiety affects 60-75% of PD patients and frequently co-occurs with depression, panic attacks and phobia. It is also well documented after STN DBS surgery [185,186]. Management of anxiety is often accomplished with benzodiazepines, selective serotonin reuptake inhibitor agents (SSRI) and cognitive behavioral therapy.

Apathy is a well reported complication after STN DBS therapy seen approximately in 12-25% of cases, mostly in PD [108]. Apathy is brought about either by lowering of dopaminergic medications or maybe related to natural progression of the disease similar to that seen with depression.

Depression in PD is frequent and is seen in more than 50% of cases. However, it may present as a DBS related complication in nearly 25% of cases [108, 178]. There are several factors such as the natural history of PD, lowering of dopaminergic medications after surgery, spread of stimulation to the medial limbic system and unrealistic patient expectations that contribute to depression [187].

Apathy and depression are both managed by an increase in dopaminergic medication doses, a decrease in the stimulation amplitude and the administration of medications which are efficacious in controlling apathy and depression [107, 178]. While apathy and depression are common, hypomania also occurs in about 5-15% cases and improves with a decrease in the dose of dopaminergic medications, as well as a trial of antidepressants and mood stabilizers.

Several case reports and observational studies have suggested an association between DBS treatment and suicide attempts or completed suicides in patients with Parkinson's disease [31, 60-62]. In an international multicenter retrospective survey involving 55 centers and 5311 patients, the percentage of patients committing suicide following STN DBS surgery for Parkinson's disease was 0.5% and that of attempted suicide was 0.9%. After adjustments for expected age, gender and country, the standardized Mortality Ratio (SMR) for suicide in the first postoperative year of STN DBS surgery were 12.6–15.6 higher ($p < 0.001$) than that expected by the World Health Organization. Although prior use of antidepressant medications did not influence the prevalence of suicidal behavior however they found a larger reduction in dopaminergic medications seemed to increase the rate. Weintraub et al. examined the results of a large randomized VA study and found that suicidal ideation and behavior were similar in the DBS and best medication management cohorts when these were compared at six months follow-up. The authors postulated that a smaller reduction of dopaminergic medications seen postoperatively may have prevented the development of suicide [188]. These studies collectively suggest that significant medical and psychiatric comorbidities including the presence of pre-and postoperative depression, larger decreases in dopaminergic medications, and other general risk factors may be associated with an increased risk for suicidal behavior post-DBS surgery.

The relative rarity of these events makes it difficult to identify the associated risk factors for suicide in DBS treated patients. The mechanisms related for a putative association between DBS and suicide are not understood, and could involve in part the stimulation itself as well the decreased need for caregivers leaving the patient with less monitoring. Based on the accumulating data the careful pre-surgical evaluation by a multidisciplinary approach is the best approach to identify potential general risk factors for suicide in DBS candidates. A special recommendation for Parkinson's disease includes avoidance of sudden large decreases in dopaminergic medications and adequate treatment of medical and major psychiatric comorbidities. Patients with a history of suicide attempts or suicidality deserve closer follow up by carriers and the multidisciplinary team.

In contrast to apathy and depression after STN DBS that responds to increased doses of dopaminergic medications, impulse control disorder after STN DBS (manifesting as hypersexuality, pathological gambling, binge eating and compulsive shopping) requires a decrease in these medications.

Finally, psychosis and hallucinations are reported to develop in approximately 12-15% of cases after DBS surgery, requiring adjustment of stimulation parameters such as possibly the use of more dorsal contacts and lowering of dopaminergic medication doses [189].

Side Effects Related to Stimulation of STN in the Context of OCD

Various stimulation-related adverse events (AEs), mostly neuropsychiatric effects including anxiety, obsessions, manic symptoms, depressive symptoms, and suicidal ideation, have been reported for STN DBS in OCD [41]. Chabardes and colleagues reported that mood changes, especially hypomania, were commonly observed in the acute phase of stimulation, and that mood changes seemed to wane over time [49]. Motor contractions probably related to the stimulation of the internal capsule were reported in a recent study following chronic STN stimulation [49]. Being a small target with dense connectivity, STN DBS e has been hypothesized to contribute to cognitive impairment in OCD, similarly to what is observed after Parkinson's disease [190]. In addition, STN DBS in OCD induces mirthful laughter [191] though less frequently than VC/VS target stimulation. The smile response has not been documented or studied in detail for STN DBS.

Table 4. Side-effects related to stimulation of Gpi surrounding anatomical structures

Anatomic relation to the GPi[a]	Structure	Observed side-effects on the contralateral side
Anterior and lateral	GPe [b]	None
	Putamen (lateral and anterior to GPe)	None
Posterior and medial	Posterior limb of the internal capsule	Muscle contractions
Ventral to GPi	Optic tract	Flashing lights in the contra-lateral visual field
Dorsal to GPi	GPe	None

[a] GPi Globus pallidus interna

[b] GPe Globus pallidus externa

Side Effects Related to Stimulation of GPi

The side-effects related to the electrical current spreading to the structures surrounding the Gpi are summarized in Table 4.

Muscle Contraction

The optimal target for stimulation is located in the postero-ventro-lateral region of GPi. Since the internal capsule is located posteriorly and medially, patients can experience tonic contraction of contralateral muscles if the lead is not placed accurately or with high energy stimulation [154].

Troubleshooting

It may be important to distinguish these tonic contractions of muscles from dystonia, before stimulation amplitudes and pulse widths are lowered or there is a change in configuration. If the internal capsule continues to remain stimulated even at low thresholds, repositioning of the lead more anteriorly or laterally may be needed.

Dysarthria/Dysphagia

At our center, we retrospectively analyzed the swallowing outcomes after STN DBS and GPi DBS [192]. We found there was a significant worsening of swallowing only with STN stimulation and not with GPi. In comparison to other targets such as the STN and VIM, stimulation of GPi is less frequently associated with these complications. The speculations proposed for these differential effects of GPi and STN stimulation include 1) increased likelihood of stimulating the internal capsule since STN is a smaller target; 2) GPi and STN have opposite effects on the pedunculopontine nucleus with the former inhibiting the nucleus and the latter exhibiting excitatory effects. Indeed, the pedunculopontine nucleus has modulatory effects on the swallowing centers located in the brainstem

Troubleshooting

We recommend a trial of lowering the stimulation amplitude in combination with speech and swallowing therapy for management of this complication

Visual Phenomenon

The ventral border of GPi, consisting of the optic tract, is determined during the intraoperative microelectrode recording. Stimulation of the optic tract manifests as seeing sparkles of light (phosphenes) in the contralateral visual field. Spread of electrical current to this region is usually seen when the electrode is placed close to this region or when higher stimulation doses are used [193].

Troubleshooting

Using a more dorsal stimulation contact, lowering the total stimulation dose or repositioning the DBS electrode is required for management of this complication [27].

Neuropsychiatric Complication

The GPi DBS appears to be safe in dystonia patients who have mild to moderate depression [194] however, suicides have been documented among three male patients with dystonia, aged 26, 44 and 53 years, with DBS surgery [162, 195]. Further work is needed to clarify association between GPi DBS, depression and suicide in patients with dystonia.

Side Effects Related to Stimulation of ALIC and VC/VS

Stimulation-related adverse events may vary widely across OCD individuals undergoing DBS in this target. The differences observed in phenomena may be explained by the differences in lead locations, fiber bundle locations, and anatomic variations even though the same targeting method has been utilized. In some cases, stimulation-related adverse events are temporary and do not require a change in the stimulation parameters [46].

In VC/VS stimulation, temporary adverse events related to stimulation include muscle tightness associated with dysarthria, olfactory hallucinations, and gustatory sensations [46][66]. Olfactory and gustatory responses are associated with activation of the most ventral (deep) contacts [57] that stimulate the medial olfactory stria. Hypomania, anxiety, and fear are additional symptoms resulting with activation of the ventral contacts [57]. Euphoria and hypomania thought to be related to spread of current to the hypothalamus and possibly the amygdalo-fugal pathways [57] are the most worrisome side effects. Therefore caution is needed when programming this region and patients and caregivers require proper counselling. If the side effects develop, the use of a more dorsal stimulation contact is warranted.

Side Effects Related to Stimulation of ITP in the Context of OCD

In a single ITP DBS study in OCD, Jimenez-Ponce and colleagues reported the development of transient confusion when dorsal (upper) contacts were activated. They also reported anxiety and autonomic symptoms when the ventral (lower) contacts were chosen for stimulation [51]. According to the side effect observed, the use of a more dorsal or ventral stimulation contact is warranted.

Side Effects Related to Stimulation of CM/Pf

As discussed in previous sections, this target has been used for stimulation in Tourette's syndrome. The acute stimulation side effects of CM/Pf are usually experienced during the determination of thresholds. Many patients report nausea, dizziness, vertigo, headaches, sensation of warmth and a weird metallic taste. Some patients report tingling and numbness due to the spread of current to the sensory thalamus. Occasionally patients experience pulling sensation and heaviness with further lateral spread of stimulation into the internal capsule. Based on these side effects, the DBS programmer determines the electrode contact with the lowest threshold for inducing a benefit and the largest therapeutic width (i.e., highest threshold for side effects) for final chronic stimulation.

There are very few reports of side effects related to CM-Pf stimulation. A decrease in energy level [78, 196], sexual dysfunction [76, 78, 196] and weight loss are examples of chronic stimulation-related side effects seen with CM/Pf DBS but no clear correlation to specific anatomical structures or stimulation parameters has been established.

Conclusion

Indications for DBS surgery have shown a continual increase since its inception. The clinical effectiveness of DBS depends on several interrelated factors such as target selection, accuracy of lead location, type of stimulation selected and the expertise and experience in DBS programming. Other issues affecting clinical effectiveness such as poor patient selection, disease progression, unrealistic patient expectation and poor access to DBS programming also require due consideration. Although general guidelines for DBS programming have been laid out, there are differences pertaining to individual conditions which should be kept in mind and followed for an effective programming. DBS related complications are broadly categorized into those related to the surgical procedure, those stemming from DBS device and those seen in relation to stimulation itself. With an increasing experience in DBS, most complications in each of these categories can be managed with reasonable satisfaction if a systematic approach is followed.

Acknowledgments

This work was supported by the University of Florida, CTSI sponsored NIH KL2 TR000065 (AWS) and was supported by the program "Sciences without Borders" of Brazilian National Council for Scientific and Technology Development, CNPq: 205429/2014-9 (RW).

References

[1] Schuepbach, WM; Rau, J; Knudsen, K; Volkmann, J; Krack, P; Timmermann, L; et al. Neurostimulation for Parkinson's disease with early motor complications. *N Engl J Med*, 2013 Feb 14, 368(7), 610-22.

[2] Vidailhet, M; Vercueil, L; Houeto, JL; Krystkowiak, P; Lagrange, C; Yelnik, J; et al. Bilateral, pallidal, deep-brain stimulation in primary generalised dystonia: a prospective 3 year follow-up study. *Lancet Neurol*, 2007 Mar, 6(3), 223-9.

[3] Zhang, K; Bhatia, S; Oh, MY; Cohen, D; Angle, C; Whiting, D. Long-term results of thalamic deep brain stimulation for essential tremor. *J Neurosurg*, 2010 Jun, 112(6), 1271-6.

[4] Morishita, T; Fayad, SM; Goodman, WK; Foote, KD; Chen, D; Peace, DA; et al. Surgical neuroanatomy and programming in deep brain stimulation for obsessive compulsive disorder. *Neuromodulation*, 2014 Jun, 17(4), 312, 9, discussion 319.

[5] Schrock, LE; Mink, JW; Woods, DW; Porta, M; Servello, D; Visser-Vandewalle, V; et al. Tourette syndrome deep brain stimulation: A review and updated recommendations. *Mov Disord*, 2014 Dec 5.

[6] Williams, NR; Okun, MS. Deep brain stimulation (DBS) at the interface of neurology and psychiatry. *J Clin Invest*, 2013 Nov 1, 123(11), 4546-56.

[7] Laxton, AW; Tang-Wai, DF; McAndrews, MP; Zumsteg, D; Wennberg, R; Keren, R; et al. A phase I trial of deep brain stimulation of memory circuits in Alzheimer's disease. *Ann Neurol*, 2010 Oct, 68(4), 521-34.

[8] Torres, CV; Sola, RG; Pastor, J; Pedrosa, M; Navas, M; Garcia-Navarrete, E; et al. Long-term results of posteromedial hypothalamic deep brain stimulation for patients with resistant aggressiveness. *J Neurosurg*, 2013 Aug, 119(2), 277-87.

[9] Voges, J; Muller, U; Bogerts, B; Munte, T; Heinze, HJ. Deep brain stimulation surgery for alcohol addiction. *World Neurosurg*, 2013 Sep-Oct, 80(3-4), S28.e21-31.

[10] Zhou, H; Xu, J; Jiang, J. Deep brain stimulation of nucleus accumbens on heroin-seeking behaviors: a case report. *Biol Psychiatry*, 2011 Jun 1, 69(11), e41-2.

[11] Whiting, DM; Tomycz, ND; Bailes, J; de Jonge, L; Lecoultre, V; Wilent, B; et al. Lateral hypothalamic area deep brain stimulation for refractory obesity: a pilot study with preliminary data on safety, body weight, and energy metabolism. *J Neurosurg*, 2013 Jul, 119(1), 56-63.

[12] Lipsman, N; Woodside, DB; Giacobbe, P; Hamani, C; Carter, JC; Norwood, SJ; et al. Subcallosal cingulate deep brain stimulation for treatment-refractory anorexia nervosa: a phase 1 pilot trial. *Lancet*, 2013 Apr 20, 381(9875), 1361-70.

[13] Fisher, R; Salanova, V; Witt, T; Worth, R; Henry, T; Gross, R; et al. Electrical stimulation of the anterior nucleus of thalamus for treatment of refractory epilepsy. *Epilepsia*, 2010 May, 51(5), 899-908.

[14] Zesiewicz, TA; Elble, R; Louis, ED; Hauser, RA; Sullivan, KL; Dewey, RB, Jr; et al. Practice parameter: therapies for essential tremor: report of the Quality Standards Subcommittee of the American Academy of Neurology. *Neurology*, 2005 Jun 28, 64(12), 2008-20.

[15] Lyons, KE; Pahwa, R. Deep brain stimulation and tremor. *Neurotherapeutics*, 2008 Apr, 5(2), 331-8.

[16] Moscovich, M; Morishita, T; Foote, KD; Favilla, CG; Chen, ZP; Okun, MS. Effect of lead trajectory on the response of essential head tremor to deep brain stimulation. *Parkinsonism Relat Disord*, 2013 Sep, 19(9), 789-94.

[17] Martinez-Ramirez, D; Morishita, T; Zeilman, PR; Peng-Chen, Z; Foote KD; Okun, MS. Atrophy and other potential factors affecting long term deep brain stimulation response: a case series. *PLoS One*, 2014 Oct 31, 9(10), e111561.

[18] Benabid, AL; Pollak, P; Gao, D; Hoffmann, D; Limousin, P; Gay, E; et al. Chronic electrical stimulation of the ventralis intermedius nucleus of the thalamus as a treatment of movement disorders. *J Neurosurg*, 1996 Feb, 84(2), 203-14.

[19] Sydow, O; Thobois, S; Alesch, F; Speelman, JD. Multicentre European study of thalamic stimulation in essential tremor: a six year follow up. *J Neurol Neurosurg Psychiatry*, 2003 Oct, 74(10), 1387-91.

[20] Pilitsis, JG; Metman, LV; Toleikis, JR; Hughes, LE; Sani, SB; Bakay, RA. Factors involved in long-term efficacy of deep brain stimulation of the thalamus for essential tremor. *J Neurosurg*, 2008 Oct, 109(4), 640-6.

[21] Favilla, CG; Ullman, D; Wagle Shukla, A; Foote, KD; Jacobson, CE; 4th; Okun, MS. Worsening essential tremor following deep brain stimulation: disease progression versus tolerance. *Brain*, 2012 May, 135(Pt 5), 1455-62.

[22] Kumar, R. Methods for programming and patient management with deep brain stimulation of the globus pallidus for the treatment of advanced Parkinson's disease and dystonia. *Mov Disord*, 2002, 17 Suppl 3, S198-207.

[23] Volkmann, J; Moro, E; Pahwa, R. Basic algorithms for the programming of deep brain stimulation in Parkinson's disease. *Mov Disord*, 2006 Jun, 21 Suppl 14, S284-9.

[24] Volkmann, J; Herzog, J; Kopper, F; Deuschl, G. Introduction to the programming of deep brain stimulators. *Mov Disord*, 2002, 17 Suppl 3, S181-7.

[25] Favilla, CG; Topiol, DD; Zesiewicz, TA; Wagle Shukla, A; Foote, KD; Jacobson, CE; 4th; et al. Impact of discontinuing tremor suppressing medications following thalamic deep brain stimulation. *Parkinsonism Relat Disord*, 2013 Feb, 19(2), 171-5.

[26] Okun, MS; Tagliati, M; Pourfar, M; Fernandez, HH; Rodriguez, RL; Alterman, RL; et al. Management of referred deep brain stimulation failures: a retrospective analysis from 2 movement disorders centers. *Arch Neurol*, 2005 Aug, 62(8), 1250-5.

[27] Deuschl, G; Herzog, J; Kleiner-Fisman, G; Kubu, C; Lozano, AM; Lyons, KE; et al. Deep brain stimulation: postoperative issues. *Mov Disord*, 2006 Jun, 21 Suppl 14, S219-37.

[28] Connolly, BS; Lang, AE. Pharmacological treatment of Parkinson disease: a review. *JAMA*, 2014 Apr 23-30, 311(16), 1670-83.

[29] Wagle Shukla, A; Okun MS. Surgical Treatment of Parkinson's Disease: Patients, Targets, Devices, and Approaches. *Neurotherapeutics*, 2013 Nov 7.

[30] Lang, AE; Houeto, JL; Krack, P; Kubu, C; Lyons, KE; Moro, E; et al. Deep brain stimulation: preoperative issues. *Mov Disord*, 2006 Jun, 21 Suppl 14, S171-96.

[31] Burke, RE; Fahn, S; Marsden, CD. Torsion dystonia: a double-blind, prospective trial of high-dosage trihexyphenidyl. *Neurology*, 1986 Feb, 36(2), 160-4.

[32] Thenganatt, MA; Jankovic, J. Treatment of dystonia. *Neurotherapeutics*, 2014 Jan, 11(1), 139-52.

[33] Ostrem, JL; Starr, PA. Treatment of dystonia with deep brain stimulation. *Neurotherapeutics*, 2008 Apr, 5(2), 320-30.

[34] Iansek, R; Porter, R. The monkey globus pallidus: neuronal discharge properties in relation to movement. *J Physiol*, 1980 Apr, 301, 439-55.

[35] Bejjani, BP; Damier, P; Arnulf, I; Papadopoulos, S; Bonnet, AM; Vidailhet, M; et al. Deep brain stimulation in Parkinson's disease: opposite effects of stimulation in the pallidum. *Mov Disord*, 1998 Nov, 13(6), 969-70.

[36] Tisch, S; Zrinzo, L; Limousin, P; Bhatia, KP; Quinn, N; Ashkan, K; et al. Effect of electrode contact location on clinical efficacy of pallidal deep brain stimulation in primary generalised dystonia. *J Neurol Neurosurg Psychiatry*, 2007 Dec, 78(12), 1314-9.

[37] Vayssiere, N; van der Gaag, N; Cif, L; Hemm, S; Verdier, R; Frerebeau, P; et al. Deep brain stimulation for dystonia confirming a somatotopic organization in the globus pallidus internus. *J Neurosurg*, 2004 Aug, 101(2), 181-8.

[38] Kupsch, A; Tagliati, M; Vidailhet, M; Aziz, T; Krack, P; Moro, E; et al. Early postoperative management of DBS in dystonia: programming, response to stimulation, adverse events, medication changes, evaluations, and troubleshooting. *Mov Disord*, 2011 Jun, 26 Suppl 1, S37-53.

[39] Starr, PA; Turner, RS; Rau, G; Lindsey, N; Heath, S; Volz, M; et al. Microelectrode-guided implantation of deep brain stimulators into the globus pallidus internus for dystonia: techniques, electrode locations, and outcomes. *J Neurosurg*, 2006 Apr, 104(4), 488-501.

[40] Isaias, IU; Alterman, RL; Tagliati, M. Deep brain stimulation for primary generalized dystonia: long-term outcomes. *Arch Neurol*, 2009 Apr, 66(4), 465-70.

[41] Mallet, L; Polosan, M; Jaafari, N; Baup, N; Welter, ML; Fontaine, D; et al. Subthalamic nucleus stimulation in severe obsessive-compulsive disorder. *N Engl J Med*, 2008 Nov 13, 359(20), 2121-34.

[42] Nuttin, B; Cosyns, P; Demeulemeester, H; Gybels, J; Meyerson, B. Electrical stimulation in anterior limbs of internal capsules in patients with obsessive-compulsive disorder. *Lancet*, 1999 Oct 30, 354(9189), 1526.

[43] Voorn, P; Brady, LS; Berendse, HW; Richfield, EK. Densitometrical analysis of opioid receptor ligand binding in the human striatum--I. Distribution of mu opioid receptor defines shell and core of the ventral striatum. *Neuroscience*, 1996 Dec, 75(3), 777-92.

[44] Anderson, D; Ahmed, A. Treatment of patients with intractable obsessive-compulsive disorder with anterior capsular stimulation. Case report. *J Neurosurg*, 2003 May, 98(5), 1104-8.

[45] Abelson, JL; Curtis, GC; Sagher, O; Albucher, RC; Harrigan, M; Taylor, SF; et al. Deep brain stimulation for refractory obsessive-compulsive disorder. *Biol Psychiatry*, 2005 Mar 1, 57(5), 510-6.

[46] Greenberg, BD; Malone, DA; Friehs, GM; Rezai, AR; Kubu, CS; Malloy, PF; et al. Three-year outcomes in deep brain stimulation for highly resistant obsessive-compulsive disorder. *Neuropsychopharmacology*, 2006 Nov, 31(11), 2384-93.

[47] Goodman, WK; Foote, KD; Greenberg, BD; Ricciuti, N; Bauer, R; Ward, H; et al. Deep brain stimulation for intractable obsessive compulsive disorder: pilot study using a blinded, staggered-onset design. *Biol Psychiatry*, 2010 Mar 15, 67(6), 535-42.

[48] Fontaine, D; Mattei, V; Borg, M; von Langsdorff, D; Magnie, MN; Chanalet, S; et al. Effect of subthalamic nucleus stimulation on obsessive-compulsive disorder in a patient with Parkinson disease. Case report. *J Neurosurg*, 2004 Jun, 100(6), 1084-6.

[49] Chabardes, S; Polosan, M; Krack, P; Bastin, J; Krainik, A; David, O; et al. Deep brain stimulation for obsessive-compulsive disorder: subthalamic nucleus target. *World Neurosurg*, 2013 Sep-Oct, 80(3-4), S31.e1-8.

[50] Jimenez, F; Velasco, F; Salin-Pascual, R; Velasco, M; Nicolini, H; Velasco, AL; et al. Neuromodulation of the inferior thalamic peduncle for major depression and obsessive compulsive disorder. *Acta Neurochir*, Suppl 2007, 97(Pt 2), 393-8.

[51] Jimenez-Ponce, F; Velasco-Campos, F; Castro-Farfan, G; Nicolini, H; Velasco, AL; Salin-Pascual, R; et al. Preliminary study in patients with obsessive-compulsive disorder treated with electrical stimulation in the inferior thalamic peduncle. *Neurosurgery.*, 2009 Dec, 65(6 Suppl), 203, 9, discussion 209.

[52] Huff, W; Lenartz, D; Schormann, M; Lee, SH; Kuhn, J; Koulousakis, A; et al. Unilateral deep brain stimulation of the nucleus accumbens in patients with treatment-

resistant obsessive-compulsive disorder: Outcomes after one year. *Clin Neurol Neurosurg*, 2010 Feb, 112(2), 137-43.

[53] Aouizerate, B; Guehl, D; Cuny E; Rougier A; Bioulac B; Tignol J; et al. Pathophysiology of obsessive-compulsive disorder: a necessary link between phenomenology, neuropsychology, imagery and physiology. *Prog Neurobiol*, 2004 Feb, 72(3), 195-221.

[54] Aouizerate, B; Cuny, E; Bardinet, E; Yelnik, J; Martin-Guehl, C; Rotge, JY; et al. Distinct striatal targets in treating obsessive-compulsive disorder and major depression. *J Neurosurg*, 2009 Oct, 111(4), 775-9.

[55] Kopell, BH; Greenberg, B; Rezai, AR. Deep brain stimulation for psychiatric disorders. *J Clin Neurophysiol*, 2004 Jan-Feb, 21(1), 51-67.

[56] Greenberg, BD; Gabriels, LA; Malone, DA, Jr; Rezai, AR; Friehs, GM; Okun, MS; et al. Deep brain stimulation of the ventral internal capsule/ventral striatum for obsessive-compulsive disorder: worldwide experience. *Mol Psychiatry*, 2010 Jan, 15(1), 64-79.

[57] Okun, MS; Mann, G; Foote, KD; Shapira, NA; Bowers, D; Springer, U; et al. Deep brain stimulation in the internal capsule and nucleus accumbens region: responses observed during active and sham programming. *J Neurol Neurosurg Psychiatry*, 2007 Mar, 78(3), 310-4.

[58] Benabid, AL; Pollak, P; Gervason, C; Hoffmann, D; Gao, DM; Hommel, M; et al. Long-term suppression of tremor by chronic stimulation of the ventral intermediate thalamic nucleus. *Lancet*, 1991 Feb 16, 337(8738), 403-6.

[59] Kuncel, AM; Cooper, SE; Wolgamuth, BR; Grill, WM. Amplitude- and frequency-dependent changes in neuronal regularity parallel changes in tremor With thalamic deep brain stimulation. *IEEE Trans Neural Syst Rehabil Eng*, 2007 Jun, 15(2), 190-7.

[60] Lippitz, BE; Mindus, P; Meyerson, BA; Kihlstrom, L; Lindquist, C. Lesion topography and outcome after thermocapsulotomy or gamma knife capsulotomy for obsessive-compulsive disorder: relevance of the right hemisphere. *Neurosurgery*, 1999 Mar, 44(3), 452, 8, discussion 458-60.

[61] Lehman, JF; Greenberg, BD; McIntyre, CC; Rasmussen, SA; Haber, SN. Rules ventral prefrontal cortical axons use to reach their targets: implications for diffusion tensor imaging tractography and deep brain stimulation for psychiatric illness. *J Neurosci*, 2011 Jul 13, 31(28), 10392-402.

[62] Denys, D; Mantione, M; Figee, M; van den Munckhof, P; Koerselman, F; Westenberg, H; et al. Deep brain stimulation of the nucleus accumbens for treatment-refractory obsessive-compulsive disorder. *Arch Gen Psychiatry*, 2010 Oct, 67(10), 1061-8.

[63] Sturm, V; Lenartz, D; Koulousakis, A; Treuer, H; Herholz, K; Klein, JC; et al. The nucleus accumbens: a target for deep brain stimulation in obsessive-compulsive- and anxiety-disorders. *J Chem Neuroanat*, 2003 Dec, 26(4), 293-9.

[64] Nuttin, BJ; Gabriels, LA; Cosyns, PR; Meyerson, BA; Andreewitch, S; Sunaert, SG; et al. Long-term electrical capsular stimulation in patients with obsessive-compulsive disorder. *Neurosurgery*, 2003 Jun, 52(6), 1263, 72, discussion 1272-4.

[65] Haq, IU; Foote, KD; Goodman, WG; Wu, SS; Sudhyadhom, A; Ricciuti, N; et al. Smile and laughter induction and intraoperative predictors of response to deep brain stimulation for obsessive-compulsive disorder. *Neuroimage*, 2011 Jan, 54 Suppl 1, S247-55.

[66] Okun, MS; Bowers, D; Springer, U; Shapira, NA; Malone, D; Rezai, AR; et al. What's in a "smile?" Intra-operative observations of contralateral smiles induced by deep brain stimulation. *Neurocase*, 2004 Aug, 10(4), 271-9.

[67] Kuhn, J; Lenartz, D; Mai, JK; Huff, W; Lee, SH; Koulousakis, A; et al. Deep brain stimulation of the nucleus accumbens and the internal capsule in therapeutically refractory Tourette-syndrome. *J Neurol*, 2007 Jul, 254(7), 963-5.

[68] Heimer, L. Basal forebrain in the context of schizophrenia. *Brain Res Brain Res Rev*, 2000 Mar, 31(2-3), 205-35.

[69] Martinez-Torres, I; Hariz, MI; Zrinzo, L; Foltynie, T; Limousin P. Improvement of tics after subthalamic nucleus deep brain stimulation. *Neurology*, 2009 May 19, 72(20), 1787-9.

[70] Hariz, MI; Robertson, MM. Gilles de la Tourette syndrome and deep brain stimulation. *Eur J Neurosci*, 2010 Oct, 32(7), 1128-34.

[71] Bloch, MH; Panza KE; Landeros-Weisenberger A; Leckman JF. Meta-analysis: treatment of attention-deficit/hyperactivity disorder in children with comorbid tic disorders. *J Am Acad Child Adolesc Psychiatry*, 2009 Sep, 48(9), 884-93.

[72] Cheung, MY; Shahed, J; Jankovic, J. Malignant Tourette syndrome. *Mov Disord*, 2007 Sep 15, 22(12), 1743-50.

[73] Vandewalle, V; van der Linden, C; Groenewegen, HJ; Caemaert, J. Stereotactic treatment of Gilles de la Tourette syndrome by high frequency stimulation of thalamus. *Lancet*, 1999 Feb 27, 353(9154), 724.

[74] Houeto, JL; Karachi, C; Mallet, L; Pillon, B; Yelnik, J; Mesnage, V; et al. Tourette's syndrome and deep brain stimulation. *J Neurol Neurosurg Psychiatry*, 2005 Jul, 76(7), 992-5.

[75] Maciunas, RJ; Maddux, BN; Riley, DE; Whitney, CM; Schoenberg, MR; Ogrocki, PJ; et al. Prospective randomized double-blind trial of bilateral thalamic deep brain stimulation in adults with Tourette syndrome. *J Neurosurg*, 2007 Nov, 107(5), 1004-14.

[76] Welter, ML; Mallet, L; Houeto, JL; Karachi, C; Czernecki, V; Cornu, P; et al. Internal pallidal and thalamic stimulation in patients with Tourette syndrome. *Arch Neurol*, 2008 Jul, 65(7), 952-7.

[77] Ackermans, L; Duits, A; van der Linden, C; Tijssen, M; Schruers, K; Temel, Y; et al. Double-blind clinical trial of thalamic stimulation in patients with Tourette syndrome. *Brain*, 2011 Mar, 134(Pt 3), 832-44.

[78] Visser-Vandewalle, V; Temel, Y; Boon, P; Vreeling, F; Colle, H; Hoogland, G; et al. Chronic bilateral thalamic stimulation: a new therapeutic approach in intractable Tourette syndrome. Report of three cases. *J Neurosurg*, 2003 Dec, 99(6), 1094-100.

[79] Ackermans, L; Neuner, I; Temel, Y; Duits, A; Kuhn, J; Visser-Vandewalle, V. Thalamic deep brain stimulation for Tourette syndrome. *Behav Neurol*, 2013, 27(1), 133-8.

[80] Bajwa, RJ; de Lotbiniere, AJ; King, RA; Jabbari, B; Quatrano, S; Kunze, K; et al. Deep brain stimulation in Tourette's syndrome. *Mov Disord*, 2007 Jul 15, 22(9), 1346-50.

[81] Diederich, NJ; Kalteis, K; Stamenkovic, M; Pieri, V; Alesch, F. Efficient internal pallidal stimulation in Gilles de la Tourette syndrome: a case report. *Mov Disord*, 2005 Nov, 20(11), 1496-9.

[82] Gallagher, CL; Garell, PC; Montgomery, EB, Jr. Hemi tics and deep brain stimulation. *Neurology*, 2006 Feb 14, 66(3), E12.

[83] Dehning, S; Mehrkens, JH; Muller, N; Botzel, K. Therapy-refractory Tourette syndrome: beneficial outcome with globus pallidus internus deep brain stimulation. *Mov Disord*, 2008 Jul 15, 23(9), 1300-2.

[84] Shahed, J; Poysky, J; Kenney, C; Simpson, R; Jankovic, J. GPi deep brain stimulation for Tourette syndrome improves tics and psychiatric comorbidities. *Neurology*, 2007 Jan 9, 68(2), 159-60.

[85] Flaherty, AW; Williams, ZM; Amirnovin, R; Kasper, E; Rauch, SL; Cosgrove, GR; et al. Deep brain stimulation of the anterior internal capsule for the treatment of Tourette syndrome: technical case report. *Neurosurgery*, 2005 Oct, 57(4 Suppl), E403, discussion E403.

[86] Burdick, A; Foote, KD; Goodman, W; Ward, HE; Ricciuti, N; Murphy, T; et al. Lack of benefit of accumbens/capsular deep brain stimulation in a patient with both tics and obsessive-compulsive disorder. *Neurocase*, 2010 Aug, 16(4), 321-30.

[87] Neuner, I; Podoll, K; Lenartz, D; Sturm, V; Schneider, F. Deep brain stimulation in the nucleus accumbens for intractable Tourette's syndrome: follow-up report of 36 months. *Biol Psychiatry*, 2009 Feb 15, 65(4), e5-6.

[88] Zabek, M; Sobstyl, M; Koziara, H; Dzierzecki, S. Deep brain stimulation of the right nucleus accumbens in a patient with Tourette syndrome. Case report. *Neurol Neurochir Pol*, 2008 Nov-Dec, 42(6), 554-9.

[89] Piedimonte, F; Andreani, JC; Piedimonte, L; Graff, P; Bacaro, V; Micheli, F; et al. Behavioral and motor improvement after deep brain stimulation of the globus pallidus externus in a case of Tourette's syndrome. *Neuromodulation*, 2013 Jan-Feb, 16(1), 55, 8, discussion 58.

[90] Servello, D; Sassi, M; Brambilla, A; Porta, M; Haq, I; Foote, KD; et al. De novo and rescue DBS leads for refractory Tourette syndrome patients with severe comorbid OCD: a multiple case report. *J Neurol*, 2009 Sep, 256(9), 1533-9.

[91] Eddy, CM; Cavanna, AE; Gulisano, M; Agodi, A; Barchitta, M; Cali, P; et al. Clinical correlates of quality of life in Tourette syndrome. *Mov Disord*, 2011 Mar, 26(4), 735-8.

[92] Cavanna, AE; David, K; Bandera, V; Termine, C; Balottin, U; Schrag, A; et al. Health-related quality of life in Gilles de la Tourette syndrome: a decade of research. *Behav Neurol*, 2013, 27(1), 83-93.

[93] Bronstein, JM; Tagliati, M; Alterman, RL; Lozano, AM; Volkmann, J; Stefani, A; et al. Deep brain stimulation for Parkinson disease: an expert consensus and review of key issues. *Arch Neurol*, 2011 Feb, 68(2), 165.

[94] Deuschl, G; Schade-Brittinger, C; Krack, P; Volkmann, J; Schafer, H; Botzel, K; et al. A randomized trial of deep-brain stimulation for Parkinson's disease. *N Engl J Med*, 2006 Aug 31, 355(9), 896-908.

[95] Follett, KA; Weaver, FM; Stern, M; Hur, K; Harris, CL; Luo, P; et al. Pallidal versus subthalamic deep-brain stimulation for Parkinson's disease. *N Engl J Med*, 2010 Jun 3, 362(22), 2077-91.

[96] Kupsch, A; Benecke, R; Muller, J; Trottenberg, T; Schneider, GH; Poewe, W; et al. Pallidal deep-brain stimulation in primary generalized or segmental dystonia. *N Engl J Med*, 2006 Nov 9, 355(19), 1978-90.

[97] Volkmann, J; Mueller, J; Deuschl, G; Kuhn, AA; Krauss, JK; Poewe, W; et al. Pallidal neurostimulation in patients with medication-refractory cervical dystonia: a randomized, sham-controlled trial. *Lancet Neurol*, 2014 Sep, 13(9), 875-84.

[98] Odekerken, VJ; van Laar, T; Staal, MJ; Mosch, A; Hoffmann, CF; Nijssen, PC; et al. Subthalamic nucleus versus globus pallidus bilateral deep brain stimulation for advanced Parkinson's disease (NSTAPS study), a randomised controlled trial. *Lancet Neurol*, 2013 Jan, 12(1), 37-44.

[99] Weaver, FM; Follett, K; Stern, M; Hur, K; Harris, C; Marks, WJ, Jr; et al. Bilateral deep brain stimulation vs best medical therapy for patients with advanced Parkinson disease: a randomized controlled trial. *JAMA*, 2009 Jan 7, 301(1), 63-73.

[100] Okun, MS; Gallo, BV; Mandybur, G; Jagid, J; Foote, KD; Revilla, FJ; et al. Subthalamic deep brain stimulation with a constant-current device in Parkinson's disease: an open-label randomised controlled trial. *Lancet Neurol*, 2012 Feb, 11(2), 140-9.

[101] Deep-Brain Stimulation for Parkinson's Disease Study Group. Deep-brain stimulation of the subthalamic nucleus or the pars interna of the globus pallidus in Parkinson's disease. *N Engl J Med*, 2001 Sep 27, 345(13), 956-63.

[102] Voges, J; Hilker, R; Botzel, K; Kiening, KL; Kloss, M; Kupsch, A; et al. Thirty days complication rate following surgery performed for deep-brain-stimulation. *Mov Disord*, 2007 Jul 30, 22(10), 1486-9.

[103] Beric, A; Kelly, PJ; Rezai, A; Sterio, D; Mogilner, A; Zonenshayn, M; et al. Complications of deep brain stimulation surgery. *Stereotact Funct Neurosurg*, 2001, 77(1-4), 73-8.

[104] Bhatia, S; Oh, M; Whiting, T; Quigley, M; Whiting, D. Surgical complications of deep brain stimulation. A longitudinal single surgeon; single institution study. *Stereotact Funct Neurosurg*, 2008, 86(6), 367-72.

[105] Binder, DK; Rau, GM; Starr, PA. Risk factors for hemorrhage during microelectrode-guided deep brain stimulator implantation for movement disorders. *Neurosurgery*, 2005 Apr, 56(4), 722, 32, discussion 722-32.

[106] Chan, DT; Zhu, XL; Yeung, JH; Mok VC; Wong E; Lau C; et al. Complications of deep brain stimulation: a collective review. *Asian J Surg*, 2009 Oct, 32(4), 258-63.

[107] Herzog, J; Volkmann, J; Krack, P; Kopper, F; Potter, M; Lorenz, D; et al. Two-year follow-up of subthalamic deep brain stimulation in Parkinson's disease. *Mov Disord*, 2003 Nov, 18(11), 1332-7.

[108] Krack, P; Batir, A; Van Blercom, N; Chabardes, S; Fraix, V; Ardouin, C; et al. Five-year follow-up of bilateral stimulation of the subthalamic nucleus in advanced Parkinson's disease. *N Engl J Med*, 2003 Nov 13, 349(20), 1925-34.

[109] Bauman, JA; Church, E; Halpern, CH; Danish, SF; Zaghloul, KA; Jaggi, JL; et al. Subcutaneous heparin for prophylaxis of venous thromboembolism in deep brain stimulation surgery: evidence from a decision analysis. *Neurosurgery*, 2009 Aug, 65(2), 276, 80, discussion 280.

[110] Maldonado, IL; Roujeau, T; Cif, L; Gonzalez, V; El-Fertit, H; Vasques, X; et al. Magnetic resonance-based deep brain stimulation technique: a series of 478 consecutive implanted electrodes with no perioperative intracerebral hemorrhage. *Neurosurgery*, 2009 Dec, 65(6 Suppl), 196, 201, discussion 201-2.

[111] Patel, NK; Plaha, P; Gill, SS. Magnetic resonance imaging-directed method for functional neurosurgery using implantable guide tubes. Neurosurgery 2007 Nov, 61(5 Suppl 2), 358, 65, discussion 365-6.

[112] Umemura, A; Jaggi, JL; Hurtig, HI; Siderowf, AD; Colcher, A; Stern, MB; et al. Deep brain stimulation for movement disorders: morbidity and mortality in 109 patients. *J Neurosurg*, 2003 Apr, 98(4), 779-84.

[113] Ben-Haim, S; Asaad, WF; Gale, JT; Eskandar, EN. Risk factors for hemorrhage during microelectrode-guided deep brain stimulation and the introduction of an improved microelectrode design. *Neurosurgery*, 2009 Apr, 64(4), 754, 62, discussion 762-3.

[114] Chhabra, V; Sung, E; Mewes, K; Bakay, RA; Abosch, A; Gross, RE. Safety of magnetic resonance imaging of deep brain stimulator systems: a serial imaging and clinical retrospective study. *J Neurosurg*, 2010 Mar, 112(3), 497-502.

[115] Fenoy, AJ; Simpson, RK; Jr. Risks of common complications in deep brain stimulation surgery: management and avoidance. *J Neurosurg*, 2014 Jan, 120(1), 132-9.

[116] Goodman, RR; Kim, B; McClelland, S; 3rd. Senatus, PB; Winfield, LM; Pullman, SL; et al. Operative techniques and morbidity with subthalamic nucleus deep brain stimulation in 100 consecutive patients with advanced Parkinson's disease. *J Neurol Neurosurg Psychiatry*, 2006 Jan, 77(1), 12-7.

[117] Kenney, C; Simpson, R; Hunter, C; Ondo, W; Almaguer, M; Davidson, A; et al. Short-term and long-term safety of deep brain stimulation in the treatment of movement disorders. *J Neurosurg*, 2007 Apr, 106(4), 621-5.

[118] Khatib, R; Ebrahim, Z; Rezai, A; Cata, JP; Boulis, NM; John Doyle, D; et al. Perioperative events during deep brain stimulation: the experience at cleveland clinic. *J Neurosurg Anesthesiol*, 2008 Jan, 20(1), 36-40.

[119] Ory-Magne, F; Brefel-Courbon, C; Simonetta-Moreau, M; Fabre, N; Lotterie, JA; Chaynes, P; et al. Does ageing influence deep brain stimulation outcomes in Parkinson's disease? *Mov Disord*, 2007 Jul 30, 22(10), 1457-63.

[120] Sansur, CA; Frysinger, RC; Pouratian, N; Fu, KM; Bittl, M; Oskouian, RJ; et al. Incidence of symptomatic hemorrhage after stereotactic electrode placement. *J Neurosurg*, 2007 Nov, 107(5), 998-1003.

[121] Seijo, F; Alvarez de Eulate Beramendi, S; Santamarta Liebana, E; Lozano Aragoneses, B; Saiz Ayala, A; Fernandez de Leon, R; et al. Surgical adverse events of deep brain stimulation in the subthalamic nucleus of patients with Parkinson's disease. The learning curve and the pitfalls. *Acta Neurochir*, (Wien) 2014 Aug, 156(8), 1505, 12, discussion 1512.

[122] Terao, T; Takahashi, H; Yokochi, F; Taniguchi, M; Okiyama, R; Hamada, I. Hemorrhagic complication of stereotactic surgery in patients with movement disorders. *J Neurosurg*, 2003 Jun, 98(6), 1241-6.

[123] Zrinzo, L; Foltynie, T; Limousin, P; Hariz, MI. Reducing hemorrhagic complications in functional neurosurgery: a large case series and systematic literature review. *J Neurosurg*, 2012 Jan, 116(1), 84-94.

[124] DeLong, MR; Huang, KT; Gallis, J; Lokhnygina, Y; Parente, B; Hickey, P; et al. Effect of advancing age on outcomes of deep brain stimulation for Parkinson disease. *JAMA Neurol*, 2014 Oct, 71(10), 1290-5.

[125] Palur, RS; Berk, C; Schulzer, M; Honey, CR. A metaanalysis comparing the results of pallidotomy performed using microelectrode recording or macroelectrode stimulation. *J Neurosurg*, 2002 Jun, 96(6), 1058-62.
[126] Hariz, MI; Fodstad, H. Do microelectrode techniques increase accuracy or decrease risks in pallidotomy and deep brain stimulation? A critical review of the literature. *Stereotact Funct Neurosurg*, 1999, 72(2-4), 157-69.
[127] Gorgulho, A; De Salles, AA; Frighetto, L; Behnke, E. Incidence of hemorrhage associated with electrophysiological studies performed using macroelectrodes and microelectrodes in functional neurosurgery. *J Neurosurg*, 2005 May, 102(5), 888-96.
[128] Broderick, J; Connolly, S; Feldmann, E; Hanley, D; Kase, C; Krieger, D; et al. Guidelines for the management of spontaneous intracerebral hemorrhage in adults: 2007 update: a guideline from the American Heart Association/American Stroke Association Stroke Council, High Blood Pressure Research Council, and the Quality of Care and Outcomes in Research Interdisciplinary Working Group. *Circulation*, 2007 Oct 16, 116(16), e391-413.
[129] van den Bergh, WM; van der Schaaf, I; van Gijn, J. The spectrum of presentations of venous infarction caused by deep cerebral vein thrombosis. *Neurology*, 2005 Jul 26, 65(2), 192-6.
[130] Ferro, JM; Canhao, P. Acute treatment of cerebral venous and dural sinus thrombosis. *Curr Treat Options Neurol*, 2008 Mar, 10(2), 126-37.
[131] Ferro, JM; Canhao, P; Bousser, MG; Stam, J; Barinagarrementeria, F; ISCVT Investigators. Early seizures in cerebral vein and dural sinus thrombosis: risk factors and role of antiepileptics. *Stroke*, 2008 Apr, 39(4), 1152-8.
[132] Pouratian, N; Reames, DL; Frysinger, R; Elias, WJ. Comprehensive analysis of risk factors for seizures after deep brain stimulation surgery. Clinical article. *J Neurosurg*, 2011 Aug, 115(2), 310-5.
[133] Schmidt, D; Schachter, SC. Drug treatment of epilepsy in adults. *BMJ*, 2014 Feb 28, 348, g254.
[134] Muriel, A; Jimenez, D; Aujesky, D; Bertoletti, L; Decousus, H; Laporte, S; et al. Survival effects of inferior vena cava filter in patients with acute symptomatic venous thromboembolism and a significant bleeding risk. *J Am Coll Cardiol*, 2014 Apr 29, 63(16), 1675-83.
[135] Aminoff, MJ; Christine, CW; Friedman, JH; Chou, KL; Lyons, KE; Pahwa, R; et al. Management of the hospitalized patient with Parkinson's disease: current state of the field and need for guidelines. *Parkinsonism Relat Disord*, 2011 Mar, 17(3), 139-45.
[136] Carlson, JD; Neumiller, JJ; Swain, LD; Mark, J; McLeod, P; Hirschauer, J. Postoperative delirium in Parkinson's disease patients following deep brain stimulation surgery. *J Clin Neurosci*, 2014 Jul, 21(7), 1192-5.
[137] Oh, MY; Abosch, A; Kim, SH; Lang, AE; Lozano, AM. Long-term hardware-related complications of deep brain stimulation. *Neurosurgery*, 2002 Jun, 50(6), 1268, 74, discussion 1274-6.
[138] Sillay, KA; Larson, PS; Starr, PA. Deep brain stimulator hardware-related infections: incidence and management in a large series. *Neurosurgery*, 2008 Feb, 62(2), 360, 6, discussion 366-7.

[139] Levy, RM; Lamb, S; Adams, JE. Treatment of chronic pain by deep brain stimulation: long term follow-up and review of the literature. *Neurosurgery*, 1987 Dec, 21(6), 885-93.

[140] Seal, LA; Paul-Cheadle, D. A systems approach to preoperative surgical patient skin preparation. *Am J Infect Control*, 2004 Apr, 32(2), 57-62.

[141] Lyons KE; Wilkinson SB; Overman J; Pahwa R. Surgical and hardware complications of subthalamic stimulation: a series of 160 procedures. *Neurology*, 2004 Aug 24, 63(4), 612-6.

[142] Miyagi, Y; Shima, F; Ishido, K. Implantation of deep brain stimulation electrodes in unshaved patients. Technical note. *J Neurosurg*, 2002 Dec, 97(6), 1476-8.

[143] Masterson, TM; Rodeheaver, GT; Morgan, RF; Edlich, RF. Bacteriologic evaluation of electric clippers for surgical hair removal. *Am J Surg*, 1984 Sep, 148(3), 301-2.

[144] Hariz, MI; Johansson, F. Hardware failure in parkinsonian patients with chronic subthalamic nucleus stimulation is a medical emergency. *Mov Disord*, 2001 Jan, 16(1), 166-8.

[145] Blomstedt, P; Hariz, MI. Hardware-related complications of deep brain stimulation: a ten year experience. *Acta Neurochir*, (Wien) 2005 Oct, 147(10), 1061, 4, discussion 1064.

[146] Yianni, J; Nandi, D; Shad, A; Bain, P; Gregory, R; Aziz, T. Increased risk of lead fracture and migration in dystonia compared with other movement disorders following deep brain stimulation. *J Clin Neurosci*, 2004 Apr, 11(3), 243-5.

[147] Okun, MS; Rodriguez, RL; Foote, KD; Sudhyadhom, A; Bova, F; Jacobson, C; et al. A case-based review of troubleshooting deep brain stimulator issues in movement and neuropsychiatric disorders. *Parkinsonism Relat Disord*, 2008 Nov, 14(7), 532-8.

[148] Favre, J; Taha, JM; Steel, T; Burchiel, KJ. Anchoring of deep brain stimulation electrodes using a microplate. Technical note. *J Neurosurg*, 1996 Dec, 85(6), 1181-3.

[149] Sherif, C; Dorfer, C; Kalteis, K; Thun, C; Kaiser, I; Gibson, D; et al. Deep brain pulse-generator and lead-extensions: subjective sensations related to measured parameters. *Mov Disord*, 2008 May 15, 23(7), 1036-40.

[150] Burdick, AP; Okun, MS; Haq, IU; Ward, HE; Bova, F; Jacobson, CE; et al. Prevalence of Twiddler's syndrome as a cause of deep brain stimulation hardware failure. *Stereotact Funct Neurosurg*, 2010, 88(6), 353-9.

[151] Geissinger, G; Neal, JH. Spontaneous twiddler's syndrome in a patient with a deep brain stimulator. *Surg Neurol*, 2007 Oct, 68(4), 454, 6, discussion 456.

[152] Farris, S; Vitek, J; Giroux, ML. Deep brain stimulation hardware complications: the role of electrode impedance and current measurements. *Mov Disord*, 2008 Apr 15, 23(5), 755-60.

[153] Dursun, I; Yesildag, O; Soylu, K; Yilmaz, O; Yasar, E; Meric, M. Late pacemaker twiddler syndrome. *Clin Res Cardiol*, 2006 Oct, 95(10), 547-9.

[154] Ashby, P; Kim, YJ; Kumar, R; Lang, AE; Lozano, AM. Neurophysiological effects of stimulation through electrodes in the human subthalamic nucleus. *Brain*, 1999 Oct, 122 (Pt 10)(Pt 10), 1919-31.

[155] Alesch, F; Pinter, MM; Helscher, RJ; Fertl, L; Benabid, AL; Koos, WT. Stimulation of the ventral intermediate thalamic nucleus in tremor dominated Parkinson's disease and essential tremor. *Acta Neurochir*, (Wien) 1995, 136(1-2), 75-81.

[156] Kiss, ZH; Anderson, T; Hansen, T; Kirstein, D; Suchowersky, O; Hu, B. Neural substrates of microstimulation-evoked tingling: a chronaxie study in human somatosensory thalamus. *Eur J Neurosci*, 2003 Aug, 18(3), 728-32.

[157] Albanese, A; Nordera, GP; Caraceni, T; Moro, E. Long-term ventralis intermedius thalamic stimulation for parkinsonian tremor. Italian Registry for Neuromodulation in Movement Disorders. *Adv Neurol*, 1999, 80, 631-4.

[158] Kumar, K; Kelly, M; Toth, C. Deep brain stimulation of the ventral intermediate nucleus of the thalamus for control of tremors in Parkinson's disease and essential tremor. *Stereotact Funct Neurosurg*, 1999, 72(1), 47-61.

[159] Limousin, P; Speelman, JD; Gielen, F; Janssens, M. Multicentre European study of thalamic stimulation in parkinsonian and essential tremor. *J Neurol Neurosurg Psychiatry*, 1999 Mar, 66(3), 289-96.

[160] Tamma, F; Caputo, E; Chiesa, V; Egidi, M; Locatelli, M; Rampini, P; et al. Anatomo-clinical correlation of intraoperative stimulation-induced side-effects during HF-DBS of the subthalamic nucleus. *Neurol Sci*, 2002 Sep, 23 Suppl 2, S109-10.

[161] Borretzen, MN; Bjerknes, S; Saehle, T; Skjelland, M; Skogseid, IM; Toft, M; et al. Long-term follow-up of thalamic deep brain stimulation for essential tremor - patient satisfaction and mortality. *BMC Neurol*, 2014 Jun 5, 14, 120, 2377-14-120.

[162] Burkhard, PR; Vingerhoets, FJ; Berney, A; Bogousslavsky, J; Villemure, JG; Ghika, J. Suicide after successful deep brain stimulation for movement disorders. *Neurology*, 2004 Dec 14, 63(11), 2170-2.

[163] Krack, P; Fraix, V; Mendes, A; Benabid, AL; Pollak, P. Postoperative management of subthalamic nucleus stimulation for Parkinson's disease. *Mov Disord*, 2002, 17 Suppl 3, S188-97.

[164] Krack, P; Pollak, P; Limousin, P; Benazzouz, A; Deuschl, G; Benabid, AL. From off-period dystonia to peak-dose chorea. The clinical spectrum of varying subthalamic nucleus activity. *Brain*, 1999 Jun, 122 (Pt 6)(Pt 6), 1133-46.

[165] Limousin, P; Pollak, P; Hoffmann, D; Benazzouz, A; Perret, JE; Benabid, AL. Abnormal involuntary movements induced by subthalamic nucleus stimulation in parkinsonian patients. *Mov Disord*, 1996 May, 11(3), 231-5.

[166] Moro, E; Esselink, RJ; Benabid, AL; Pollak, P. Response to levodopa in parkinsonian patients with bilateral subthalamic nucleus stimulation. *Brain*, 2002 Nov, 125(Pt 11), 2408-17.

[167] Tavella, A; Bergamasco, B; Bosticco, E; Lanotte, M; Perozzo, P; Rizzone, M; et al. Deep brain stimulation of the subthalamic nucleus in Parkinson's disease: long-term follow-up. *Neurol Sci*, 2002 Sep, 23 Suppl 2, S111-2.

[168] Ramig, LO; Sapir, S; Countryman, S; Pawlas, AA; O'Brien, C; Hoehn, M; et al. Intensive voice treatment (LSVT) for patients with Parkinson's disease: a 2 year follow up. *J Neurol Neurosurg Psychiatry*, 2001 Oct, 71(4), 493-8.

[169] Burchiel, KJ; Anderson, VC; Favre, J; Hammerstad, JP. Comparison of pallidal and subthalamic nucleus deep brain stimulation for advanced Parkinson's disease: results of a randomized, blinded pilot study. *Neurosurgery*, 1999 Dec, 45(6), 1375, 82, discussion 1382-4.

[170] Ghika, J; Villemure, JG; Fankhauser, H; Favre, J; Assal, G; Ghika-Schmid, F. Efficiency and safety of bilateral contemporaneous pallidal stimulation (deep brain

stimulation) in levodopa-responsive patients with Parkinson's disease with severe motor fluctuations: a 2-year follow-up review. *J Neurosurg*, 1998 Nov, 89(5), 713-8.

[171] Defebvre, LJ; Krystkowiak, P; Blatt, JL; Duhamel, A; Bourriez, JL; Perina, M; et al. Influence of pallidal stimulation and levodopa on gait and preparatory postural adjustments in Parkinson's disease. *Mov Disord*, 2002 Jan, 17(1), 76-83.

[172] Loher, TJ; Burgunder, JM; Pohle, T; Weber, S; Sommerhalder, R; Krauss, JK. Long-term pallidal deep brain stimulation in patients with advanced Parkinson disease: 1-year follow-up study. *J Neurosurg*, 2002 May, 96(5), 844-53.

[173] Spiegel, Ea; Wycis, Ht; Szekely, Eg; Soloff, L; Adams, J; Gildenberg, P; et al. Stimulation of Forel's Field during Stereotaxic Operations in the Human Brain. *Electroencephalogr Clin Neurophysiol*, 1964 Jun, 16, 537-48.

[174] Kleiner-Fisman, G; Fisman, DN; Sime, E; Saint-Cyr, JA; Lozano, AM; Lang, AE. Long-term follow up of bilateral deep brain stimulation of the subthalamic nucleus in patients with advanced Parkinson disease. *J Neurosurg*, 2003 Sep, 99(3), 489-95.

[175] Tozlovanu, V; Forget, R; Iancu, A; Boghen, D. Prolonged orbicularis oculi activity: a major factor in apraxia of lid opening. *Neurology*, 2001 Sep 25, 57(6), 1013-8.

[176] Forget, R; Tozlovanu, V; Iancu, A; Boghen, D. Botulinum toxin improves lid opening delays in blepharospasm-associated apraxia of lid opening. *Neurology*, 2002 Jun 25, 58(12), 1843-6.

[177] Martinez-Martin, P; Valldeoriola, F; Tolosa, E; Pilleri, M; Molinuevo, JL; Rumia, J; et al. Bilateral subthalamic nucleus stimulation and quality of life in advanced Parkinson's disease. *Mov Disord*, 2002 Mar, 17(2), 372-7.

[178] Volkmann, J; Allert, N; Voges, J; Weiss, PH; Freund, HJ; Sturm, V. Safety and efficacy of pallidal or subthalamic nucleus stimulation in advanced PD. *Neurology*, 2001 Feb 27, 56(4), 548-51.

[179] Macia, F; Perlemoine, C; Coman, I; Guehl, D; Burbaud, P; Cuny, E; et al. Parkinson's disease patients with bilateral subthalamic deep brain stimulation gain weight. *Mov Disord*, 2004 Feb, 19(2), 206-12.

[180] Barichella, M; Marczewska, AM; Mariani, C; Landi, A; Vairo, A; Pezzoli, G. Body weight gain rate in patients with Parkinson's disease and deep brain stimulation. *Mov Disord*, 2003 Nov, 18(11), 1337-40.

[181] Gironell, A; Pascual-Sedano, B; Otermin, P; Kulisevsky, J. Weight gain after functional surgery for Parkinsons disease. *Neurologia*, 2002 Jun-Jul, 17(6), 310-6.

[182] Bejjani, BP; Gervais, D; Arnulf, I; Papadopoulos, S; Demeret, S; Bonnet, AM; et al. Axial parkinsonian symptoms can be improved: the role of levodopa and bilateral subthalamic stimulation. *J Neurol Neurosurg Psychiatry*, 2000 May, 68(5), 595-600.

[183] Romito, LM; Scerrati, M; Contarino, MF; Bentivoglio, AR; Tonali, P; Albanese, A. Long-term follow up of subthalamic nucleus stimulation in Parkinson's disease. *Neurology*, 2002 May 28, 58(10), 1546-50.

[184] Castelli, L; Perozzo, P; Genesia, ML; Torre, E; Pesare, M; Cinquepalmi, A; et al. Sexual well being in parkinsonian patients after deep brain stimulation of the subthalamic nucleus. *J Neurol Neurosurg Psychiatry*, 2004 Sep, 75(9), 1260-4.

[185] Hariz, MI; Johansson, F; Shamsgovara, P; Johansson, E; Hariz, GM; Fagerlund, M. Bilateral subthalamic nucleus stimulation in a parkinsonian patient with preoperative deficits in speech and cognition: persistent improvement in mobility but increased dependency: a case study. *Mov Disord*, 2000 Jan, 15(1), 136-9.

[186] Houeto, JL; Mesnage, V; Mallet, L; Pillon, B; Gargiulo, M; du Moncel, ST; et al. Behavioural disorders; Parkinson's disease and subthalamic stimulation. *J Neurol Neurosurg Psychiatry*, 2002 Jun, 72(6), 701-7.
[187] Voon, V; Kubu, C; Krack, P; Houeto, JL; Troster, AI. Deep brain stimulation: neuropsychological and neuropsychiatric issues. *Mov Disord*, 2006 Jun, 21 Suppl 14, S305-27.
[188] Weintraub, D; Duda, JE; Carlson, K; Luo, P; Sagher, O; Stern, M; et al. Suicide ideation and behaviours after STN and GPi DBS surgery for Parkinson's disease: results from a randomized, controlled trial. *J Neurol Neurosurg Psychiatry*, 2013 May 10.
[189] Schupbach, WM; Chastan, N; Welter, ML; Houeto, JL; Mesnage, V; Bonnet, AM; et al. Stimulation of the subthalamic nucleus in Parkinson's disease: a 5 year follow up. *J Neurol Neurosurg Psychiatry*, 2005 Dec, 76(12), 1640-4.
[190] Morishita, T; Foote, KD; Burdick, AP; Katayama, Y; Yamamoto, T; Frucht, SJ; et al. Identification and management of deep brain stimulation intra- and postoperative urgencies and emergencies. *Parkinsonism Relat Disord*, 2010 Mar, 16(3), 153-62.
[191] Okun, MS; Fernandez, HH; Wu, SS; Kirsch-Darrow, L; Bowers, D; Bova, F; et al. Cognition and mood in Parkinson's disease in subthalamic nucleus versus globus pallidus interna deep brain stimulation: the COMPARE trial. *Ann Neurol*, 2009 May, 65(5), 586-95.
[192] Troche, MS; Brandimore, AE; Foote, KD; Morishita, T; Chen, D; Hegland, KW; et al. Swallowing outcomes following unilateral STN vs. GPi surgery: a retrospective analysis. *Dysphagia*, 2014 Aug, 29(4), 425-31.
[193] Kirschman, DL; Milligan, B; Wilkinson, S; Overman, J; Wetzel, L; Batnitzky, S; et al. Pallidotomy microelectrode targeting: neurophysiology-based target refinement. *Neurosurgery*, 2000 Mar, 46(3), 613, 22, discussion 622-4.
[194] Jahanshahi, M; Czernecki, V; Zurowski, AM. Neuropsychological, neuropsychiatric, and quality of life issues in DBS for dystonia. *Mov Disord*, 2011 Jun, 26 Suppl 1, S63-78.
[195] Foncke, EM; Schuurman, PR; Speelman, JD. Suicide after deep brain stimulation of the internal globus pallidus for dystonia. *Neurology*, 2006 Jan 10, 66(1), 142-3.
[196] Ackermans, L; Duits, A; Temel, Y; Winogrodzka, A; Peeters, F; Beuls, EA; et al. Long-term outcome of thalamic deep brain stimulation in two patients with Tourette syndrome. *J Neurol Neurosurg Psychiatry*, 2010 Oct, 81(10), 1068-72.

INDEX

#

A

B

C

D

E

F

G

H

I

J

K

L

M

N

O

P

Q

R

S

T

U

V

W